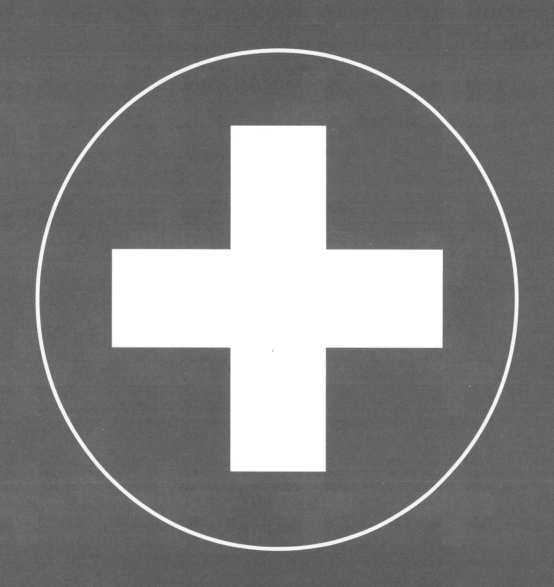

PRACTICAL
FIRST AID

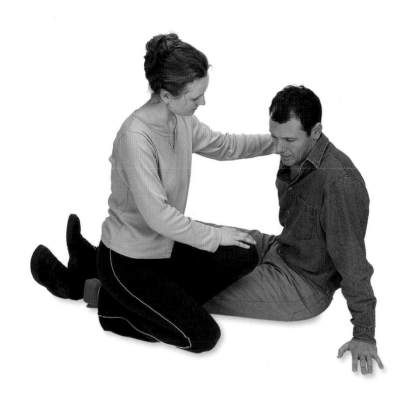

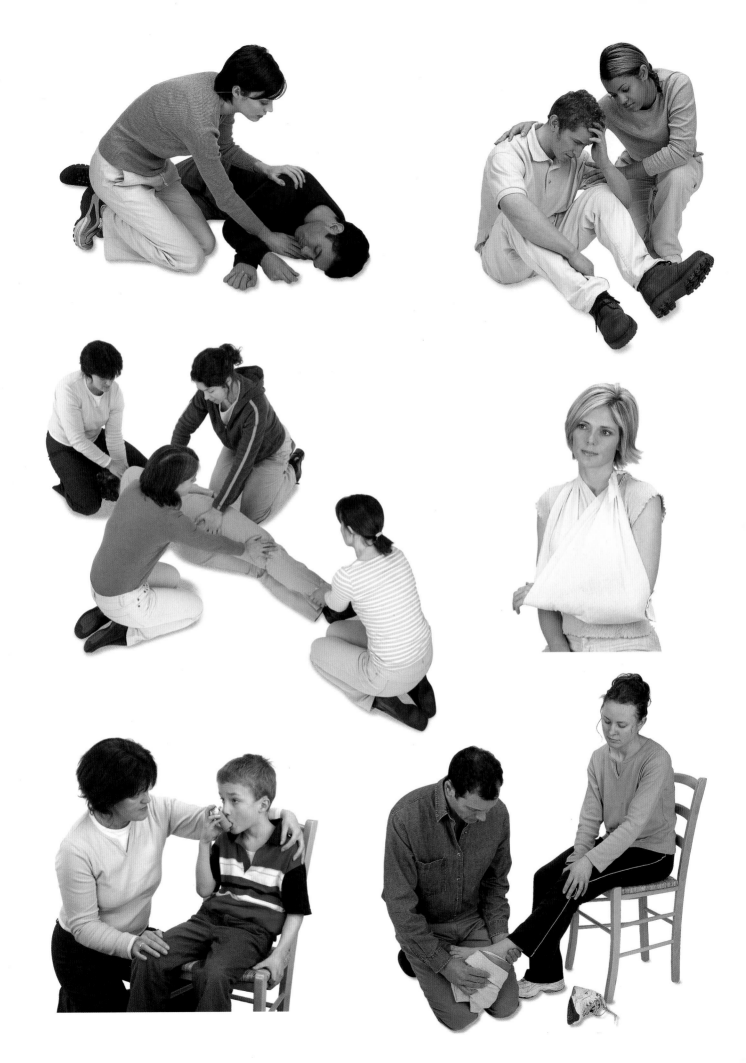

PRACTICAL FIRST AID

WHAT TO DO IN AN EMERGENCY

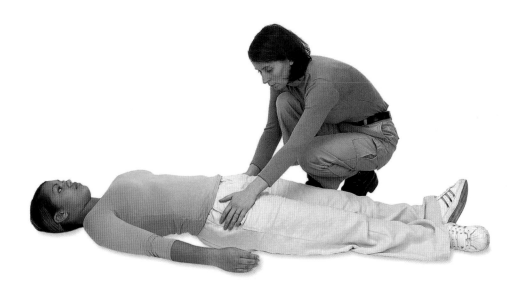

Clear step-by-step techniques • How to deal with accidents in the home, workplace and outdoors

Dr Pippa Keech MB ChB MRCGP

Editorial consultants: Anne Charlish, Sheena Meredith

LORENZ BOOKS

This edition is published by Lorenz Books
an imprint of Anness Publishing Limited
info@anness.com
www.lorenzbooks.com
www.annesspublishing.com

© Anness Publishing Ltd 2021

A CIP catalogue record for this book is available from the British Library.

Publisher: Joanna Lorenz
Editorial Director: Helen Sudell
Project Editors: Melanie Halton, Ann Kay
Editorial Consultant/Additional Text: Anne Charlish, Sheena Meredith
Text Editors: Sue Barraclough, Kim Davies, Tracey Kelly, Mary Lindsay, Nikki Sims
Designer: Lisa Tai
Cover Design: Nigel Partridge
Photographer: Mark Wood
Special effects make-up: Dauphine's of Bristol
Illustrations: Samantha Elmhurst
Production Controller: Ben Worley
Editorial Reader: Penelope Goodare

Publisher's Note:

While this book provides information and instructions for treating life-threatening and emergency
situations, any person with a condition or symptoms requiring medical attention should consult a
fully qualified medical practitioner as early as possible. Although the advice and information
in this book are believed to be accurate and true at the time of going to press, neither the authors
nor the publisher can accept any legal responsibility or liability for any errors or omissions that
may be made, nor for any inaccuracies nor for any harm or injury that comes about from following
instructions or advice in the book.

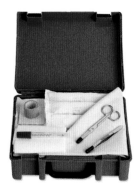

A skill for life

These days, we are constantly bombarded with health advice. It is easy to pick up inaccurate, distorted or partially digested information or to give up altogether and think that only the experts have any chance of knowing what to do in any kind of medical situation – especially in first-aid scenarios.

However, we all need to acquire a certain level of health understanding as a basic life skill – to stay as healthy and fit as we can be and enjoy our lives to the full, to prevent ourselves and others getting into more serious problems and to protect our loved ones. What we need for this is a basic fund of solid, up-to-date information combined with practical, common sense advice. Whether we are soothing a child's headache or attempting resuscitation, we often underestimate just how far common sense can help us and sometimes literally be a life-saver.

The good news is that this book goes a long way towards providing just such a sensible approach. It has been devised to be your companion through all kinds of day-to-day and emergency situations, as well as offering general advice on a healthy lifestyle and highlighting preventative tips along the way. Remember, however, that nothing replaces a good first-aid course, which gives you the skills needed to tackle emergencies confidently and calmly, and also that you should always consult a medical practitioner when faced with anything other than the most minor of conditions. That said, health is perhaps the most fascinating of subjects, so enjoy reading about your precious body while learning some essential skills.

Dr Pippa Keech
MB ChB MRCGP

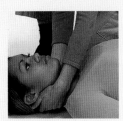 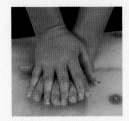 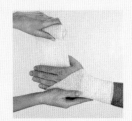 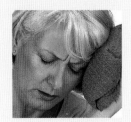

Contents

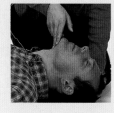
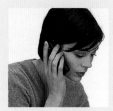
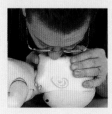
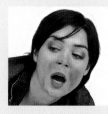
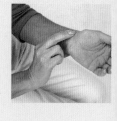
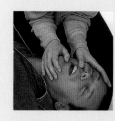
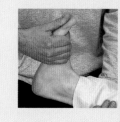
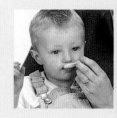

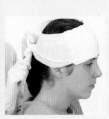

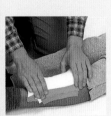

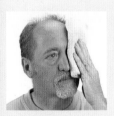

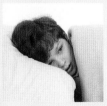

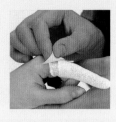

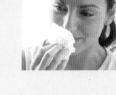
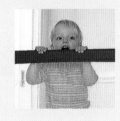

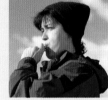
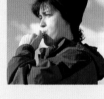

Introduction

Understanding the basics of first aid will help you to stay calm and in control in an emergency. This is vital in a crisis, regardless of the level of your specific knowledge. It is also enormously reassuring to the casualty, whatever the eventual outcome, and will often inspire bystanders to offer assistance. Remember, even those with no training can do something really useful, such as phoning for help or comforting the casualty.

FIRST PRINCIPLES

Here are a few first principles that anyone attempting to help out in an emergency must be aware of; many of them are elaborated upon throughout the book:

- Do not delay in calling for emergency help, it may take some time to arrive.
- Do not put yourself in any danger – if you get hurt, you won't be helping anyone.
- Remember that you may make matters worse if you act too impulsively.

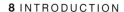

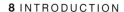
◁ Improvising a dressing for an injured hand.

WHAT TO EXPECT AT THE ACCIDENT AND EMERGENCY DEPARTMENT

You may well end up going to hospital with a casualty. If you know what to expect in an accident and emergency (A&E) department, you will cope more calmly when you get there. You will also be able to talk to the casualty about what to expect, which should in turn help to reduce their anxiety.

A nurse may be the first person you see after you register at the accident and emergency desk. The nurse's job is to assess what immediate treatment is needed and how urgently the casualty needs to be seen. This is called "triaging". Casualties who need immediate care are often moved to a room called the "resuscitation room". Cases such as possible heart attacks and severe asthma attacks will be classed as urgent.

After this the triage nurse will deal with people who need a bed to lie on, usually classified as a major casualty; the more minor casualties will need to wait a little longer to be treated.

When appropriate, the nurse may ask the casualty to undress and put on a hospital gown. This makes it much easier for medical personnel to examine the patient.

In some hospitals, there may be a separate pediatric emergency department, and this spares them the distressing scenes that are often played out in a hospital's emergency department.

- If you find yourself in charge, try to formulate an overall plan of action.
- Look around the accident site for hazards such as flammable substances, but leave dangerous situations to be dealt with by professionals.
- Be aware of your limitations. Do not try clambering up a rock face to help someone if you are terrified of heights. Do not attempt mouth-to-mouth if you have no idea what to do – summon help as an urgent priority.
- Tackle aggressive casualties cautiously – get trained help as fast as possible.
- Protect yourself in whatever way you can from body fluids, especially blood.

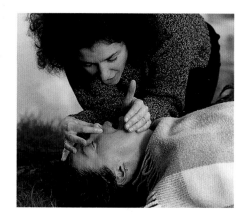
△ Carrying out resuscitation procedures on a victim of drowning at the water's edge.

- If you were the first to turn up at an incident, but other helpers come to your aid and seem better qualified to help, then forgo your pride and defer to them. That in itself will have been an immensely helpful thing to do.
- If you are in charge and a large crowd gathers, try to get everyone out of the way except for close friends or relatives and those who are giving actual aid.
- Remember that it is often a good idea to

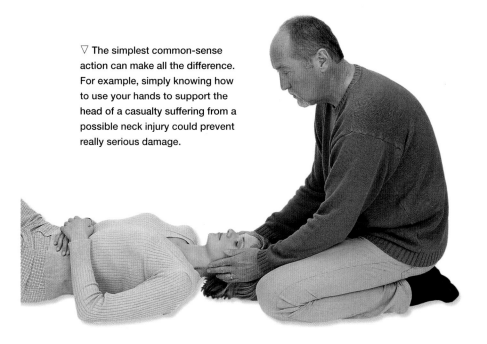

△ The simplest common-sense action can make all the difference. For example, simply knowing how to use your hands to support the head of a casualty suffering from a possible neck injury could prevent really serious damage.

FIRST-AID PRIORITIES

➤ Don't panic.

➤ Assess the situation quickly and calmly and try to identify the problem.

➤ Waste no time in summoning any professional help.

➤ Give medical aid if you feel you can; do nothing if in doubt.

➤ Comfort a conscious casualty.

➤ Stay with the casualty until help arrives.

"debrief" after an emergency event – talking to family and friends, or to a counsellor if necessary. You may be more shaken up than you realize.

WHEN YOU SHOULD DO NOTHING

It is sometimes better to do nothing than to risk doing the wrong thing. In one example, a man dealt with an elderly lady who had collapsed in the street by kneeling beside her and gathering her up so that he was cradling her slumped against his chest. In this position, her head lolled forwards, making her breathing tortuous. He meant well, but he was actually compromising her breathing – and her chances of survival.

Also, you should never put yourself in danger – there is no point trying to help if that just creates a second casualty for the emergency services to deal with. Know your limitations. Do not try to swim out to someone in distress at sea if you cannot swim, or attempt a first-aid procedure if you have no idea what you are doing.

BE PREPARED

Another important part of being a potential first-aider, especially when helping people within your circle of family and friends, is thinking through in advance what would need to be done in an emergency. This means, for example, that if a crisis arises, you don't end up having to take four children and the family dog to the accident and emergency department.

Advance preparation means that you will be able to cope with whatever happens more confidently. It might mean thinking about which family members or friends are close enough to look after the children at short notice, having a list of medication to hand that you or a potential casualty needs, or discussing with a neighbour whether they would feed your animals in a crisis.

Keeping the following two lists on your mobile or near your landline will help enormously if sudden emergencies arise:

1 A list of important telephone numbers – neighbours, friends and relatives who live close by, plus your doctor and the emergency services.
2 A list of medication taken by any members of the household (this may be quite extensive in the case of an elderly person). Also make sure you have a record of any allergies – this might be invaluable to a doctor or paramedic.

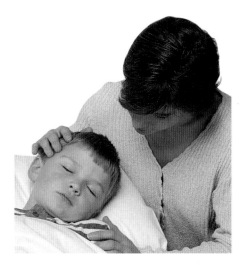

△ With children, it can be hard to distinguish mild from serious problems. Learning to recognize tell-tale symptoms is a vital skill.

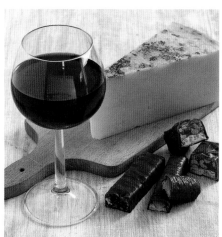

△ It is important to understand the kinds of substances that may trigger adverse reactions, from certain foods and drinks to dust and pollen.

How to use this book

This essential guide has been specially arranged to help readers target the precise kind of information they need at any one time. The introductory chapters offer special guides explaining how to cope with emergencies and how to formulate a life-saving action plan. Other chapters highlight a vast range of vital topics – from children's health to sports injuries – while some deal with a specific body system, placing problems in their proper anatomical context. Each chapter closes with a helpful Skills Checklist – handy summaries that can be ticked off by the reader.

First-aid procedures are presented throughout in a clear step-by-step style, featuring helpful colour photographs and straightforward, jargon-free text, supported where necessary by fully annotated colour artworks. A range of special features, from flow charts to symptoms boxes, has also been used, in order to help readers access vital facts as readily as possible – these are explained below.

See Also boxes
These refer readers to related topics in the book. Cross-references may be to whole chapters (in capital letters), or to specific pages.

Flow charts
Lilac-coloured flow charts appear regularly throughout, summarizing the essential steps to follow in all kinds of situations.

Step-by-step sequences
Wherever relevant, procedures are broken down into numbered steps, where techniques can be seen clearly in full-colour photographs.

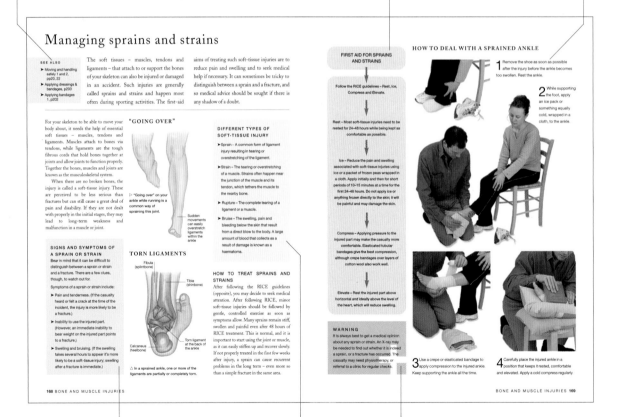

Signs and Symptoms boxes
These blue boxes pick out the major symptoms of each condition, making them easily accessible to first-aiders.

Information boxes
Beige-tinted boxes contain a range of valuable supporting information, from prevention advice and action checklists to useful facts and figures.

Warning boxes
These green-tinted boxes with white crosses alert readers to matters of particular importance. *Always* pay good attention to this advice.

1

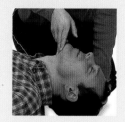

ACTION AT AN EMERGENCY

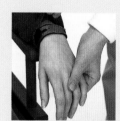

The action that you take at an emergency may have a lasting effect on the casualty. You will need to think quickly and make the correct decisions. Your assessment and examination of the casualty are all-important. This chapter takes you through those initial stages and shows you how to move and handle a casualty who may be badly injured and/or unconscious safely without causing further injury. In many cases, if you are in any doubt at all about what to do or how to do it, it may be best to do nothing: simply to call the emergency services and do what you can to reassure the casualty and keep them warm and safe from further injury. However, in the case of a suspected cardiac arrest, your actions could be life-saving and you should never do nothing.

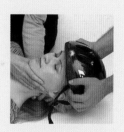

CONTENTS

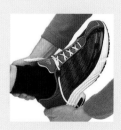

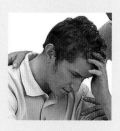

What is first aid?

SEE ALSO
➤ Responsiveness
and the airway, p28
➤ Chest
compressions, p30
➤ Full resuscitation
sequence, p33

First aid is literally the very FIRST assistance you give someone who is ill or has been injured. All of us should know basic first-aid techniques, in the home, at the office or when out and about. One in three of all accidents takes place in our homes, the majority involving children and the elderly. Knowing what to do first and recognizing how potentially serious a casualty's condition is may speed recovery and even prove vital to saving a life. Please note that the text on these two pages is a summary and is expanded in detail over subsequent chapters.

First aid help can cover an extremely varied range of scenarios – from simple reassurance after a small accident to dealing with a life-threatening emergency. A speedy response is crucial. Emergency workers refer to the first hour after an accident as the golden hour: the more help given within this hour, the better the outcome for the patient.

THE GOALS OF FIRST AID

- To summon urgent medical help when necessary.
- To keep the casualty alive. The ABC of life support – Airway, Breathing and Circulation – constitutes the absolute top priority of first aid.
- To stop the casualty getting worse.
- To promote their recovery.
- To provide reassurance and comfort to the casualty.

THE DRABC CODE

Remembering and acting on these can save lives:

D for DANGER
R for RESPONSE
A for AIRWAY
B for BREATHING
C for CIRCULATION

WHAT TO DO IN AN EMERGENCY

First, STAY CALM. Secondly, ASSESS THE SITUATION promptly. Now carry out the "DRABC" sequence, as follows:

1 DANGER

Your assessment should have alerted you to any potential hazards. Now you should:

- Keep yourself out of any danger.
- Keep passers-by out of danger.
- Make safe any hazards, if you can do so without endangering yourself or others. Only move the casualty away from danger in extreme circumstances.

2 RESPONSE

Try to establish the responsiveness level.

- If the casualty appears unconscious or semi-conscious, speak loudly to them – as in "Can you hear me?".
- If this fails to get a response, tap them firmly on the shoulders (or elsewhere if they have a shoulder injury).

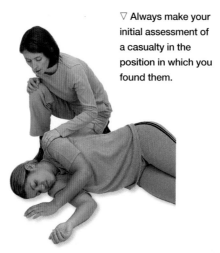

▽ Always make your initial assessment of a casualty in the position in which you found them.

◁ Always try to get help from passers-by. Ideally, ask someone to call the emergency services while you stay with the casualty; keep them warm until trained aid arrives.

3 AIRWAY

Now determine whether the airway (the passage from the mouth to the lungs) is clear enough to allow proper breathing.

- Check the mouth and remove any visible obvious obstructions, such as food, that are at the front of the mouth only.
- Tilt the casualty's head back gently to prevent the tongue from falling back and blocking the airway. Place a hand on the forehead/top of head and two fingers under the jaw. Tilt back gently until a natural stop is reached.

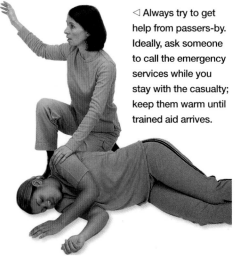

▷ Tilt the head using a hand on the forehead/top of head and two fingers under the jaw. This casualty was found on his back. Avoid moving a casualty on to their back unless you need to start resuscitation.

4 BREATHING

Is the casualty breathing?

- LOOK to see if the chest is moving.
- LISTEN for breathing sounds – put your ear against their mouth.
- FEEL for expired air by placing your cheek or ear close to their face.
- CHECK for breathing for about 10 seconds. If these checks are negative... CALL FOR AN AMBULANCE; ideally get someone else to do so. Make sure you tell the emergency services that the person is not breathing.
- Without delay, start CPR (cardio-pulmonary resuscitation) with chest compressions alone, or if trained and willing to do so, with rescue breaths as well as chest compressions. The emergency dispatcher may be able to tell you if there is a public access defibrillator nearby. If so, or if you know of one's location, send someone to get it if you can. If you are alone, do not stop CPR in order to fetch it yourself.

5 CIRCULATION

Look for signs of a working circulation.

- If you have established that the person is breathing, check for signs of severe bleeding by looking systematically down the body, on both sides.
- Treat severe bleeding promptly by compressing with a dressing or clothing or gloved hand. CALL FOR AN AMBULANCE, and monitor for shock.
- If there is no severe bleeding, then check for other injuries or illnesses.

GETTING HELP

If the casualty is inside a building and other people are present, ask someone to stand outside the building in order to guide the emergency services.

DON'T MOVE THEM!

There are good reasons for leaving a casualty in place until more skilled personnel arrive. Injuries to the spine, especially to the neck, are possible after accidents and falls, and further movement

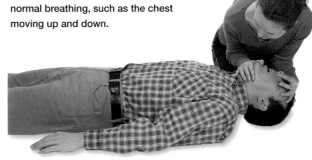

▽ Look, listen and feel for any signs of normal breathing, such as the chest moving up and down.

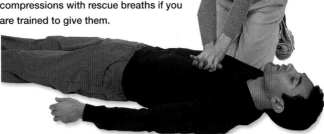

▽ If there are no signs of breathing, start CPR: chest compressions only or chest compressions with rescue breaths if you are trained to give them.

INFORMATION FOR THE EMERGENCY SERVICES

- ➤ Your location (ideally the postal or zip code, but a landmark will do if you know no more) and the phone number you are calling from.
- ➤ What the problem is and what time it happened.

This is sufficient for the emergency operator to send an ambulance if required. While waiting, other information that may be helpful may include:

- ➤ Whether the casualty is conscious and breathing, and if they have any chest pain.
- ➤ The patient's age, sex and any medical history you know.
- ➤ If it is relevant, how many casualties there are, and their sex and approximate age.
- ➤ Any hazards, such as ice on the road or hazardous substances.

The operator may ask further questions and is trained to give instructions over the phone for potentially life-saving procedures. Don't hang up the telephone until the authorities tell you to do so.

can cause serious damage to the spinal cord. You may have to use some movement to deal with an injury, but the golden rule after an accident is not to move an injured person unless they are in danger, need to be resuscitated, or are unconscious and should be put into the recovery position. If moving a casualty is unavoidable, you must be extremely careful with their neck.

▽ If someone falls from a height, keep them warm and do not move them – unless it is necessary for resuscitation.

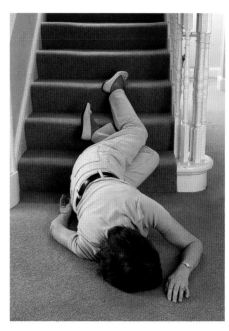

Making your assessment

SEE ALSO

➤ What is first aid?, p12
➤ Examining the casualty, p16
➤ Moving and handling safely 1 and 2, pp20, 22

Your initial assessment may be of major importance to the outcome of an accident. Remember DR (Danger, Response) and ABC (Airway, Breathing, Circulation). Together these form DRABC, which you can also remember as the "DR.ABC". Once you know a casualty is conscious and breathing, you can start to identify the nature of the problem. Ask if they can remember what happened. Look around for clues to the accident. Appearing as calm as possible will help to give vital reassurance to the casualty.

Once you have checked DRABC and established that breathing and circulation are functioning, you have more time to address the casualty's specific problems. They may be simple and the remedy straightforward. If the situation is less clear, however, the "Signs and Symptoms" box indicates what you should look out for.

In general, after completing DRABC, a first-aider should call for emergency aid if needed, then gather initial information (what has happened, plus vital medical facts such as whether the casualty is diabetic), and locate and treat – as far as possible – any obvious physical injury. They may then go on to gather more information from the casualty about the incident and their medical history, and carry out a more thorough examination – by looking, feeling, and questioning the casualty.

TAKING A HISTORY

This involves gathering information by asking questions and listening. Remember that it is very reassuring for everyone concerned to see that something is being done for a friend or relative, and this information may be vital for the ambulance and medical staff later on. Begin by questioning the casualty; if their answers are vague or unhelpful, ask anyone else who may know something useful.

1 Ask their name. It is very comforting to be called by name, and useful to use if the casualty starts to lose consciousness.

2 Ask children their age and, if they are old enough to have the information, ask them how you can contact a parent or carer.

3 What is the problem? Let the casualty talk for a while. They may end up telling you not only what their current problem is, but also useful details about previous similar episodes and what their causes were. If they are still vague, you may find it useful to ask about possible symptoms relating to different systems of the body such as the:
- **Nervous system** – Headache, dizziness, weakness of arms or legs, tingling, pins and needles, loss of movement or sensation.
- **Chest** – Cough, shortness of breath, wheeze, pains in the chest – especially on taking a deep breath.
- **Heart** – Chest pains, pain moving to the left arm or jaw, swollen ankles.
- **Abdomen** – Vomiting, diarrhoea, stomach or pelvic pain.

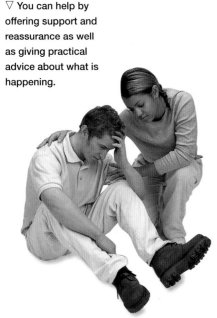

▽ You can help by offering support and reassurance as well as giving practical advice about what is happening.

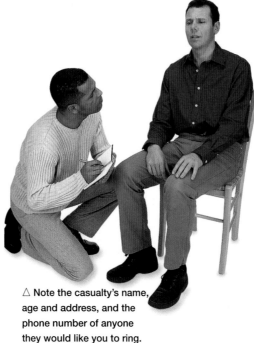

△ Note the casualty's name, age and address, and the phone number of anyone they would like you to ring.

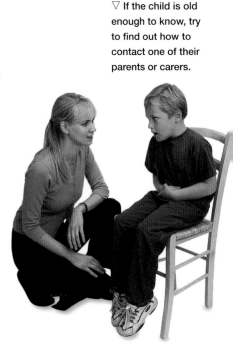

▽ If the child is old enough to know, try to find out how to contact one of their parents or carers.

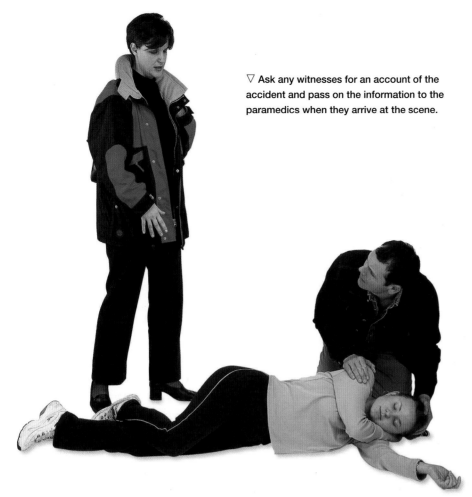

▽ Ask any witnesses for an account of the accident and pass on the information to the paramedics when they arrive at the scene.

SIGNS AND SYMPTOMS

➤ **Symptoms** – What can the casualty tell you about their injury or illness? Are they in pain or stiff, feeling anxious, hot, cold, dizzy, nauseous, faint or thirsty? Is there a sensation of tingling, weakness or memory loss?

➤ **Visual signs** – What can you see in relation to the casualty's condition? Anxious or painful expression, unusual chest movement, burns, sweating, bleeding, bruising, abnormal skin colour, swelling, deformity, vomiting or incontinence? Look for foreign bodies and objects related to substance abuse, such as aerosol cans and small plastic bags. Check for a medical ID tag.

➤ **Other signs** – What can you feel, hear or smell in relation to the casualty? Dampness, abnormal temperature, groaning, sucking sound, alcohol, acetone, solvents or glue, gas or fumes, vomit, urine or faeces?

➤ **Vital signs** – In what state are the casualty's pulse, respiration, colour and temperature? Sum up their general condition.

4 Ask about known medical problems such as diabetes, heart attacks or strokes, which may give you a clue as to what has happened this time.

5 Ask for information about any medication they are currently taking and whether they have any known allergies.

6 Ask when they last ate. If they are going to need emergency surgery, this is a very important question, and it may also be vital if they have diabetes.

GATHERING INFORMATION

Never underestimate how useful bystanders' information can be. People often become ill when they are out by themselves, and passers-by may see what has happened but don't accompany the casualty to hospital; the information is then lost. Exact sequences of events are vitally useful to the medical staff, because they often give big clues about the cause of a collapse or illness.

Sick or injured people may be very vague about what has happened to them, and will not know if, for example, they had a convulsion while they were unconscious. They may not know that one side of their face drooped for a short time, or that they lost their speech. These events will determine what investigations are carried out at the hospital. Ultimately, longer-term outcomes – such as whether they will be allowed to drive home or not – may depend very much on what actually happened. Any information you can gather and relay to the emergency services is very useful.

IDENTIFICATION DEVICES

If a casualty is wearing one, a medical ID tags, which is usually worn as a necklace or bracelet, can be life-saving. One side often features a staff-and-snake emblem (an international medical symbol), and the other will have useful information about the casualty, for example if they suffer from diabetes or epilepsy. Tell the emergency services about the information on the tag.

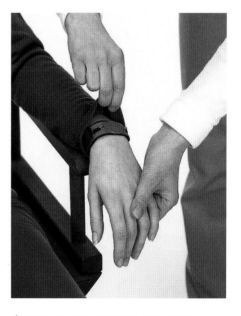

△ Always check a casualty's neck, wrists and ankles for a medical ID tag and pass on the information it carries to the paramedics.

Examining the casualty

SEE ALSO
➤ What is first aid?, p12
➤ Removing clothing and helmets, p18
➤ Responsiveness and the airway, p28
➤ The recovery position, p36

Once you are happy that a casualty is conscious and breathing, try to identify the problem by carrying out an examination. One of the first steps is to look at their face – are they very pale, for example? Don't move them at this stage, especially the neck or back. Now check the body for injury. Start with the head and finish with the arms and legs. Unless they are unresponsive, always gain a casualty's consent before starting an examination ("I just need to examine you to check for injuries, OK?") and keep the casualty and any friends or relatives informed as you go along.

You can tell a lot from looking at people, even before you touch them. Remember that ensuring a casualty's airway is clear is a top priority before any physical check. The feel and colour of skin is another hint. People in shock have pale, cold, clammy skin; a fever makes skin hot, dry and often flushed. Blue skin and lips suggest a heart that is not pumping well, or breathing problems that are preventing enough oxygen from reaching the blood.

Examine people in a systematic, gentle but businesslike way. If there is any possibility of a head or spinal injury, do not move the casualty unless you need to start CPR. Otherwise, place unconscious but breathing casualties in the recovery position (see page 36 (adults) and page 48 (children)) before examining them. If you suspect any injuries that may worsen with movement, especially spinal injuries, examine them first. Always ensure that you protect the casualty's spine when moving them.

WHAT TO CHECK FOR

➤ Bruising, swelling, puncture wounds, burns and tender or painful areas.

➤ Changes in the casualty's appearance, breathing or state of consciousness.

➤ The presence of a medical ID tag.

➤ Any medication carried by the casualty, such as an inhaler or adrenaline injector.

VITAL NOTE: Anyone with a suspected spinal injury (see Step 5) must be kept as still as possible (especially the head) as you check. Ideally, hold them still while a helper checks areas other than the back.

HEAD-TO-TOE EXAMINATION

1 HEAD
Check the scalp for injury – swelling, depressions, cuts and bleeding. Also look out for blood or clear fluids leaking from the nose or ears. Check the mouth for any objects or fluids

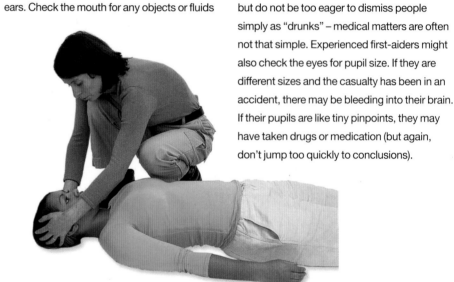

(such as vomit) that could obstruct breathing and remove if very easy to do (only remove dentures that are loose or broken and easy to extract). Smell the casualty's breath for alcohol, but do not be too eager to dismiss people simply as "drunks" – medical matters are often not that simple. Experienced first-aiders might also check the eyes for pupil size. If they are different sizes and the casualty has been in an accident, there may be bleeding into their brain. If their pupils are like tiny pinpoints, they may have taken drugs or medication (but again, don't jump too quickly to conclusions).

2 NECK
Make sure clothing is not tight, and check for a medical ID tag. Working very gently, feel along the back of the neck, without moving the head, for swelling or tenderness. Some people who have undergone a tracheotomy have a surgical opening called a stoma at the front of the neck that acts as an airway, so make sure that nothing obvious is blocking it.

3 CHEST

Is the chest moving normally? Are there very tender places over the ribs (these may be rib fractures)? If there is an object (such as a knife) stuck in the chest, do not remove it. Feel the collarbones for swelling and tenderness. In some cases, it may be necessary to remove clothing to look at the chest, to check for obvious lacerations or bruises, for example. Typically, you might do this if the emergency services are delayed, but always proceed with sensitivity.

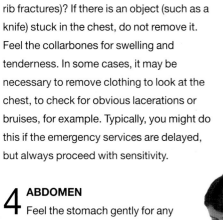

4 ABDOMEN

Feel the stomach gently for any large swellings or tender places. If the casualty is conscious, they will flinch, moan or cry out if you touch an area that is painful.

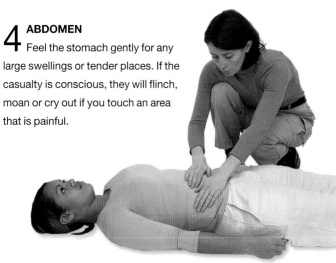

5 LOWER BACK

If you suspect a spinal injury, from the circumstances of the accident or from what the casualty says, do not try examining the back – even the tiniest amount of movement could risk further damage (see also What to Check For box). If you do not suspect spinal injury, gently feel the back for any tender areas.

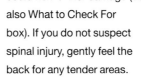

6 PELVIS

Note any tender places over the hips. Maintain a very light touch because a pelvic injury can be excruciatingly painful.

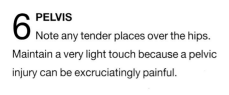

7 ARMS AND LEGS

Look for injuries. Now test the limbs' function by asking whether the casualty can feel you touching their arms and legs. Ask them to grip your hand with theirs and to try tensing their leg muscles.

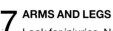

Removing clothing and helmets

SEE ALSO
➤ Examining the casualty, p16
➤ Moving and handling safely 1 and 2, pp20, 22

Removing a casualty's clothing should not be an automatic reaction. It is often unnecessary, especially if the casualty will soon be seen at a hospital, and can make people feel anxious and vulnerable, as well as exposing them to the elements. The movement required may also cause further injury. Only remove clothing if it is absolutely essential in order to treat the casualty effectively, for instance to look at a wounded site that is hidden by clothing in order to assess and deal with the injury. Seek consent from a conscious casualty and respect people's privacy.

Do not remove clothing that is stuck to the skin. Be very careful in the case of chemical contamination of clothes – wear gloves to protect yourself, cut away clothing, rather than pulling it over head or limbs, and flood the affected area with clean water as quickly as possible.

POINTS TO CONSIDER

➤ People can get upset at having their clothes removed by a stranger. Unless it is absolutely necessary, it is best to wait until they reach hospital. Remember, you can often feel injuries adequately through clothing.

➤ If you are in any doubt about removing an item of clothing or footwear, or if you are causing the casualty increased pain, it is best to wait for the paramedics.

➤ If they are conscious, seek the casualty's consent for your actions and explain what you are doing.

➤ Remove clothes and shoes with the minimum of movement, to avoid further injury and pain – never pull at clothing.

➤ The injured area may be very sensitive, so try to keep clothing away from it.

➤ Be careful that cutting clothes does not injure the skin, especially if you are using scissors not designed for this job.

➤ The easiest route for cutting is often along the seams.

➤ With leg and foot injuries, try to take off shoes or boots before the leg and ankle become so swollen that it is more painful to remove the footwear.

SWEATERS AND T-SHIRTS

If the injury is in the upper part of the body, then you may need to remove the casualty's top garment. Make sure that you do not attempt to do this if there is any chance that the casualty may have sustained a spinal injury. If there is chemical contamination of clothing do not pull garments off over the head as this risks spreading the chemical to unaffected areas of skin.

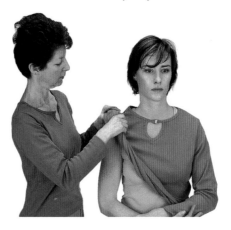 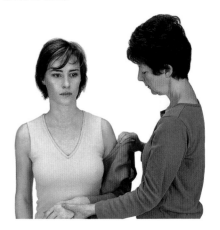

1 Release the uninjured arm carefully, before trying to undress the injured arm. Roll the garment up to the shoulder.

2 Pull the garment over the head, then slowly and very gently pull it down over the injured arm and smoothly off the hand.

SHOES

Removing shoes can be tricky because the foot or ankle may have become swollen. Undo the shoe entirely and support the foot under the ankle with one hand, while gently sliding the shoe off the heel and then over the toes with the other hand.

▽ Make sure that the laces are loose before you attempt to remove shoes.

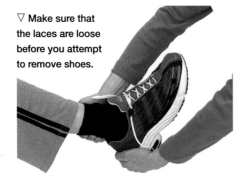

SOCKS

The tight fit of socks causes problems for removal. If there is no swelling or pain you can try rolling the sock down over the foot. If the ankle or foot is very swollen, it is easier to cut off the sock. Pull the material away from the skin as you cut.

▽ You should cut the sock off an injured foot rather than trying to pull it off.

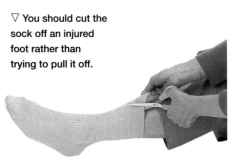

TROUSERS

If trousers are too tight to pull up from the ankle to reach a leg wound, you may need to cut them along the seam.

▽ Hold the trousers clear of a leg injury while pulling them up.

▽ You may have to cut the trousers and socks off the injured leg in order to avoid causing any further pain.

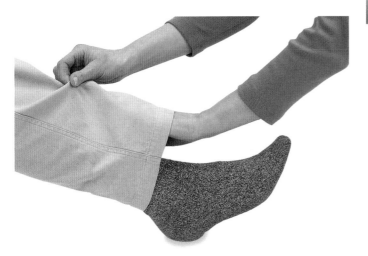

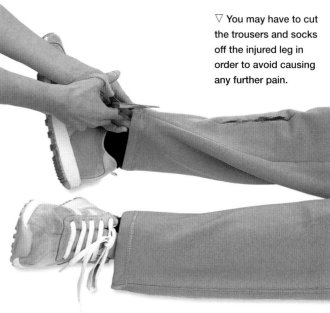

HELMETS

Only remove helmets as a last resort – as a rule of thumb, do so only if they are direly impeding a casualty's breathing. If the casualty is breathing and has an unrestricted airway, leave removal to the experts. If you have to proceed urgently, get someone to assist you so that the neck is supported, in a straight line with the head and spine while the helmet is taken off.

Full-face helmets

Two people are needed to remove a full-face helmet. One person is in charge of supporting the casualty's neck and holding on to the lower jaw; the second person undoes (or cuts) the straps and places their fingers under the helmet's rim. Sitting behind the casualty's head, the second person starts to ease off the helmet. The first person must keep the head still. The helmet may have to be tilted back to get it over the chin, and then forwards in order to lift it over the back of the head.

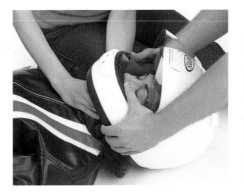

1 One helper firmly supports the casualty's neck and jaw while the other carefully undoes the straps and eases the helmet up.

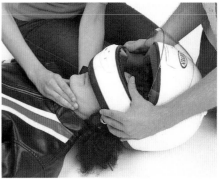

2 The first helper maintains neck and jaw support while the other helper slowly lifts the helmet over the chin and over the head.

Helmets with an emergency quick release system (EQRS)

These have two red tabs underneath the chin, one on each side. One rescuer sits behind the casualty's head holding the helmet while the second rescuer releases or cuts the chin strap, as above, then pulls firmly on the red tabs, one at a time, to remove the cheek pads. This allows more room and enables the helmet to be removed with minimal load on the neck.

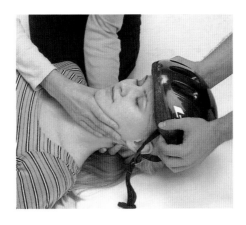

◁ Open-face helmets

These helmets should also be removed by two people, if possible. One person supports the neck and jaw while the second person undoes (or cuts) the chin strap. The second person then grips the sides of the helmet from the inside and pulls the straps apart. The helmet can then be lifted off without causing pain or further injury. This type of helmet is often used by cyclists.

Moving and handling safely 1

SEE ALSO

➤ Moving and handling safely 2, p22

➤ WOUNDS AND BLEEDING, p125

➤ BONE AND MUSCLE INJURIES, p147

Generally, its best not to move a sick or injured person, and you should never move a casualty if there is any chance that they could have a spinal injury, especially in the neck area. Sometimes, however, you will have no choice in the matter – the injured person may not be breathing and the airway must always take first priority, although you should still take care to protect the neck during movement and resuscitation. Very rarely, it may be vital to move the casualty away from danger into a safer environment, perhaps because of fire or danger of explosion, or to get the casualty away from poisonous fumes.

Causing further injury is always a risk with moving people, so doing nothing may be wise – it is a question of weighing up the relative perils. If you have to, you need to know how to move a casualty without causing further injury or endangering yourself. Always observe the rules of safe lifting, listed below. Also, think laterally and don't automatically rush to drag people all over the place. It may be easier to remove the danger from the casualty than the other way around. So, if a casualty is lying in a busy road, you might be able to park your car so that others will drive around the incident area.

SAFE MOVING

If moving another adult, you must be certain that this is necessary and that you are strong enough to do so. It is vital to protect your own back, so always remember to:

• Lift or move someone only if you are trained or if it is a dire emergency.
• Get the casualty to move himself or herself if possible.
• Keep your feet slightly apart.
• Bend from the knees and use your legs to lift, not your back.
• Do not twist or turn as you lift.
• Keep your back straight and locked.
• Keep the weight that is being lifted close to your body.

MOVING A CASUALTY SINGLE-HANDEDLY

The moving techniques shown below and on the opposite page are for when there is just one rescuer at the accident scene. Here the options for moving a casualty are more limited than if there are two or more rescuers. Careful thought must be given to the technique you choose: consider your strength and fitness, the weight of the casualty, whether they are conscious and whether there could be a spinal injury.

Unconscious casualty

An unconscious person is unable to protect their airway so you must ensure there is no danger of their head flopping forwards and blocking their airway when you move them. Dragging by either the arms or legs (if there is no injury) is the best way to move the casualty in this instance. Dragging can also be used when the casualty is too heavy to lift.

Mobile casualty

If the casualty can still walk in a limited way you can try the human crutch. This helps to stabilize their walking.

Immobile casualty

If the casualty cannot move, they may have a spinal injury. If there is any risk of this, never move a casualty – call the emergency services immediately.

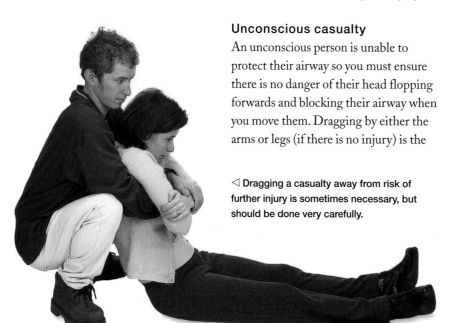

◁ **Dragging a casualty away from risk of further injury is sometimes necessary, but should be done very carefully.**

DRAGGING

You may have to drag a casualty away from the risk of further injury, such as in a fire. Bend down at the knees, lock your arms around the casualty's chest and keep them as close to you as possible as you move back. Do not drag the casualty sideways.

THE HUMAN CRUTCH

If the casualty is still at all mobile, this highly useful "assisted walk" technique allows the casualty to use your body as a crutch, to give them greater stability. Place a supporting arm firmly around their waist and grasp their nearest hand in your other hand. Make sure that you tell them about any obstacles in their path or changes in floor level, and take only small steps.

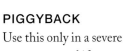

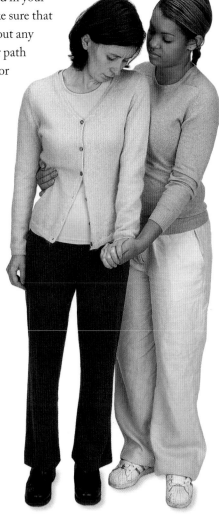

CRADLE CARRY

This method works particularly well with children and helps them to feel reassured and safe. Never attempt this lift on someone unless they are a great deal lighter than you, as you may damage your back; there is also the danger of dropping the casualty and causing further injury.

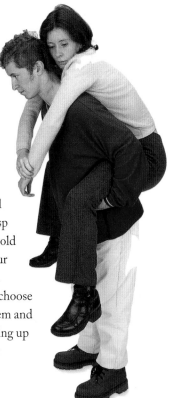

PIGGYBACK

Use this only in a severe emergency and if confident of your strength. Your approach will vary depending on how tall, heavy and strong you are in relation to the casualty. With your back to the casualty, bend forward and get the casualty to put both arms over your shoulders. Pull them on to your back and grasp their thighs. If you can, take hold of their hands. Try to keep your knees slightly bent. If lifting a small, light casualty, you may choose to crouch down in front of them and grasp their thighs before coming up gradually with your back kept straight.

WHICH SINGLE-HANDED CARRY TO USE

➤ Try to use the human crutch wherever possible, especially if you are small and light. This excellent technique poses minimum risk to the rescuer, and little risk of damaging the casualty's internal organs. Ideally, the cradle and piggyback carries are usually best left for lifting someone about half your weight or less, making them particularly suitable for children.

➤ Avoid the "fireman's lift" (where the casualty is carried over the rescuer's shoulder), as this is tricky to do well and safely and could potentially cause severe damage to the casualty.

Moving and handling safely 2

MOVING A CASUALTY WITH TWO OR MORE HELPERS

It is much easier and less likely to cause further injury if you can move or lift a casualty with two or more people helping. This is because you have more control over the move, and your combined strength means you are sharing the burden of weight. At the scene of an accident, always try to enlist help from any bystanders before attempting to move the casualty single-handedly. Explain step-by-step exactly what you intend to do and ensure they understand the importance of coordinating every move.

you can attempt a fore and aft carry. This can also be used if the person is conscious, but it should be avoided if there is any possibility of a spinal injury or if the arms, shoulders or ribs are injured. If four helpers are available and you have a blanket or piece of cloth handy, a blanket lift provides a safe, supportive method of transporting an injured person – except when spinal injury is suspected, in which case, avoid it. If there is an immediate risk to life, such as fire or water, that outweighs the danger of movement, very carefully roll the victim

away from the danger with as many helpers as possible supporting and controlling the body with the head and spine kept in a straight line to minimize damage. All helpers must act in sync when rolling the casualty.

Conscious casualty

The two-hand seat carry can be used if the casualty is conscious and able to move into a sitting position. If the casualty is extremely heavy, then do not try to lift them – leave this to the experts.

Unconscious casualty

If the casualty is unconscious or is immobilized as a result of their injuries,

FORE AND AFT CARRY

With an unconscious or immobile casualty and two helpers, the stronger should take the upper body and the other the legs. Make sure you synchronize your actions and move in the same direction. Move slowly and carefully and watch out for any obstacles such as steps or stairs.

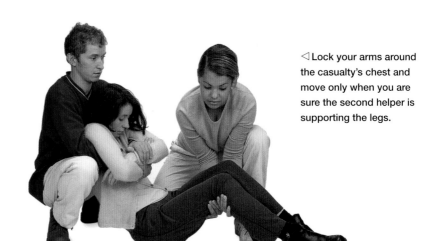

◁ Lock your arms around the casualty's chest and move only when you are sure the second helper is supporting the legs.

TWO-HAND SEAT

This move should be used when the casualty is conscious. Squat one on each side of the casualty and cross arms across their back. Hold on to the casualty's clothes, then pass your other hands under the casualty's knees and grip each other's wrists. Keep close to the casualty and lift together, keeping knees bent.

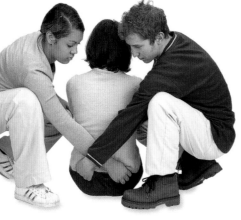

1 Get as close to the casualty as you possibly can in order to reduce strain on your own back. Bend at the knees and take hold of the casualty's clothes, on or just above the buttocks, with your hands crossed.

△ Detail of hand grip.

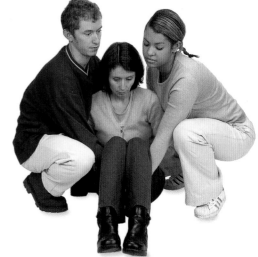

2 With your other hands, support the casualty's legs. Lock wrists with the other helper and lift, keeping your back straight.

BLANKET LIFT

This rudimentary "stretcher" is the safest, easiest way of moving an unconscious or immobile casualty if there is no possibility of spinal injury and if there are at least four helpers – doing it with fewer risks further injury. You need a strong blanket, sheet, rug or any large piece of fabric that is long enough to support the casualty's entire body. Use this to carry the casualty a short way or to transfer them to a proper stretcher. All helpers must move the casualty in a synchronized action.

Note that you should never attempt to improvise any kind of stretcher if you are uncertain what to do.

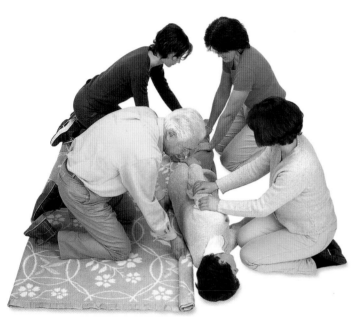

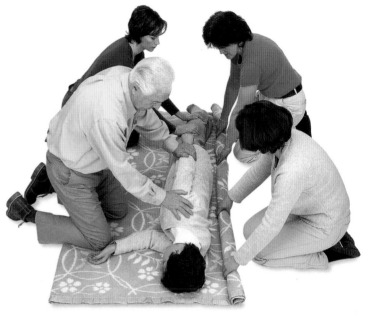

1 With the casualty placed on their side, and the blanket edge rolled up lengthways, position the roll against the casualty's back.

2 Move the casualty over the rolled edge, on to their other side. Make sure the casualty's head isn't close to the edge.

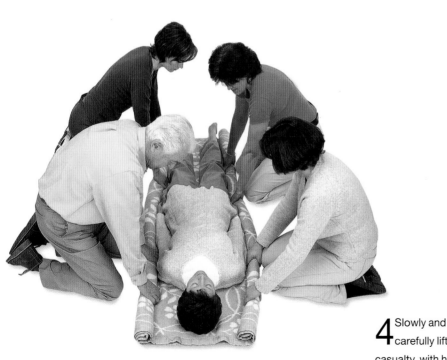

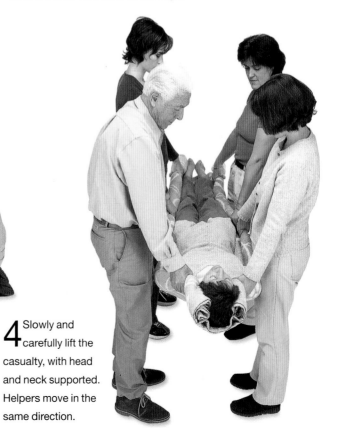

3 Roll up the other long edge of the blanket. The two helpers on either side of the casualty grasp the roll firmly with both hands.

4 Slowly and carefully lift the casualty, with head and neck supported. Helpers move in the same direction.

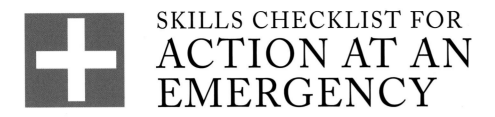

SKILLS CHECKLIST FOR
ACTION AT AN EMERGENCY

KEY POINTS

- Always do the DRABC ☐

- Assess the situation promptly but with thought – do not rush in impulsively ☐

- Do not move the casualty before the paramedics arrive unless it is absolutely necessary ☐

- Always treat casualties with respect; seek permission for actions of a personal nature where possible, and keep them well informed of what you are doing ☐

SKILLS LEARNED

- The principal rules of approaching and dealing with emergencies safely and effectively ☐

- The basics of life-saving: what the DRABC of Danger, Response, Airway, Breathing, Circulation is all about ☐

- Assessing the nature of the problem ☐

- When and how to remove clothing and helmets, without causing further injury ☐

- Handling and moving a casualty safely ☐

LIFE-SAVING PRIORITIES

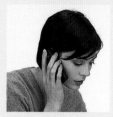

For the best possible outcome, it is essential that life-saving techniques are carried out in the correct order. Once you have assessed DRABC (see the previous chapter), until help arrives you need to concentrate on issues such as continuing resuscitation, possibly moving the casualty into the recovery position, or deciding which technique is best to use for choking, depending on whether the casualty is conscious or unconscious. You must also consider the impact of shock on any casualty. In first aid terms this means 'surgical shock', a serious condition due to insufficient blood flow to organs and tissues, which constitutes a medical emergency. It is not the same as emotional shock, though obviously you should do your best to calm and reassure the casualty at every stage of the emergency.

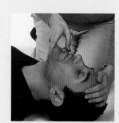

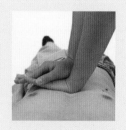

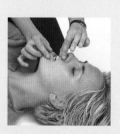

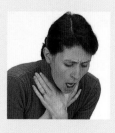

Understanding resuscitation

SEE ALSO

➤ Responsiveness and the airway, p28
➤ Rescue breathing, p32
➤ Chest compressions, p30
➤ The recovery position, p36

You could save someone's life by applying basic resuscitation skills. Using CPR (cardio-pulmonary resuscitation), you should be able to maintain a person's breathing and circulation until the emergency services arrive, so ensuring that oxygen gets into the lungs and that oxygenated blood gets to the brain. Since once the heart has stopped, the casualty will die if circulation is not restored, you should always attempt resuscitation using the techniques that are explained in this chapter: in the case of cardiac arrest, it is always better to do something than nothing.

WHAT IS CARDIOPULMONARY RESUSCITATION (CPR)?

CPR is the technique of providing basic life support by using chest compressions, and sometimes accompanied by artificial ventilation. The latter is also called "the kiss of life", mouth-to-mouth resuscitation, or rescue breathing. Although resuscitation techniques have been used for over 50 years, it was not until the 1970s that the idea of training the public in these skills began.

CPR is needed after a cardiac arrest, that is, when the heart suddenly stops beating and circulation of the blood around the body ceases. A person who has had a cardiac arrest is unresponsive to voice or touch, is not breathing normally and has no pulse. Since two-thirds of cardiac arrests occur unexpectedly and not in hospitals, it makes sense for members of the public to be able to carry out resuscitation.

After only 3–4 minutes without oxygen, the brain can suffer irreversible damage, and this can be fatal, so a bystander who recognises cardiac arrest and immediately calls for emergency medical help and starts effective CPR before the ambulance arrives can significantly improve a victim's chance of survival.

(There have been some instances of successful resuscitation up to 40 minutes after cardiac arrest when it occurred in cold water, but this is the exception.) In most cases, a little knowledge and training can definitely save lives.

NORMAL CIRCULATION

Blood flows through the blood vessels in one direction at a fairly constant rate. The heart is at the centre of the circulatory system, pumping blood around the body. The heart pumps blood to the lungs where it absorbs oxygen and gives up the carbon dioxide collected as it travels around the body. The blood then returns to the heart, and the oxygenated blood is sent to all parts of the body including the brain. The brain controls all body functions, including those of the heart and lungs, and the working of these three organs is closely linked. If any one fails, it does not take long for the other two organs to fail too.

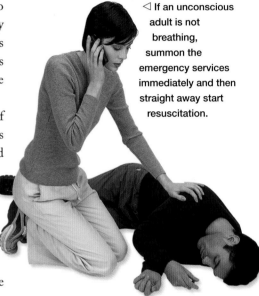

◁ If an unconscious adult is not breathing, summon the emergency services immediately and then straight away start resuscitation.

HOW CPR WORKS

Keeping the casualty's airway open and doing chest compressions to simulate the pumping action of the heart means that an oxygenated blood supply continues to reach their brain. This "buys" really valuable time for the casualty by keeping their brain alive until more specialized help is available.

CHEST COMPRESSIONS

The blood is kept circulating by the use of external pressure on the chest cavity. By pressing down on the breastbone, blood is forced out of the heart and forced into the rest of the casualty's body. When pressure is released, the heart fills up with more blood, ready for the next compression, and so on. This is done at a rate of 100-120 compressions per minute.

▷ If the person is unconscious but breathing, place them in the recovery position unless a spinal injury is suspected.

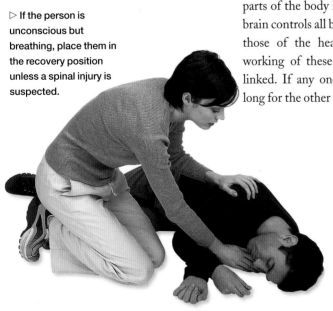

DEFIBRILLATORS

An automatic external defibrillator (AED) is a device that applies an electric shock to the chest in order to re-start the heart, so buying valuable time for a victim of cardiac arrest. The device analyses the heart rhythm and delivers a shock where necessary. AEDs may be life-saving, particularly if the ambulance takes more than five minutes to arrive.

Portable versions of these life-saving machines are now frequently available in public locations such as shopping malls, sports and fitness facilities, education institutions, public buildings, and public parks, as well as in many workplaces. They may also be known as public access defibrillators (PAD) or community defibrillators. The devices are designed for use by untrained people and are very simple to use. Emergency operators may know the location of your nearest AED and how to access it, and can give instructions on using it.

In some places, trained non-medical first responders may be alerted to arrive with an AED before the emergency services. You can download various apps that give registered AED locations nationwide. In most states in the United States, specific legislation or general 'Good Samaritan laws' provide immunity from legal liability for any harm resulting from the use of an AED in good faith by a lay person.

IMPROVING SURVIVAL

Because early initiation of chest compressions vastly improves survival rates, experts now recommend that bystanders should perform compression-only CPR in cases of adult cardiac arrest, and attempt rescue breaths ('kiss of life') as well only if trained and willing to do so. The use of chest compressions alone gives survival rates at least similar to those of traditional CPR with compressions plus artificial ventilation.

Note the position is different in children (see page 44).

BASIC LIFE SUPPORT PRINCIPLES FOR AN UNRESPONSIVE ADULT WHO IS NOT BREATHING NORMALLY

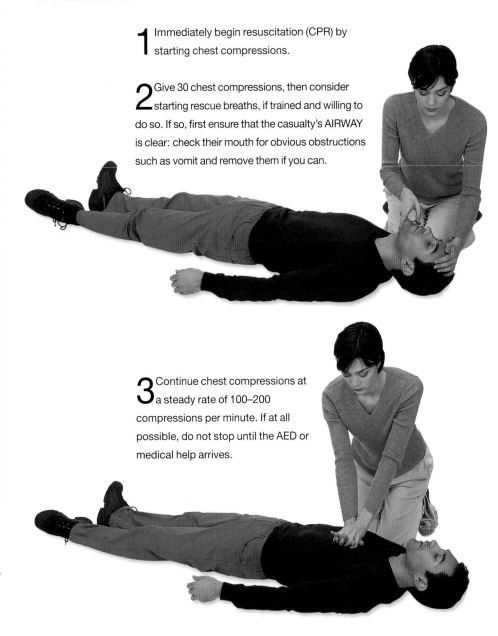

1 Immediately begin resuscitation (CPR) by starting chest compressions.

2 Give 30 chest compressions, then consider starting rescue breaths, if trained and willing to do so. If so, first ensure that the casualty's AIRWAY is clear: check their mouth for obvious obstructions such as vomit and remove them if you can.

3 Continue chest compressions at a steady rate of 100–200 compressions per minute. If at all possible, do not stop until the AED or medical help arrives.

△ Defibrillators (AEDs) can be found at many public locations, such as sports grounds, shopping centres and even in village telephone boxes. Emergency operators can advise how to access the device and how to use it.

Public access bleed control kits may also be available in some areas.

Responsiveness and the airway

SEE ALSO
➤ What is first aid?, p12
➤ Moving and handling safely 1 and 2, pp20, 22
➤ Coping with neck injuries, p156 (for "log roll" technique)

You must assess a casualty's responsiveness before acting. In the first instance, obtain basic responsiveness information that will tell you whether or not a casualty is conscious and breathing – look for signs of life and try for a verbal response – this should take no more than a few seconds. If a casualty is unresponsive and not breathing, you should start chest compressions without delay (see pages 30–31 for adults and 46–47 for children). If a casualty has any level of response, then they don't need to be resuscitated but maintain a vigilant watch.

Should the casualty stop breathing at any time, start resuscitation at once. Otherwise, treat other injuries, consider whether you should move a breathing but unconscious casualty into the recovery position, and make sure to keep their airway open. If the person is conscious, offer reassurance and keep them warm while you wait for the paramedics to arrive.

People who have collapsed may have different levels of consciousness, from fully alert to a deep coma. Once you have dealt with the immediate dangers (DRABC and assessed the extent of any injuries), you might try to determine this level – such additional responsiveness information may be useful, and you can pass it on to the paramedics when they arrive. Professionals use the letters AVPU for the levels of consciousness – Alert, Verbal, Pain and Unresponsive.

RESPONSIVENESS ASSESSMENT IN DETAIL – THE AVPU CODE

ALERT

An alert casualty is awake and will be able to talk to you spontaneously. Reassure them that help is on the way and that you will do all you can to make them comfortable. Then try to find out exactly what happened.

VERBAL

The casualty may seem to be unconscious but will respond to a verbal prompt. Shout "Are you OK?" close to their ear, and they will respond as if being roused from sleep. You could also try tapping them on the shoulder, or even giving them a gentle shake (but not if there is any possibility of a spinal injury).

PAIN

If shouting and gentle tapping or shaking does not wake the casualty, they might respond to a painful stimulus such as rubbing hard on their breastbone with your knuckles or giving a gentle pinch. Do not do anything that could draw blood, such as pricking them with a pin or sharp object.

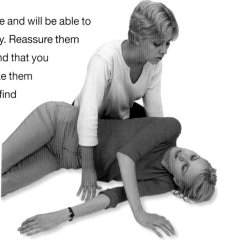

UNRESPONSIVE

This is when the casualty does not respond at all, in any way – you may well have decided this when going through DRABC initially. If you run through A, V and P, and none of these techniques works, then the casualty is considered unresponsive.

SHOULD YOU MOVE AN UNRESPONSIVE CASUALTY?

Always make your first assessment of a casualty in the position in which you find them. If, while following the DRABC procedures, your initial conclusion is that a casualty is unresponsive and not breathing, then you must commence CPR at once, if necessary moving them onto their back on a flat surface in order to do so. Only move them if absolutely necessary – if this is the only way to keep them clear of danger, perform CPR or keep their airway unobstructed.

If there is any likelihood at all of injury, take great care to protect the injured person's spine if you move them. Ideally, move them by using the log-roll technique – although at least three helpers are needed to do this safely.

1 If it is essential to move an unresponsive casualty on to their back (most notably, to perform resuscitation), first straighten the casualty's legs and put their arms as close to their sides as possible. Make sure their airway is always kept clear by ensuring the head does not drop down towards their chest.

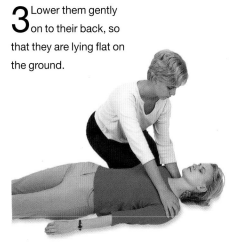

2 Cradle the head and neck with one hand, while holding the lower shoulder with your other hand.

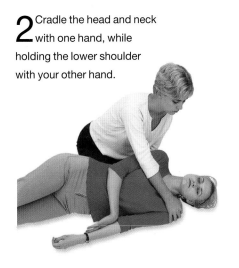

3 Lower them gently on to their back, so that they are lying flat on the ground.

KEEPING THE AIRWAY CLEAR

The airway is just that – a passage through which air passes. This passage stretches from the nose and mouth, through the throat (pharynx), then into the windpipe (trachea), and down to the lungs. Food also passes through the upper part of this tube – the mouth and throat. The airway must be clear for the casualty to be able to breathe, either alone or during resuscitation.

The most common things that block a casualty's airway are the tongue, blood and vomit. When checking an airway, look in the mouth. Do not sweep your finger around blindly, don't risk getting your fingers bitten, and avoid the throat area altogether; never risk pushing something further in. Scoop out objects such as sweets and food with two fingers. If an obstruction is likely to slip further down, or if there is liquid in the mouth, turn the person on their side in order to remove it.

Opening the airway

In an unconscious casualty, the tongue may flop to the back of the throat and block the airway. To prevent this, provided there is no possibility of a spinal injury, put your hand on their forehead and tilt the head back; with two fingers under the chin and thumb on top, lift the jaw. If the casualty is upright, you can support their neck and tilt their head back to open the airway.

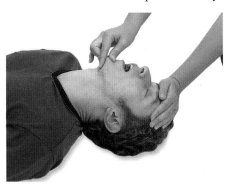

△ Carrying out the simple move of opening the airway can be enough to save someone's life.

If there is a possibility of spinal injury, you must adapt your manoeuvre. Your priority is to get a person breathing, so if they cannot breathe and have a possible neck injury, it is important to open the airway without further injury.

Instead of tilting the head back, lift the jaw forwards by pushing upwards at the angle of the jaw.

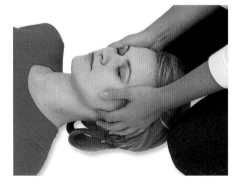

△ In a suspected neck injury, push up at the sides of the jaw, as shown, to open the airway.

Chest compressions

SEE ALSO

➤ What is first aid?, p12

➤ Understanding resuscitation, p26

➤ Full resuscitation sequence, p33

Chest compressions are also known as cardiac compressions, or as cardiac/chest/heart massage. These compressions form part of the CIRCULATION stage of DRABC. If you are faced with a casualty who is not responding and not breathing properly, you must immediately start to give compressions to initiate cardiopulmonary resuscitation (CPR). You do not need to give mouth-to-mouth respiration unless you are trained and willing to do so: CPR using chest compressions alone greatly increases the survival rate after cardiac arrest.

For chest compressions to be effective, the casualty should be lying flat on their back on a firm surface such as the floor – or the ground if they are outside. Although it is a good idea to practise finding the CPR compression site before you need to act in an emergency, never carry out practice compressions on conscious volunteers, as you may cause harm. Always use a first aid dummy.

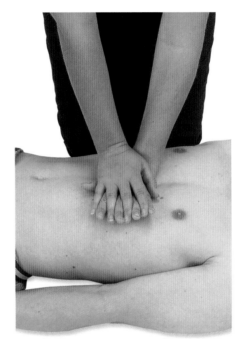

▷ When carrying out chest compressions, the heel of only one of your hands should come into contact with the compression site.

WARNING

In general, do not check for a pulse when assessing a person unless you are highly trained and can check it rapidly, without wasting vital seconds. It is not easy to find a pulse, even for trained people. People can die when first-aiders mistakenly feel a non-existent pulse, and fail to resuscitate. Instead of checking for a pulse, check the casualty's responsiveness and whether they are breathing normally. This should take no more than a few seconds. Remember, occasional gasps are not effective breathing.

HOW TO FIND THE COMPRESSION SITE

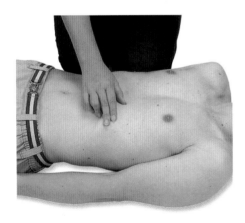

1 Kneel beside the casualty and run the fingers of your hand nearest the waist along the lower ribs until they meet the breastbone at the centre of the ribcage.

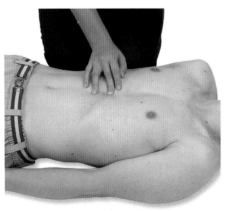

2 Keeping your middle finger at this notch, place the index finger of the same hand over the lower end of the breastbone.

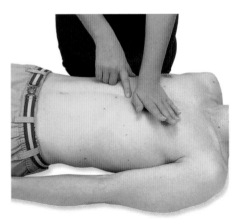

3 Place the heel of the other hand on the breastbone, and slide it down to lie beside the index finger already there. The heel of your hand is now on the compression site.

HOW TO GIVE CARDIAC MASSAGE

1 Kneel down at right angles to the casualty, so that you are positioned roughly halfway between their shoulders and waist.

2 Locate the compression site, and place the heel of one hand over this area. Place the heel of the other hand on top with both sets of fingers interlaced. The heels of your hands are going to do the work; your fingers should not touch the chest. Keep your elbows locked and arms straight all the time.

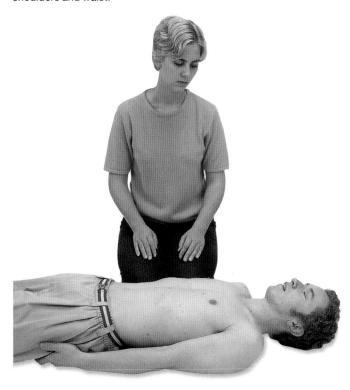

3 Place your shoulders directly over your hands so you are leaning over the casualty. This will concentrate pressure at the compression site. Compress the chest wall down by about 5–6cm (2–2⅓in). Release the pressure without taking your hands off the chest or bending your elbows.

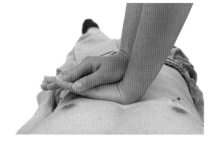

4 Using your body weight as well as your arms, push down on the chest at a rate of 100–120 compressions per minute – about twice per second. A helpful way to get the rate right is to pace your compressions to the imagined soundtrack of the Bee Gee's 'Staying Alive', or Queen's 'Another One Bites the Dust'. Keep your hands on the chest and release the pressure in between pushes.

5 Continue giving compressions until help arrives. If there is more than one bystander, take turns if you can, but keep the compressions going with minimal interruption.

WARNING
Do not stop compressions because you are worried about hurting the casualty, for instance by cracking a rib. Once the heart has stopped the person will die without your help – they are better off alive and with a broken rib.

Rescue breathing

Rescue breathing (also called "kiss of life", mouth-to-mouth respiration and artificial ventilation) is a technique that supplies oxygen to the lungs of a person who is not breathing. Usually performed mouth to mouth, it may be done mouth to nose (if the mouth is damaged), mouth to mouth and nose (for babies) or mouth to stoma (a hole in the neck seen in people who have had a tracheotomy). Never let hygiene fears hold you back – infection is unlikely. If you have not been trained in giving rescue breaths, stick to chest compressions only.

Although first aiders used to be encouraged to use rescue breaths in addition to chest compressions, many experts now recommend that they should use compression-only CPR unless they have been properly trained to give rescue breaths.

Compression-only CPR has been shown to be as effective as traditional CPR with compressions and rescue breathing, and bystanders are more likely to start compression-only CPR during the crucial life-saving minutes following a cardiac arrest.

HOW DOES IT WORK?

As well as replacing the pumping action of the heart to propel blood around the body, giving chest compressions acts like a pair of bellows, drawing air into the lungs and allowing it to be released, simulating breathing. The air supplies oxygen to the blood that is being pumped through the heart by the compressions. In addition, surrounding air contains higher levels of oxygen than exhaled air, and using compression-only CPR means that compressions need not be interrupted to give rescue breaths.

Bystander CPR using compressions only has been shown to have the same statistical odds of saving a life as traditional CPR with compressions and rescue breathing.

SIGNS AND SYMPTOMS OF AGONAL BREATHING

➤ Agonal breathing often occurs in the first few minutes following cardiac arrest. It is not normal breathing and does not mean that the casualty is getting any oxygen.

➤ Symptoms include short, sporadic breaths or gasping inhalations. The skin may turn from pink to blue and then grey

➤ Should Agonal breathing occur, CPR should be performed immediately.

◁ ▽ If, at any point, the casualty starts to breathe spontaneously, turn them on to their side into the recovery position. This keeps the airway open and ensures that if they vomit or regurgitate, the vomit will not block their airway. On their side, it should naturally drain out of the mouth.

Full resuscitation sequence

SEE ALSO
➤ Understanding resuscitation, p26
➤ Rescue breathing, p32
➤ Chest compressions, p30
➤ The recovery position, p36

Here, all of the component skills of cardiopulmonary resuscitation are shown in action together, to give the complete CPR sequence. Remember that CPR can buy valuable time for a casualty before paramedics arrive. You are keeping the casualty's brain alive by performing chest compressions to keep the blood circulating and air flowing in and out of the lungs.

There are many high quality videos on the internet demonstrating how to successfully give chest compressions: you can learn the technique in 90 seconds or less. If you would like to go further as a first aider, a formal first aid course will enable you to practise your technique on a dummy mannequin and, in addition, learn how to give rescue breaths if you wish.

HOW TO RESUSCITATE

The DRABC resuscitation sequence should be followed exactly, with no short cuts or changes of order. Each step has been described in detail separately, but this sequence shows how all the individual elements fit together.

CHECK for danger
· Do not put yourself at risk, for example by running into the road to help an accident victim without first checking for oncoming traffic.
· Keep bystanders away from hazards such as electrical accidents or chemical spills.
· Make the scene safe if you can, for example by switching off a vehicle ignition.
· Only move the victim if they are in immediate danger, for instance from fire.

CHECK responsiveness
Remember AVPU: Alert, Vocal, Pain, Unresponsive. To check for breathing:
· Look for chest movement.
· Listen at the mouth for breath sounds.
· Feel for breath on your cheek.
Checking responsiveness and breathing should take nor more than a few seconds. If an unresponsive victim is not breathing normally, they need urgent CPR. If the

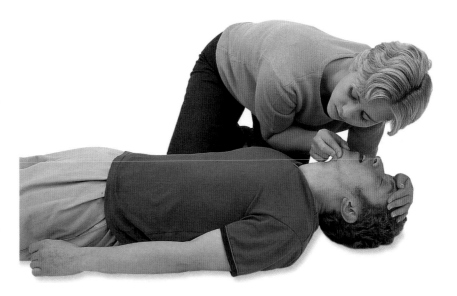

△ Check for breathing by looking for chest movements, listening for breath sounds and feeling for breath on your cheek.

casualty is unconscious but breathing, put them into the recovery position (see pages 36–37).

CALL for help
· Call an ambulance immediately or ask someone else to do so as you start CPR.
· Keep the line open, preferably on speaker.
· If you have a helper and know the location of a nearby automated external defibrillator (AED), send them to fetch it to you.

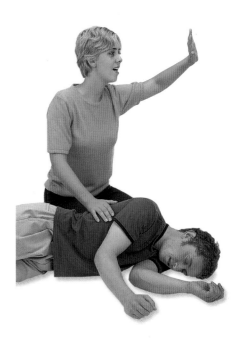

▷ Call for help at the earliest opportunity.

CARE for the victim
CPR

- Start CPR at once if the person is unresponsive and not breathing normally. Remember agonal gasps are not effective breathing.
- Place the casualty face-up on a firm surface. Kneel so that you are positioned beside their chest.
- Perform chest compressions at a rate of 100–120 a minute.
- If you are trained, do 30 compressions followed by 2 rescue breaths. If not, continue with chest compressions only. Continue CPR until help arrives.
- As soon as an AED arrives, turn it on and follow the instructions. A public access defibrillator (PAD) can be used by anyone: you do not need training.

.

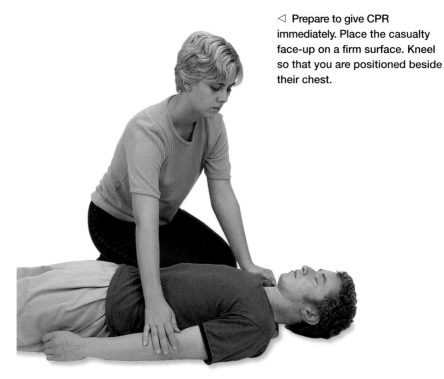

◁ Prepare to give CPR immediately. Place the casualty face-up on a firm surface. Kneel so that you are positioned beside their chest.

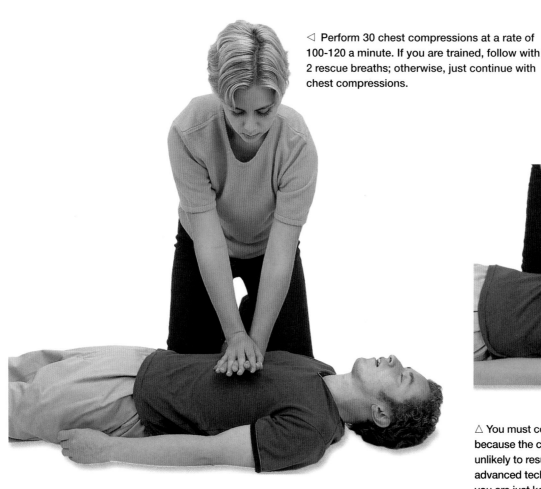

◁ Perform 30 chest compressions at a rate of 100-120 a minute. If you are trained, follow with 2 rescue breaths; otherwise, just continue with chest compressions.

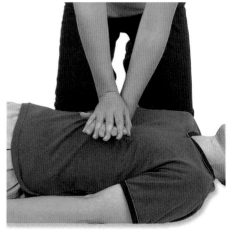

△ You must continue until aid arrives because the casualty's circulation is very unlikely to resume functioning without advanced techniques such as defibrillation – you are just keeping things going until help arrives with specialized equipment.

Airway and breathing

- Once you are sure that the victim has a working circulation, check that their airway is clear, to allow proper breathing.
- Check the mouth for obstructions and remove them if you can do so easily. Tilt the head back gently, by placing one hand on their forehead and the other on their chin, to keep the airway open.

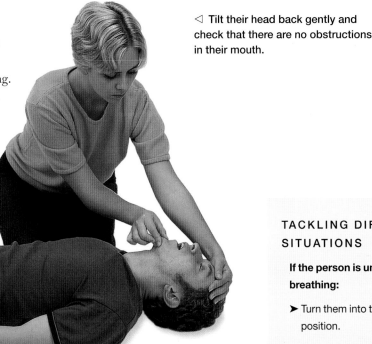

◁ Tilt their head back gently and check that there are no obstructions in their mouth.

Bleeding

- Next, treat any severe bleeding promptly by compression and monitor for signs of shock until the ambulance arrives – see pages 68–69 (shock) and 138–139 (bleeding).
- If there is no severe bleeding, and help has still not arrived, then check for and treat any other injuries or illnesses.

SPECIAL SITUATIONS

- If you are alone and treating an infant or child, give CPR for 2 minutes before you call for help (see pages 46–47).
- If you are treating a victim of choking or drowning, the first aid sequence may differ – see the specific sections on these problems (pages 38–41 (choking) and 60–61 (drowning).
- If you know or strongly suspect that an unconscious casualty is under the influence of an opioid drug, call 999 and, if you are willing to do so, give 2 rescue breaths before starting chest compressions, then continue with cycles of 30 chest compressions to 2 rescue breaths. Inform the emergency despatcher, as the person may need naloxone (which reverses the effects of the drugs) as well as an AED. If you have

access to naloxone (also known as Narcan®), administer it yourself according to the package instructions. Opioid drugs include heroin, fentanyl, oxycodone (OxyContin®), hydrocodone (Vicodin®) and morphine.

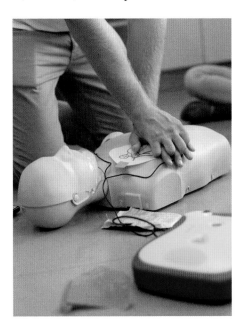

△ If you are interested in becoming a more experienced first aider there are plenty of first aid courses you can attend that will teach you how to conduct CPR manually and how to use an automated external defibrillator device, AED, as well as how to cope with other life-threatening situations.

TACKLING DIFFERENT SITUATIONS

If the person is unconscious but breathing:

➤ Turn them into the recovery position.

You should be able to see the chest rising visibly as you give rescue breaths. If it is not rising:

➤ Recheck the mouth for any obvious obstructions in the airway and use your fingers to hook or sweep them out carefully, but try not to put your fingers past the teeth and don't risk pushing objects down the throat.

➤ Recheck that the head is tilted back and the chin lifted up so that the airway is clear.

➤ Check that there is a good mouth-to-mouth seal, and pinch the nostrils together.

If the person has signs of a circulation:

➤ If you notice movement suggesting that they have a circulation but they are not breathing, continue with rescue breathing until they start breathing again or medical help arrives.

➤ Check for signs of a circulation every 10 breaths. If the person resumes breathing spontaneously, turn them into the recovery position and continue to monitor and record their breathing, circulation and level of response.

The recovery position

SEE ALSO
➤ What is first aid?, p12
➤ Understanding resuscitation, p26
➤ Responsiveness and the airway, p28

This is for casualties who are unconscious but breathing. An unconscious casualty is not in control of their airway and, because of this, it can easily become blocked. If the airway remains blocked for more than a few minutes, the lack of oxygen will quickly lead to a cardiac arrest. To ensure that this does not happen, it is best to place the casualty on their side, so that their tongue falls forwards and any fluids, such as vomit or blood, drain out of their mouth instead of down their airway. This is known in first aid as the recovery position.

PLACING A CASUALTY IN THE RECOVERY POSITION

Placing a casualty in the recovery position means that they are in a secure pose that ensures an open airway for easier breathing, and also allows any fluid to drain out of their mouth. Plan the direction in which you will roll the casualty in such a way that they remain accessible to help and are not exposed to potential further injury.

MODIFIED RECOVERY POSITION

In the following situations, you may have to alter the recovery position:

➤ If you feel that there is any possibility at all that the casualty has sustained a spinal injury, then keep them in the position in which you found them, if they are breathing. However, if you think they are in danger of inhaling vomit, then you must roll them on to their side, making sure that their head is kept in alignment with the rest of their body and not twisted or bent at the neck.

➤ If the limbs have been injured and cannot be bent, use rolled-up blankets or similar rolls of material, or even paper, in order to support them in a secure position.

➤ If the casualty's condition suggests multiple injuries and you have extra helpers available, use them to support the casualty and prevent them from toppling over.

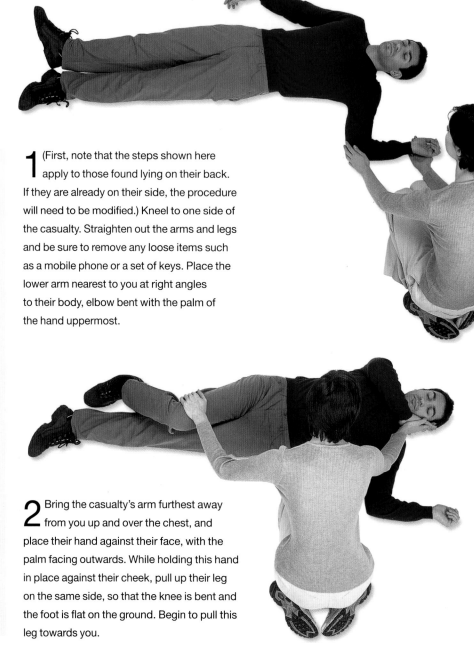

1 (First, note that the steps shown here apply to those found lying on their back. If they are already on their side, the procedure will need to be modified.) Kneel to one side of the casualty. Straighten out the arms and legs and be sure to remove any loose items such as a mobile phone or a set of keys. Place the lower arm nearest to you at right angles to their body, elbow bent with the palm of the hand uppermost.

2 Bring the casualty's arm furthest away from you up and over the chest, and place their hand against their face, with the palm facing outwards. While holding this hand in place against their cheek, pull up their leg on the same side, so that the knee is bent and the foot is flat on the ground. Begin to pull this leg towards you.

3 Continuing to support their hand against their face, pull them by the leg towards you, until their bent knee touches the ground. You can use your knees to stop them rolling all the way over on to their front.

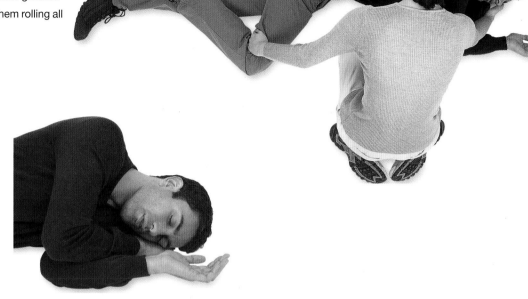

4 Check the airway, tilting their head back to keep the airway open. You may need to adjust the hand under their cheek, so that it is in the correct position to keep their airway open.

5 Adjust the leg so that the thigh is at right angles to the hip, as shown, and the casualty is completely stable. The knee acts as a prop and prevents them rolling forwards.

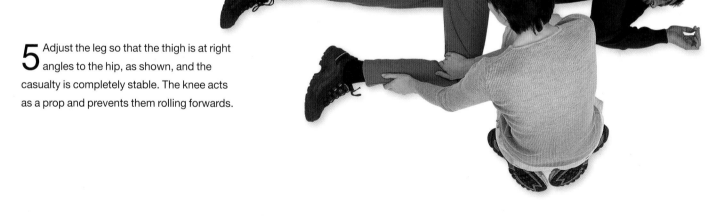

6 This is the recovery position. Note that you may need to separate out the arms if you feel that they are in a position where the circulation might be impeded. You should, ideally, have called the emergency services by now, if you have followed DRABC. However, if you are alone and do need to leave the casualty for any reason, then the recovery position is a safe and secure one in which to leave them. On your return, continue to check their airway, breathing and circulation every few minutes until expert help arrives.

Coping with choking 1

SEE ALSO

➤ Rescue breathing, p32
➤ Chest compressions, p30
➤ Coping with choking 2, p40

This common hazard can cause death if prompt action is not taken. The brain can suffer irreversible damage if it is deprived of oxygen for as little as 3–4 minutes. Choking is most likely when people are eating, particularly if they are talking or laughing at the same time. Some people are more at risk of choking, particularly children who have a narrower windpipe, those with dentures making proper chewing difficult, or someone who has had a stroke that has affected their swallowing abilities. All choking victims are best checked out at a hospital even if the object has been successfully expelled, as it may have harmed the airway lining.

Although food is most often the culprit, any foreign body may partially or completely block the airway if it is stuck at the back of the throat. The airway may also be obstructed by the tongue dropping back, especially in people who are unconscious.

COMPLETE OBSTRUCTION

Someone with a completely blocked airway will be unable to speak or cough. They may clutch their neck, or point frantically at their throat, and open their mouth wide. Initially the victim will be red-faced as they struggle for air; then they will become pale and their lips will turn blue as oxygen fails to reach their lungs. Eventually they will lose consciousness, and all chest movements will stop as they cease breathing. An effective circulation will quickly stop unless the airway is cleared and air starts getting through to the lungs once again.

INCOMPLETE OBSTRUCTION

A person may be choking but still be able to get air past the obstruction and into their lungs – this is an incomplete or partial obstruction. Do not interfere with their breathing efforts in any way, apart from encouraging them to cough. If they can cough, there must be enough room around the foreign body for air to pass, and a sharp cough might dislodge and expel it. You may decide to keep the victim seated, in order to reduce the body's demand on an imperfect supply of oxygen.

Other signs of partial blockage include:
• Snoring, gurgling and wheezing.
• Blue or grey lips, earlobes and tongue, even though the person is breathing.
• Breathing that alternates between normal and difficult/laboured.

CLEARING THE AIRWAY

There are three principal ways in which the first-aider should deal with a blocked airway, depending in the first instance on whether the person who is choking is conscious or unconscious:
FOR CONSCIOUS CASUALTIES:
• Encourage coughing.
• Back slaps, if coughing alone will not shift the obstruction.
• Abdominal thrusts (the Heimlich manoeuvre) if back slaps do not work.

FOR UNCONSCIOUS CASUALTIES:
• CPR.
These techniques can be used singly or in combination, depending on the circumstance.

Whichever technique you need to use, keep reassuring the person who is choking and stay as calm as possible yourself, as people who are choking tend to panic, quite understandably, and this makes breathing difficulties much worse. If the casualty loses consciousness, open the airway and check for breathing: as the muscles relax this may start spontaneously. If not, you will need to attempt rescue breaths and begin chest compressions.

CLEARING THE AIRWAY OF A CONSCIOUS CASUALTY

1. BACK SLAPS

This simple method is often an instinctive reaction when people see someone choking. First encourage them to lean forwards and cough sharply and deeply in order to help move the foreign body. If this proves ineffective, stand to the side and slightly behind the casualty. Making sure they are leaning forwards, support their chest with one hand and with your other hand flat, give up to 5 hard slaps between the shoulder blades. If this fails, or you are not sure about the technique, move on to abdominal thrusts.

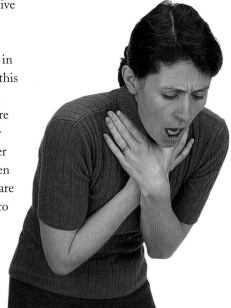

▷ People who think they are choking can panic very easily. Try to keep them calm.

2. ABDOMINAL THRUSTS

This is the main technique used with conscious casualties, but it should never be used on babies under age one and needs to be modified for pregnant women. It relies on pressing sharply and forcefully into the abdomen to cause an artificial cough, which may force enough air against the blockage to shift it. This method can be used whether the casualty is standing up or sitting down. It is often referred to as the Heimlich manoeuvre.

If someone is too large for you to get your arms around their abdomen, or for pregnant women, perform chest thrusts instead, using the same technique but with your hands a little higher, at the base of the person's breastbone, just above where the lowest ribs join it.

Alternate between back slaps and abdominal thrusts until the object is dislodged. Call for emergency help after five cycles, and continue until help arrives.

SELF-HELP

If you're alone and choking, the Heimlich manoeuvre can also be performed on

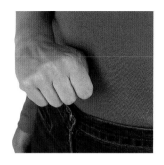

△ Stand behind the person who is choking. Now slide your arms around the victim and wrap them around their trunk just below the bottom of the ribcage. Clench one fist and place it thumb-side in between their navel and lower ribs, as shown above.

▷ Wrap the other hand on top of the wrist. Pull sharply inwards and upwards towards yourself. You may have to repeat the procedure several times. Give up to five thrusts and if the object has not dislodged, call an ambulance. Keep cycling five back blows with five abdominal thrusts until help arrives.

yourself. Call for an ambulance first if you are able to speak. Place your fist slightly above your navel and grasp it with your other hand. Bend over a hard edge, such as a countertop or chair back and pull your fist sharply inwards and upwards.

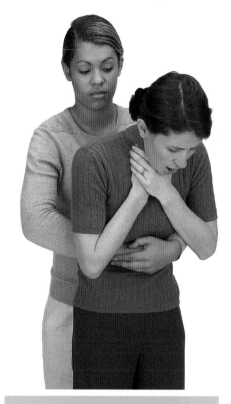

WARNING
Abdominal thrusts can cause serious injuries and even if you clear the airway quickly, the casualty should be checked over by a doctor afterwards.

CLEARING THE AIRWAY OF AN UNCONSCIOUS CASUALTY

If the choking victim becomes unconscious, lower them to the floor and check the mouth for a visible blockage. Don't poke around if you can't see one, and be very careful not to push any object farther down. If you can't clear the airway, immediately start CPR.

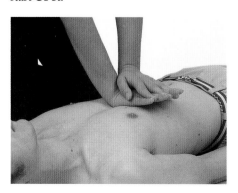

CHOKING IN CHILDREN

For children over one year old, perform the Heimlich manoeuvre as for adults, but with extra care to avoid pressure on the lower ribcage.

For babies under one year, lie the baby face down along the length of a thigh, supporting the head with your hand. Give up to five sharp blows with the heel of one hand in the centre of the back between the shoulder blades.

If this does not clear the obstruction, turn the baby face upwards and place two fingers of one hand on the breastbone in the

◁ Chest compressions can help to dislodge objects stuck in the airway of an unconscious casualty.
▷ To give a baby back blows, lay the baby face down along your thigh, supported by your arm, with their head low down.

middle of the chest. Give five sharp chest thrusts, aiming to compress the chest by about one-third of its depth. Reassess the baby after five cycles and call 999, even if the object has cleared as the baby will need to be assessed by a doctor or paramedic. Continue to perform chest thrusts until help arrives (See also page 50).

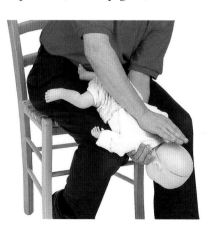

Coping with choking 2

PUTTING IT ALL TOGETHER

The individual techniques detailed in Coping with Choking 1 can now be slotted into full sequences. Time is vital when someone is choking – assess the situation and act as swiftly as possible. To recap: with conscious victims, try to calm them down – this will make your job much easier. Encourage them to dislodge the obstruction with a few deep coughs. If this fails, you will need to proceed to abdominal thrusts, if necessary. If a casualty is unconscious, or loses consciousness as you are helping them, call the emergency service and start resuscitation swiftly, as shown, using chest thrusts to shift the obstruction.

HELPING A CONSCIOUS CASUALTY

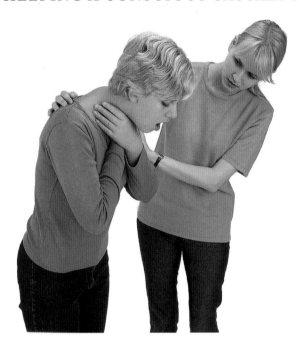

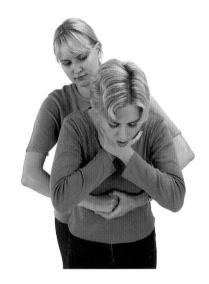

1 If the person who is choking is still managing to breathe, but feels that something is lodged in their airway, they will probably panic. Ask them to cough to try to dislodge the foreign body, but do not do anything else yet. Attempt to calm them, and summon emergency help.

2 If the situation worsens, or if the casualty cannot cough, speak or breathe and is beginning to look pale, give them 5 sharp back blows.

3 If coughing does not expel the object, give them abdominal thrusts. Continue until the foreign body has moved, or until the emergency services arrive.

HELPING AN UNCONSCIOUS CASUALTY

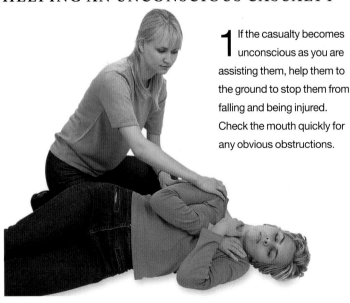

1 If the casualty becomes unconscious as you are assisting them, help them to the ground to stop them from falling and being injured. Check the mouth quickly for any obvious obstructions.

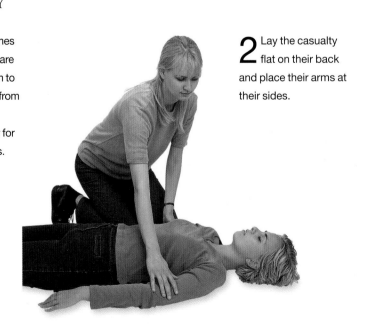

2 Lay the casualty flat on their back and place their arms at their sides.

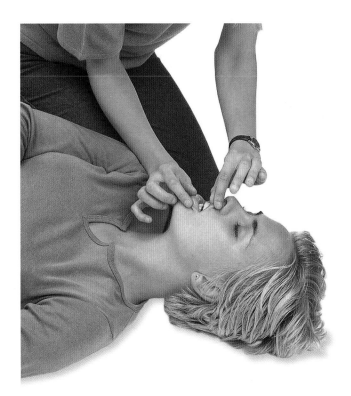

3 Recheck the casualty's mouth for any visible obstructions and remove anything you can see very carefully; do not poke your finger blindly around the mouth.

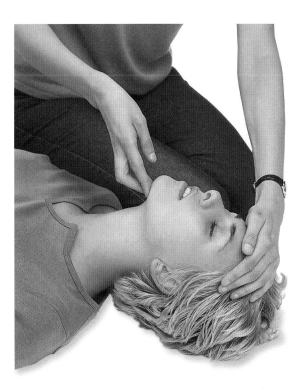

4 Open the airway by placing one hand on the forehead and two fingers of your other hand under the chin, and tilting the head back gently, as far as possible.

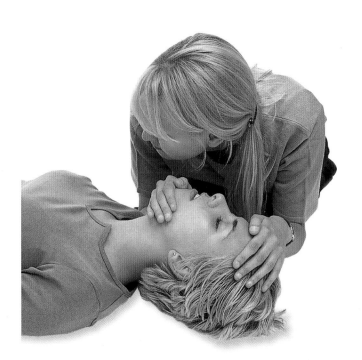

5 Check for breathing by looking, listening and feeling – as muscles relax during unconsciousness the victim may now be breathing again.

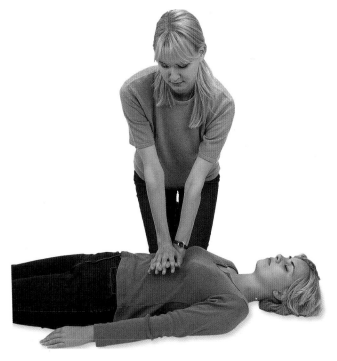

6 If the person is not breathing, get someone to call the emergency services (if you are alone, give CPR for 1 minute before going for help). Start chest compressions in an attempt to dislodge the obstruction. Give 30 compressions, at a rate of 100-120 compressions per minute. Continue until help arrives.

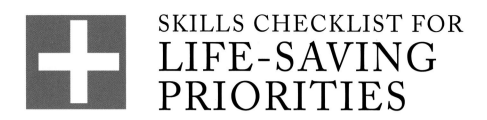

SKILLS CHECKLIST FOR
LIFE-SAVING PRIORITIES

KEY POINTS

- Don't waste time checking for a pulse unless you are highly trained in this technique. ☐

- Always stick to DRABC procedures when dealing with life-support situations . ☐

- If someone has a cardiac arrest, call an ambulance immediately and start CPR immediately. Never do nothing. ☐

- Send someone to fetch an AED if you can. ☐

- Pay plenty of attention to keeping a casualty's airway open. ☐

- The technique for helping a choking victim depends on whether the person is conscious or unconscious. ☐

SKILLS LEARNED

- Chest compression (heart massage). ☐

- Rescue breathing, also known as mouth-to-mouth respiration, artificial ventilation, or the "kiss of life". ☐

- The correct sequence of resuscitation. ☐

- The recovery position. ☐

- Back slaps to treat choking. ☐

- Abdominal thrusts to treat choking. ☐

- Chest thrusts to treat choking. ☐

CHILDREN'S LIFE SUPPORT

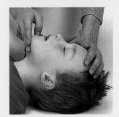

Children are notoriously accident-prone and both babies and children can get dangerously ill very rapidly, so every second counts and you must get help for a collapsed child as fast as possible. The whole story is not entirely depressing, however – children often have remarkable powers of recuperation. It is essential for first-aiders to appreciate the differences between dealing with an older child or adult and dealing with a baby or young child. Many of the basic principles remain the same as for adults, but the techniques used must be tailored to smaller, more fragile bodies.

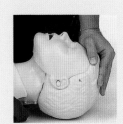

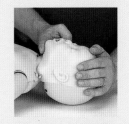

CONTENTS

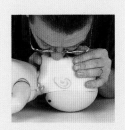

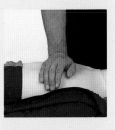

Basic life support

SEE ALSO

➤ What is first aid?, p12

➤ Resuscitating a baby or child, p46

➤ Choking in babies and children, p50

Young children are not mini-adults, but the basic life-support rules of checking airway, breathing and circulation still apply. Babies under 1 require different treatment to older children. Children over 8 can be treated as adults. One important issue to bear in mind is that adult first-aiders may feel more emotionally affected by a young casualty, and this can sometimes cloud their judgement – you must avoid this and act decisively. The elements of life support are shown below, and are then put together as a full routine on the following pages.

As in adults, basic life support in babies and children involves CPR, which is given to ensure blood carrying vital oxygen continues to circulate around the body in an emergency. However, the causes of cardiac arrest in children are very different to those in adults. Children rarely have problems with their hearts, but a healthy heart will stop if insufficient oxygen reaches other vital organs, such as the brain.

Cardiac arrest in children more often stems from causes such as choking, suffocation or strangulation; drowning; severe injuries; poisoning; infection; and medical conditions that affect breathing. The resuscitation sequence is slightly different and you should start CPR at once, before calling an ambulance. Children have a much better chance of survival if CPR is started immediately.

Children are anatomically different to adults, hence the need for different life-support techniques. They have narrower air passages and these are more prone to blockage by food or other objects. Their windpipe is more flexible and the airway may become blocked if the neck is bent back too far. In addition, a child's tongue is bigger than an adult's relative to the size of their mouth and throat, so it is more likely to block the airway, particularly if the child is unconscious.

STARTING RESUSCITATION

If you are on your own, open the child's airway and immediately carry out CPR for two minutes before calling an ambulance. If you are trained, or if you are willing to try, give two rescue breaths before commencing chest compressions. Instructions for doing this are in the next section. Even if you don't give rescue breaths you should still perform chest compressions straight away.

BREATHING

Children breathe mainly by using their diaphragms, rather than their chest muscles. Look for their abdomen rising and falling as well as their chest when checking if they are breathing. You should make a decision whether or not to start CPR within 10 seconds. If you are still in doubt after that start CPR. As with adults, gasping breaths are not normal breathing.

RESCUE BREATHING

If a baby or child is unconscious and not breathing and someone else is nearby, get them to call an ambulance while you commence CPR. Ask them to fetch a defibrillator if there is one nearby or the emergency operator tells them the nearest location.

If you decide to give rescue breaths to a child, don't blow an adult-sized breath –

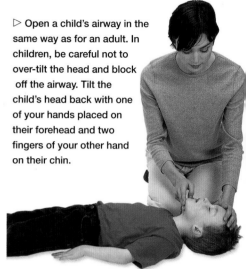

▷ Open a child's airway in the same way as for an adult. In children, be careful not to over-tilt the head and block off the airway. Tilt the child's head back with one of your hands placed on their forehead and two fingers of your other hand on their chin.

use just enough air to make their chest rise and then fall, as if they have taken a deep breath, and blow gently for about one second, watching to make sure the chest or abdomen rises each time. In a baby, it is easier to put your mouth over both their nose and mouth at the same time. Make sure you have a good seal over the infant's nose/mouth.

Open a child's airway in the same way as for an adult. In children, be careful not to over-tilt the head and block off the airway. Gently tilt the child's head back with one of your hands placed on their forehead and two fingers of your other hand on their chin.

It might be that you cannot get any air into the casualty's chest, even after trying to do so with their head in several different positions. In this case, they may have something blocking the airway. Carefully check and clear the mouth, and then if their airway still seems blocked, follow the appropriate choking procedure (see pages 50–51).

REMEMBER DRABC

Remembering and acting on these priorities will save lives:

D for DANGER

R for RESPONSE

A for AIRWAY

B for BREATHING

C for CIRCULATION

FINDING AND USING THE CPR COMPRESSION SITE IN A BABY (UNDER 1 YEAR)

1 Hold the index finger of one hand horizontally between the baby's nipples, in such a way that the centre of your finger is at the sternum, or breastbone.

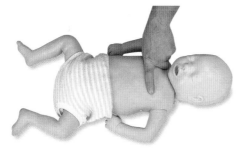

2 The correct compression site is located one finger's width beneath this line between the nipples. Position two fingertips over this site, ready to press down.

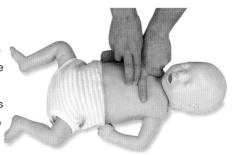

3 Using these two fingertips, compress the breastbone to a depth of 4cm (1.6in), which is approximately one-third of the depth of the infant's chest. Release. After initial rescue breaths, if you are willing to do this, give 30 compressions at the rate of about 100–120 a minute. For every 30 compressions performed, give 2 rescue breaths. Continue to give the infant chest compression and rescue breaths at a ratio of 30:1 until help arrives.

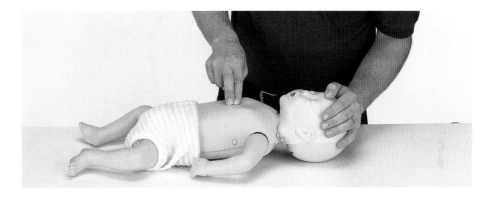

FINDING AND USING THE CPR COMPRESSION SITE IN A CHILD (1–8 YEARS)

1 Place the heel of one hand on the lower third of the child's breastbone, one finger's width above the point where the ribs join in the middle.

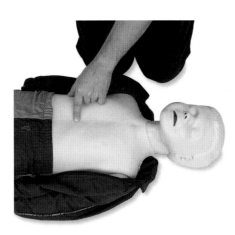

2 Lift your fingers to avoid putting pressure on the ribs.

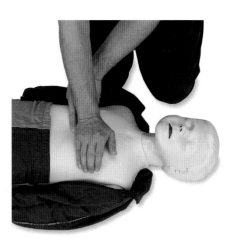

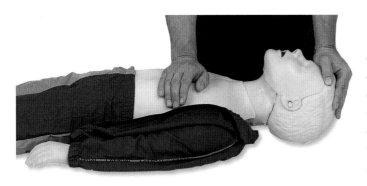

3 To give a chest compression, press down vertically with the heel of just one hand to a depth of 5cm (2in), which is one-third of the depth of the child's chest. Do this at a rate of 100-120 chest compressions per minute, as for adults (about 5 times in 3 seconds). After every 30 compressions, give 2 rescue breaths. Continue with this ratio of 30 compressions followed by 2 effective rescue breaths until help arrives.

Resuscitating a baby or child

Every second is vital when resuscitating a baby or child. Taking immediate effective action may prevent brain damage and save life. Resuscitation of a baby differs from that of an older child, so familiarize yourself with both techniques. Also, your approach will vary depending on whether you are alone or have helpers. When checking for a response, remember that you cannot rely on a verbal response from babies and young children, so look for other responsiveness clues.

RESUSCITATING A BABY (UNDER 1 YEAR)

DANGER, RESPONSE
• Make yourself and the baby safe.
• To test responsiveness, shout, tap the baby gently, or flick the soles of their feet. Never shake them.

AIRWAY
• Make sure the baby's head is in a neutral position and not tilted. Remove any obvious obstructions from the mouth. Place your hand on their forehead and tilt the head back. Using just your fingertips, push gently to lift the baby's chin. Don't push on the soft tissues below the chin as this could itself obstruct breathing.

BREATHING
• Look, listen and feel for breathing and for any signs of life, for up to 10 seconds. Gasping breaths are not normal breathing.
• If they are unconscious but breathing normally, hold them in the recovery position and call an ambulance.
• If the baby is not breathing normally after checking for up to 10 seconds, give 5 initial rescue breaths if trained or willing to do so. Seal your lips tightly around the baby's mouth and nose, and breathe lightly into the lungs until the chest rises. If your breaths do not make the chest or abdomen rise, the airway may be blocked and you should treat as for choking. Keeping the baby's head tilted back and the chin lifted, remove your mouth and watch for the chest to fall as the air is expired, then repeat for five initial breaths.

CIRCULATION
• **Look, listen and feel** for signs of circulation _ movement, coughing or breathing – for up to 10 seconds.
• If there are no definite signs, give 5 chest compressions, using two fingers.
• Making sure that the chin is up and the head back, give 2 rescue breaths.
• Continue in cycles of 30 compressions to 2 rescue breaths.
• If the baby is unconscious but breathing normally, call an ambulance and hold them in the recovery position. While waiting, make sure that the baby's head is in a neutral position and not tilted, and that their airway remains open. Monitor their condition and be prepared to start resuscitation if necessary.

WARNING
If a baby or child is not breathing, it is vital to start CPR immediately and continue to do so for two minutes before attempting to call for help. Ask someone else to call an ambulance whenever possible while you continue to administer CPR.

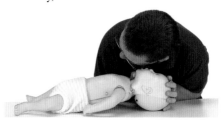

1 Look, listen and feel for signs of breathing, and vital signs such as warmth and colour, for up to 10 seconds. If the baby is breathing normally, carefully place in the recovery position and get help.

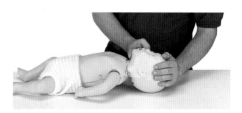

2 If the baby is not breathing, immediately start CPR. Remove blood, vomit or any other visible obstructions. Tilt the head back to open the baby's airway, avoiding the soft tissue beneath the chin.

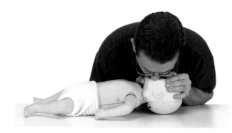

3 Place your mouth over the baby's mouth and nose. Give 2 initial rescue breaths if trained or if willing to do so.

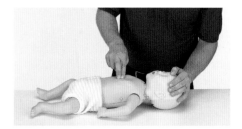

4 Now begin chest compressions: give 30 chest compressions followed by 2 rescue breaths, and continue with this ratio of 30:2. If breathing starts, hold the baby in the recovery position and monitor and record their breathing, circulation and response.

RESUSCITATING A CHILD (OVER 1 YEAR)

Follow the same rules about when to call for an ambulance (depending on whether you are alone or have helpers) as for a baby.

DANGER, RESPONSE
- Make yourself and the child safe.
- To test the child's responsiveness, shout or tap firmly on the shoulder.

AIRWAY
- Open the airway: remove any obvious obstructions and gently tilt back the head with two fingers under the chin and the other hand on the forehead.

BREATHING
- Look, listen and feel for breathing and for any signs of life, for up to 10 seconds.
- If the child is unconscious but breathing normally, place them in the recovery position and call an ambulance.
- If there are no signs of normal breathing after checking for up to 10 seconds, give an initial 5 rescue breaths if trained or willing to do so. If your breaths do not make the chest or abdomen rise, the child's airway may be blocked and you should treat as for choking.

CIRCULATION
- Look, listen and feel for signs of circulation – movement, coughing or breathing.
- If there are no definite signs give 30 chest compressions, using the heel of one hand, as previously explained.
- Making sure that the chin is up and the head back, give 2 effective breaths.
- Continue in cycles of 30 compressions to 2 rescue breaths until help arrives.

CHILDREN OVER 8 YEARS
For older children, it may be necessary to use two-handed compressions, to get sufficient depth of compression. Follow the same rules about going for help, whether you are acting alone or with helpers, as you would for a baby or younger child.

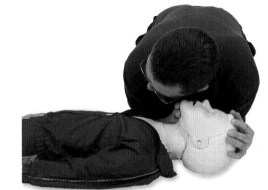

1 Look, listen and feel for signs of breathing, and vital signs such as warmth and colour, for up to 10 seconds. If the child is breathing normally, place in the recovery position and get help.

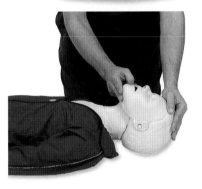

2 If breathing is absent immediately start CPR. Remove blood, vomit or any other visible obstruction from the mouth. Tilt the head back to open up the airway.

3 Place your mouth over the child's mouth. Give 2 initial rescue breaths if trained or willing to do so. If you have help, send someone to call for an ambulance as you start the rescue breathing.

4 Give 30 compressions followed by 2 rescue breaths. Continue with this ratio of 30:2. After two minutes call an ambulance if no-one has yet done so. If breathing starts, place the child in the recovery position (see pages 48–49) and monitor and record their breathing, circulation and response.

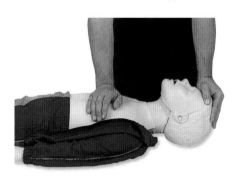

WARNING

If you have no helpers with you and a child known to have heart disease collapses suddenly (and this was not caused by an accident or poisoning), get help straight away, before starting CPR.

CONTINUE RESUSCITATING UNTIL:

➤ The baby/child shows basic signs of life (normal breathing, coughing or movement).

➤ Someone else takes over.

➤ The defibrillator arrives.

➤ Qualified professionals arrive at the scene.

➤ You are completely exhausted.

The recovery position

An unconscious child who is still breathing should be placed in the recovery position (essentially the same as for an adult). This simple procedure can be a life-saver. It keeps the airway open, allows the tongue to fall forwards so it does not block the airway and lets any fluids that could cause choking drain out of the mouth – most specifically lessening the likelihood of inhaling and choking on vomit while unconscious. This vital position should be learned by anyone who cares for or works with babies and children.

PLACING A CHILD IN THE RECOVERY POSITION

The purpose of the recovery position is to minimize the possibility of the child choking on their tongue or the contents of their stomach while you wait for professional help to arrive. The position is secure enough for you to leave the child for a short time if you need to go to summon help. The sequence shown here starts with the child on their back; the technique is shorter if the casualty is found on their side or front.

1 Kneel near the head of the unconscious child. With one hand on their forehead and the fingers of the other hand under the chin, tilt the head back to keep the airway open.

TIPS FOR DEALING WITH UNCONSCIOUS CHILDREN

➤ A child's windpipe is flexible, and it may close up if you over-extend their head when opening their airway.

➤ Keep an eye on their breathing and circulation and start resuscitating immediately if you see it has stopped.

➤ Place a breathing but unconscious child in the recovery position before you go for help.

2 Straighten the arms and legs. Place the arm nearest to you at right angles so the elbow is bent and the hand flat on the ground palm upwards.

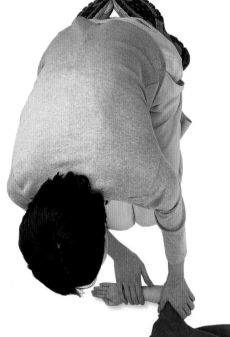

WARNING
If you suspect a spinal injury, move the child only if they are in danger. If you have to move them, do your best to keep the head, neck and trunk aligned at all times.

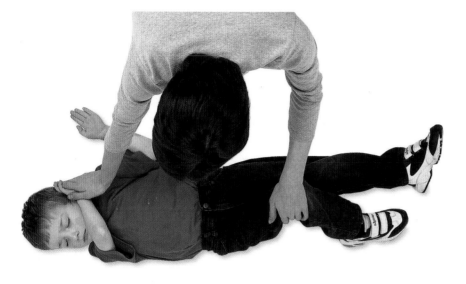

3 Move the other arm across the child's chest. Position the back of the hand against the cheek that is on the same side of the body as the bent arm. Bend the knee furthest from you and hold the leg at the thigh. Try to keep the foot of the bent leg on the ground as you do this.

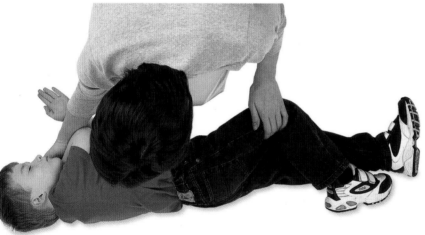

4 Hold the child's hand in position against their cheek. Pull them towards you using the bent leg to gently roll them over. The child should end up lying on their side.

PLACING A BABY IN THE RECOVERY POSITION

Infants under 1 year are too small to place in the conventional recovery position, but by keeping them on their side and with the head tilted down, the principles remain the same. Hold the baby with one hand under their head and the other under their lower back and bottom. Place their head lower than the rest of their body. Try not to press against their stomach as this may make them vomit.

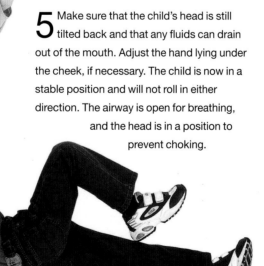

5 Make sure that the child's head is still tilted back and that any fluids can drain out of the mouth. Adjust the hand lying under the cheek, if necessary. The child is now in a stable position and will not roll in either direction. The airway is open for breathing, and the head is in a position to prevent choking.

▷ Try to remember to keep the baby's head lower than their body. This is so that, if they vomit, they will not inhale it and choke.

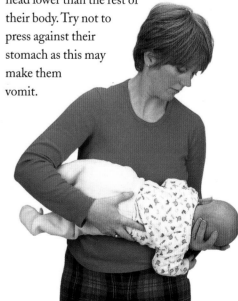

Choking in babies and children

SEE ALSO

➤ Rescue breathing, p32

➤ Basic life support, p44

➤ Safety in the home, p224

Choking is common in children because their narrow airways are easily obstructed. Very young infants are also still learning to chew and swallow properly and are fond of putting objects in their mouths. It is best to not give toys with small parts or hard foods such as nuts, hard candy or popcorn to children under four. If choking does occur, you must act decisively as there may not be enough time to wait for the emergency services. The sad fact is that significant numbers of small children die each year from choking, but it is often easy to prevent.

SIGNS AND SYMPTOMS

➤ Unable to speak or cough.

➤ Difficult or noisy breathing.

➤ Blue lips.

➤ Pale/blue/ashen skin.

➤ Loss of consciousness/collapse.

TREATMENT FOR A CHOKING BABY (UNDER 1 YEAR)

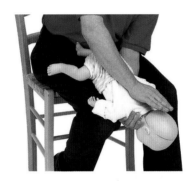

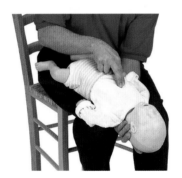

◁ Left and bottom left: to give a baby back blows (top), lay the baby face down along your thigh, supported by your arm, with their head down low. For chest thrusts (bottom), use two fingertips placed on the lower half of their breastbone, a finger's width below the nipples.

FIRST AID FOR A CHOKING CONSCIOUS BABY (UNDER 1 YEAR)

1. **Check the mouth and breathing** and remove any obvious obstruction.

2. Rest your arm on your thigh and place the baby face down along your arm with the head lower than the body.

3. **Give up to 5 back blows with the heel of your hand.**

4. Carefully turn the baby face up, and re-check their mouth and breathing. Remove any obvious obstruction.

5. If this is unsuccessful, use 2 fingers to **give 5 sharp chest thrusts**.

6. **Repeat steps 2–5** until the baby starts breathing spontaneously or becomes unconscious. Call an ambulance immediately if the first set of chest thrusts fails.

SOME BASIC ISSUES

There are certain differences between treating choking babies and choking children. There are also differences in their treatment depending on whether they are conscious or unconscious. One of the most important points to appreciate is that, whether you are dealing with a child or a baby, rescue breathing is started only once the child or baby becomes (or already is) unconscious. The airway may become clear as the muscles relax with loss of consciousness, in which case the rescue breathing will cause the chest to rise, and you should move on to basic life support measures.

FIRST AID FOR A CHOKING UNCONSCIOUS BABY (UNDER 1 YEAR)

1. **Do not grope about in the mouth**, as this may push the obstruction further down.

2. **Give 2 initial rescue breaths.** If there are no chest movements, check the mouth again and make sure that the head and chin are in the correct position. Make up to 5 attempts to give rescue breaths.

3. Place the baby on a firm surface (which could be your arm supported on your thigh) and give 30 chest compressions with 2 fingertips.

4. Check mouth and breathing again and call 911.

5. Continue giving compressions and rescue breaths at a ratio of 30:2 until help arrives.

TREATMENT FOR A CHOKING CHILD (1–8 YEARS)

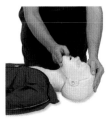

△ Unconscious child – open the airway.

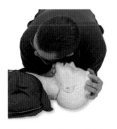

△ Unconscious child – check for breathing.

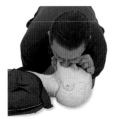

△ Unconscious child – rescue breaths.

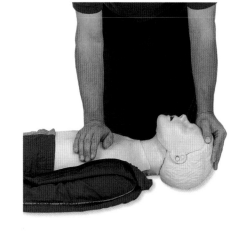

△ Unconscious child – chest compressions.

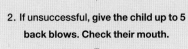

FIRST AID FOR A CHOKING CONSCIOUS CHILD (1–8 YEARS)

1. Get the child to cough.

2. If unsuccessful, give the child up to 5 back blows. Check their mouth.

3. If unsuccessful, give up to 5 abdominal thrusts: standing or kneeling behind the child, place your fist against the upper part of their abdomen above the naval. Grasp it with the other hand and pull sharply inwards and upwards, once every 3 seconds. Re-check the mouth.

4. If unsuccessful, send for help. Keep repeating back blows and abdominal thrusts, re-checking the mouth between each cycle.

6. Even if the obstruction is removed, take the child to casualty – the airway lining may be damaged.

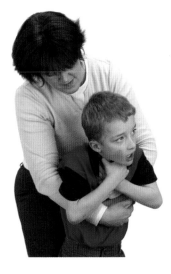

△ Abdominal thrusts on a conscious child who is choking are done from behind the victim, employing the same technique as for adults, but using less force.

IMPORTANT POINTS

➤ Never blindly sweep a finger inside anyone's mouth as it may make the obstruction worse.

➤ If the baby or child is still passing some air in and out of the lungs, and you know or suspect that an obstruction remains, do nothing and quickly call the emergency services.

➤ Any child who has collapsed and is unconscious and not breathing may have choked. Start the CPR at once. If the chest does not move with up to 5 rescue breaths. Treat for choking.

➤ Abdominal thrusts are not used at all in babies as they may damage their internal organs.

FIRST AID FOR A CHOKING UNCONSCIOUS CHILD (1–8 YEARS)

1. Remove an object from the mouth only if you can see it – do not grope around, as this may push the obstruction further down.

2. Get the child onto the floor or a firm surface and start CPR – give 30 chest compressions.

3. Give 2 rescue breaths, then continue giving compression and rescue breaths at a ratio of 30:2.

4. Continue until help arrives.

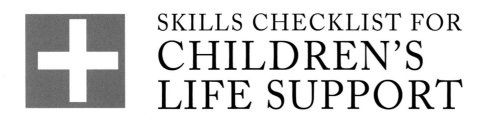

SKILLS CHECKLIST FOR
CHILDREN'S
LIFE SUPPORT

KEY POINTS

- Resuscitation is carried out differently in babies and young children from adults ☐

- Following the correct sequence of resuscitation is of the utmost importance ☐

- Speedy action is particularly important where young casualties are concerned ☐

SKILLS LEARNED

- Basic techniques of life support for babies and young children ☐

- Chest compressions for babies and young children ☐

- The correct sequence of resuscitation techniques for babies and children ☐

- The recovery position for babies and children ☐

- Coping with a choking baby or child ☐

LUNGS AND BREATHING

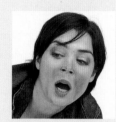

Breathing is vital for each of us to stay alive, and if anyone is not breathing they need immediate resuscitation. A basic knowledge of the parts of the respiratory system and how they work can help if you have to deal with an emergency involving breathing problems. While serious accidents can cause breathing to stop, a number of diseases and accidents directly affect the working of the breathing apparatus. These include certain respiratory conditions (such as asthma), inhalation of noxious fumes or smoke, drowning, hanging and strangulation.

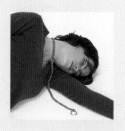

CONTENTS

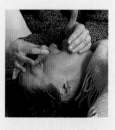

Understanding the respiratory system

SEE ALSO
➤ Understanding resuscitation, p26
➤ Responsiveness and the airway, p28
➤ Rescue breathing, p32

The technical term for breathing is respiration. With each breath, air enters the lungs and oxygen passes into the blood through the delicate tissues of the lung. Every cell in our bodies needs oxygen to work properly. Without oxygen, muscles cannot contract, nerves cannot send impulses, the heart stops and the brain cannot function. The end product of respiration is carbon dioxide, which leaves the blood in the lungs as oxygen enters it. If the lungs did not expel carbon dioxide as we breathe out, confusion, coma and death would follow.

THE BREATHING APPARATUS

The lungs form the main part of the respiratory system. The two spongy organs are surrounded and protected by a bony cage comprising the ribs, spine and sternum (breastbone). The diaphragm is a dome-shaped muscle attached to the lower ribs lying under the lungs and is the main muscle of breathing control. Other muscles that help with breathing, especially during exercise, or in times of stress or illness, are the intercostal muscles lying between each rib. Each lung is surrounded by a double membrane called the pleural sac. Together these structures form an airtight, protective cage around the lungs.

Air reaches the lungs through a series of branching airways, which become progressively more numerous and smaller. Air enters the body through the nose and mouth, and travels down the airway past the larynx, or voice box, which contains the vocal chords. The epiglottis is a flap of cartilage that covers the larynx when we swallow food, in order to prevent food from entering the trachea, or windpipe.

The air then reaches the trachea, which soon divides into two branches called bronchi – one going to the left lung and the other to the right. These branch into smaller vessels called bronchioles. The bronchioles taper into smaller and smaller branches, until they end in tiny sacs of lung tissue called alveoli. This is where gas exchange takes place. Tiny branches of veins and arteries are wrapped around the alveoli, and through their walls, oxygen and carbon dioxide are transferred in and out of the blood.

THE RESPIRATORY SYSTEM

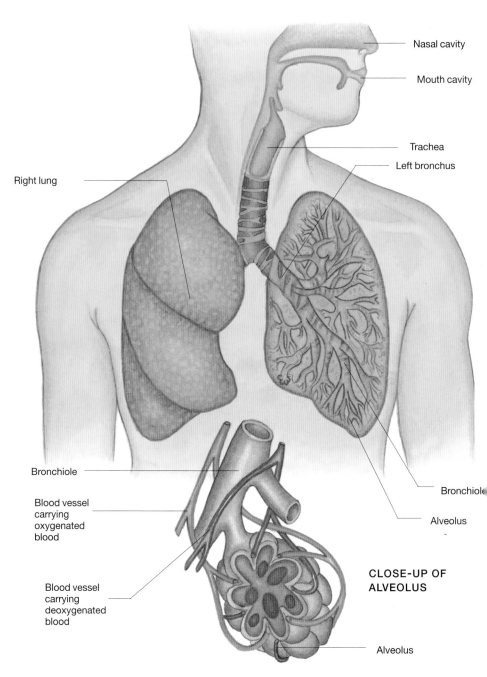

Nasal cavity

Mouth cavity

Trachea

Left bronchus

Right lung

Bronchiole

Blood vessel carrying oxygenated blood

Blood vessel carrying deoxygenated blood

Bronchiole

Alveolus

CLOSE-UP OF ALVEOLUS

Alveolus

HOW DO WE BREATHE?

We breathe automatically. Apart from being able to control how fast or deeply we breathe over a short period, our breathing is beyond our voluntary control. The respiratory centre in the brain stem controls the basic rhythm of breathing. It is from here that messages are sent to and from the nerves supplying the diaphragm and intercostal muscles. This leads to a continuous cycle of relaxation and contraction of the breathing muscles.

As the diaphragm contracts and moves down, the intercostal muscles pull the ribs up and out. This causes an increase in chest volume, which in turn results in expansion of the lungs, and the reduced pressure causes air to be sucked in – this is called inspiration. In the reverse process, the diaphragm relaxes, the ribs move down and in, and air is pushed out – this is called expiration.

In an adult, the normal rate for breathing at rest is 13–17 breaths per minute. This rate increases during exercise, which is a normal response to the body's increased demand for oxygen. An increased rate at rest or during only mild exertion can be a sign of physical illness. Psychological problems, such as extreme anxiety and panic attacks, can also increase breathing rate.

In babies and young children, breathing rate is much higher, ranging from around 50 breaths a minute in a baby under 1 year to 30 breaths a minute in children over 5 years.

PROBLEMS WITH BREATHING

All kinds of different diseases and situations can adversely affect breathing. As soon as the delicate balance between air on one side and blood on the other is upset, problems start to arise. Part of a lung may fill with fluid from a tumour or infection. A lung may collapse or burst and then become squashed due to air escaping into the space between the lungs and the chest wall. The airways may go into temporary spasm as in asthma, or become permanently narrowed, as in the chronic lung disease, emphysema.

Breathing problems may be caused by:
• Heart disease.

BREATHING IN AND OUT

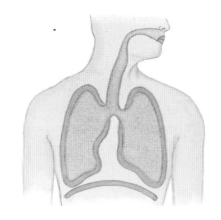

1 In between breathing in or out, the powerful diaphragm muscle found below the lungs rests in its relaxed position – in a pronounced dome shape.

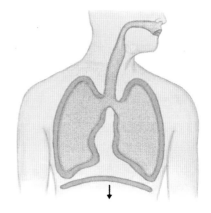

2 The diaphragm muscle now starts to contract, moving downwards as it does so. The intercostal muscles also contract, expanding the rib cage.

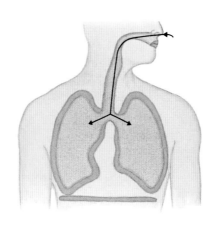

3 As the chest cavity and lungs expand, pressure in the cavity and lungs drops and air rushes in to equalize it – breathing in. At full contraction, the diaphragm lies flat.

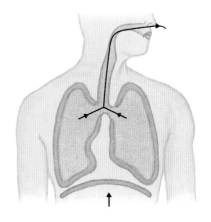

4 The diaphragm relaxes and moves up again. The intercostal muscles relax and the rib cage contracts. Pressure rises in the lungs, so air starts to rush out – breathing out.

• Chest infection.
• Lung tumour or lung disease.
• Collapsed or punctured lung.
• Asthma.
• Smoking.
• Fear, panic and anxiety.
• Inhalation of fumes.
• Choking.
• Chest injury.
• Head injury.

A person who develops breathing problems suddenly must be seen by a doctor without delay. While you are waiting for help to arrive, give any necessary first aid.

SIGNS AND SYMPTOMS OF BREATHING PROBLEMS

➤ Pale or blue face and lips.

➤ A rapid respiratory rate (this will vary with age, but the rate should be less than 20 breaths per minute in a healthy adult).

➤ Noisy breathing.

➤ Cough.

➤ Shortness of breath.

➤ Confusion and aggression.

Dealing with breathing difficulties

SEE ALSO
➤ What is first aid?, p12
➤ Coping with choking 1 and 2, pp38, 40
➤ Coping with a heart attack, p72

Breathlessness occurs in healthy people as a normal response to exercising, but it can also be a symptom of many diseases, including chronic conditions such as asthma and emphysema. Breathing difficulty should always be taken seriously, especially if it starts suddenly. Even young, fit people can be affected by conditions that cause breathing difficulty, such as a collapsed lung (pneumothorax), or a clot in the lung (pulmonary embolus). These conditions can be life-threatening, so prompt recognition and medical treatment are very important.

ACTION FOR BREATHING DIFFICULTY

Even if you do not know the cause of the breathing difficulty, act as follows:
• Sit the sufferer upright and supported.
• If they are on medication for breathing problems, get them to take it.
• Loosen clothing around the neck.
• Try to keep the sufferer calm.
• If the breathing does not return to normal, seek medical attention.

ASTHMA

At least 7 per cent of adults and 8 per cent of children suffer from chronic asthma. This is a condition in which the airways become narrowed and blocked with secretions. People with asthma typically suffer from repeated attacks of wheezing and breathlessness. They may use a quick relief or "rescue" inhaler containing short-acting medication for immediate relief in an attach, and a "preventer" inhaler containing long-acting medication to help prevent attacks in the future. A person with asthma should always carry a reliever inhaler with them to use during an attack.

Asthma tends to be triggered by factors that differ between individuals. Sufferers are often allergic to pollen, dust mites, mould, animals (particularly household pets such as cats), dust, smoke, air pollution, chemicals, foods or drugs. Asthma attacks may also be triggered by viral infections, cold temperatures, exercise, certain chemicals, stress or intense emotions.

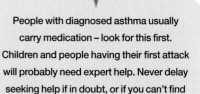

FIRST AID FOR ASTHMA

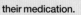

People with diagnosed asthma usually carry medication – look for this first. Children and people having their first attack will probably need expert help. Never delay seeking help if in doubt, or if you can't find their medication.

Most asthmatics will sit upright, often grasping the arms of a chair, to help them breathe. Leave them in whatever position is comfortable, as long as it is sitting up. Loosen any tight clothing, especially around the neck

The casualty should use an inhaler that will relieve symptoms, ideally with a spacer device so more drug reaches the lungs. Let the casualty take the medication themselves. Help them if necessary. If no spacer is available and they are not overly distressed, tell them to hold each inhaled puff for ten seconds. Encourage the person to take one or two puffs every one or two minutes, until they have had four puffs. If this does not relieve the wheezing, or there are signs of a serious attack, call the emergency services. Have them repeat four puffs every four minutes until the ambulance arrives. In very severe attacks use up to eight puffs every five minutes.

If hospital admission is necessary, more medication may be given, plus oxygen via a mask or tube. This treatment usually eases the attack within 12 to 24 hours.

RECOGNIZING AN ASTHMA ATTACK

As asthma can be life-threatening, it is important that symptoms are recognized and action taken as early as possible.

Signs of worsening asthma that needs medical attention:

➤ Wheezing or coughing occurs during exercise or at night.

➤ Inhaled medications are less effective at controlling symptoms.

➤ Peak-flow measurements start dropping. (A peak-flow meter is a device that many asthmatics have at home to measure the maximum volume of air that a person can breathe out.)

Signs of a very serious attack (always call the emergency services for these):

➤ Inability to finish sentences in one breath.

➤ Exhaustion from the effort of breathing.

➤ Confusion and irritability caused by lack of oxygen.

➤ Blue lips, and pale, clammy skin.

Signs of imminent respiratory arrest:

➤ Complete inability to talk.

➤ A silent chest (no wheezing) – the blocked airways cannot let air in.

➤ Weak, fast pulse.

DEALING WITH AN ASTHMA ATTACK

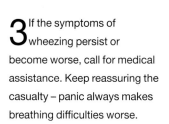

1 Make sure that a person having an asthma attack is sitting upright. They may be distressed and tense, as shown here. Comfort them and get them to relax back into their chair if possible, as relaxing conserves vital oxygen.

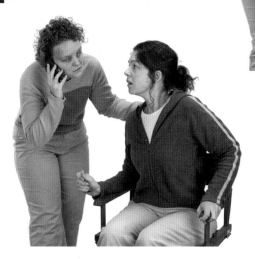

2 In the first instance, get the casualty to take the reliever medication themselves, ideally through a spacer device. If one is not available, get them to use their inhaler (shown). If absolutely necessary, help them to take it.

3 If the symptoms of wheezing persist or become worse, call for medical assistance. Keep reassuring the casualty – panic always makes breathing difficulties worse.

PANIC ATTACKS

Hyperventilation may be a sign of a panic attack, a sudden and shortlived bout of extreme anxiety. The victim may also experience a tension headache, a feeling of pressure in the chest, trembling, sweating and palpitations.

➤ Try to identify the cause of the fear and escort the victim to a quiet place.

➤ Reassure them and stay with them until they are calm. Advise them to consult a doctor to address the underlying cause of the attack.

DEALING WITH HYPERVENTILATION

Rapid breathing or over-breathing, also known as hyperventilation, is often caused by anxiety. It differs from breathing difficulty in that the sufferer has some control over the situation, although they may not feel this. Hyperventilation may cause tingling in the extremities and around the mouth, dizziness, chest pains and cramps. These symptoms make the sufferer feel even more anxious, and so they over-breathe even more.

The symptoms are caused by a lack of carbon dioxide, which the sufferer is breathing out at a very fast rate. A vicious circle ensues, with more anxiety developing as the hyperventilation worsens. Eventually, if the sufferer does not stop over-breathing, they faint, and the body resumes a normal breathing pattern. Hyperventilation can be a feature of phobias and panic attacks, both of which can be treated by psychologists.

WHAT TO DO

The most effective way of treating hyperventilation is through calm and firm reassurance. If possible, sit with the casualty in a quiet area and encourage them to stay calm and to concentrate on their breathing.

WARNING

If a casualty is hyperventilating, do not advise breathing their own air from a paper bag. Such practise has been known to cause further illness.

Tackling fume inhalation

SEE ALSO
➤ Dealing with
   breathing difficulties,
   p56
➤ Coping with
   headache, p86
➤ Managing dizziness
   and fainting, p88

Fumes inhaled into the lungs have the potential to do serious damage to the respiratory system. If you find a casualty you suspect has inhaled fumes, you must move them from the source, provided it does not put you at risk. Dangerous fumes include car exhaust, smoke, fumes from faulty domestic appliances, such as boilers, or blocked chimneys, fumes from smouldering foam-filled upholstery, such as sofas, household cleaners and industrial gases. Dry-cleaning solvents and some other chemicals also give off toxic fumes.

DAMAGE FROM FUMES

Accidental or deliberate inhalation of fumes – whether from the smoke in a burning building or glue sniffing – can be extremely dangerous. The extent of the damage depends on the length of exposure and the type of fume. The likelihood of fume inhalation increases dramatically if the fire or leakage is in an enclosed space. It is important to know that people are usually overcome by the fumes of a fire well before the flames reach them.

Children, older people and those with existing illnesses are the groups most vulnerable to fumes; children because of their size, and older people because they are generally less robust. Another problem is that injury to the casualty may not be obvious until up to 36 hours after exposure to the fumes, by which time irreparable damage to the lung tissue may have occurred.

Why are smoke and fumes from a fire harmful?

Fire eats up oxygen, as can the materials that burn in a fire, which means little is left for a casualty to breathe. The burning materials give off toxic gases such as carbon monoxide and cyanide. These not only poison the casualty as they breathe in, but also irritate the lining of their lungs, making them wheeze and cough. The heat of the fire can burn the mouth, throat and upper airways, which then swell and obstruct entry of air even more.

What to do in an emergency

As serious damage can be done by fumes, always assess the situation before rushing in to a potentially lethal scene. You should not make a rescue attempt if it puts your own life at risk; do not go into a smoke- or fume-filled building or room unless you are sure you are safe. Unless you are well protected yourself, you are likely to meet the same fate as the person you are rescuing. Never enter a room filled with smoke from a fire: do not attempt a rescue, call the emergency services who have the right equipment.

If you can do so safely, get any casualties away from the fumes as quickly as possible. Sit them upright, and if they are not too distressed, get them to take deep, slow breaths. If distressed people try to take deep breaths, they will simply become more distressed and breathless. Check for signs of fume inhalation, and also burns and any other injuries that may have been sustained in the accident. While waiting for the emergency services, check the casualty's vital signs and begin resuscitation if necessary.

SIGNS AND SYMPTOMS OF SMOKE OR FUME INHALATION

➤ A hoarse voice or no voice at all.

➤ Drooling or dribbling.

➤ Soot in the nostrils or phlegm.

➤ Singed hairs around the nostrils.

➤ Wheezing.

➤ Noisy breathing on inhaling.

➤ Burns around the mouth and neck.

➤ A large area of burns on any part of the body.

➤ Confusion.

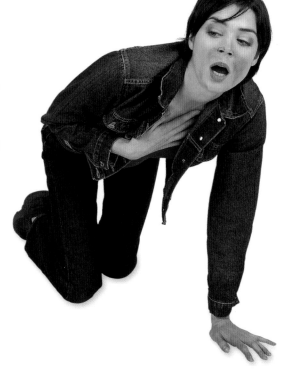

▷ A person suffering from smoke inhalation is likely to be gasping for breath, and there may be other signs such as soot around the mouth or burns on exposed parts of the body.

IS YOUR HOME SAFE?

Many cases of fire and fume inhalation occur in the home, but with a few simple safety measures the risk of an accident can be greatly reduced. Follow these guidelines to safeguard your family, friends and home-based employees:

• Fit smoke detectors. These reduce the number of deaths from fires by 60 per cent. They should be fitted on every floor of your home, including any areas, such as hallways, shared with other people. Check regularly that they work.

• Furnaces and central heating systems should be serviced by a professional boiler engineer/plumber once a year.

• Gas appliances should be checked on a regular basis.

• Motor engines should not be left on in an enclosed space, for example a car engine running in a garage or a gasoline-powered mower running in a garage.

• Tobacco smoke is a lethal cocktail containing over 4000 chemicals, all of which can injure the lungs in both the short term and the long term. Emphysema, chronic bronchitis and lung cancer are the well-known conditions associated with tobacco, but smoking is also the most common cause of fire fatalities. For people addicted to nicotine, e-cigarettes (vapes) won't start a fire if dropped near soft furnishing, so are a better option from a fire safety perspective. Never smoke near oxygen or while using paraffin-based emollient creams for skin conditions, as they could ignite.

• All soft furnishings made today must by law be fire retardant. Take extra care with old upholstered furniture, such as sofas, armchairs and beds, as they may not have been made under the latest rigorous safety standards.

• Never use aerosol sprays and dry-cleaning products in a confined area.

• Solvents burn at low temperatures, and are easily ignited. Store them away from ignition sources, properly labelled, and never smoke near them.

• Purchase a carbon monoxide monitor and keep a regular check on emissions from heating appliances.

Outside the home, make sure that there are smoke detectors at your place of work and at your child's school or day care provider, and anywhere else where they spend any length of time.

How to avoid fume damage

If you are in a situation where you have to escape from fumes, you need to employ a coordinated set of actions that, ideally, has been discussed previously with other members of the household. This should include escape routes and a place for you to meet and be accounted for outside the building. If you are away from the house during the day and your children are cared for by someone else, make sure that they know what to do in an emergency.

ESCAPING FROM FUMES

Get everyone to leave as fast as possible. Do not stop too long to find the source of the smoke – you will put yourself and others at risk of inhaling a toxic level of fumes.

As you escape, lie low on the floor and crawl below the level of the heat and fumes. Otherwise, you may be overcome by fumes before you have time to act.

Smoke inhalation causes confusion and disorientation. If the smoke is so thick that you cannot see, work your way towards a safe exit by sticking to familiar walls. Always feel a door before you open it; if it is hot, leave it shut. It will provide a barrier to fire and fumes for as long as it is closed and standing.

CARBON MONOXIDE POISONING

Carbon monoxide is one of the most toxic fumes. It has no taste or smell so is hard to detect. It is present in exhaust fumes, most types of smoke and can escape from defective gas or paraffin heaters and blocked chimney flues. A large amount of carbon monoxide is quickly fatal, but most cases of poisoning occur more gradually due to a slow leakage from a faulty appliance. Simple gauges are available to buy that indicate whether there is a leakage near a heater.

Symptoms of long-term exposure

➤ Irritability, confusion and bizarre behaviour.

➤ Headache, nausea and vomiting.

Symptoms of sudden high exposure

➤ Lips and tissues lining the mouth turn cherry red.

➤ Balance, vision and memory disturbances.

➤ Breathlessness, fast heart rate, muscle spasms, chest pain.

➤ Dizziness, abdominal pain.

➤ Distressed breathing pattern leading very quickly to a loss of consciousness.

Action in suspected carbon monoxide poisoning

➤ Get the victim out into the fresh air without delay.

➤ Loosen any tight clothing on the victim.

➤ Call an ambulance immediately. It is essential that you act quickly to obtain professional help including oxygen therapy.

Drowning: what to do

SEE ALSO

➤ What is first aid?, p12

➤ Safety in the bathroom, p228

➤ Safety in the garden, p230

Drowning is the third most common cause of accidental death worldwide. Children are particularly at risk. It can happen not only in the sea, rivers and lakes but also in swimming pools and garden ponds, even in the bath. A toddler can drown in just a few inches of water, so never leave a young child alone in the bathroom or anywhere near water, even if it is very shallow. In adults, falling asleep, being drunk or having an epileptic fit in the bath may be fatal. Knowing what to do in a drowning incident and doing it effectively can save someone's life.

Many of those who die through drowning are children and teenagers. It is not only non-swimmers who drown. Someone may have a heart attack while in the water, a boating accident may cause head injury, or a normally good swimmer may develop cramp or be overcome by a strong current or rip tide

WHAT IS DROWNING?

Drowning is submersion in water or another liquid, resulting in impaired respiration that may lead to death by suffocation as a result of brain injury from oxygen deprivation. When water enters the windpipe it provokes a muscular spasm that seals off the airway, preventing breathing and rapidly leading to unconsciousness. The airways then relax and the victim's lungs fill with water. This is what happens in most deaths from drowning. In a few cases the airway remains sealed and this eventually leads to respiratory failure and cardiac arrest even without water in the lungs. Drowning victims often cannot call for help as the vocal cords go into spasm on contact with water as well. Sometimes a casualty may survive but deteriorate later from damage caused by fluid or debris in the lungs ("secondary drowning").

The effect of cold water

Cold water can be a blessing or a curse. Sometimes, especially in children, the cold water shuts the body down; the heart rate drops and blood vessels constrict in major organs and muscles, so that heart and brain function are prioritized. Hypothermia sets in and the body's demand for oxygen drops dramatically. In this state of "hibernation" people have been resuscitated even after up to 40 minutes under water.

However, a more common reaction to cold water is for the casualty to take an automatic and involuntary gasp as they hit the water, and then start hyperventilating. They may then drown before they have a chance to swim to safety. This is known as cold shock.

SIGNS AND SYMPTOMS OF DROWNING

➤ No breathing or laboured breathing.

➤ Confusion, irritability or loss of consciousness.

➤ Cold, blue skin.

➤ Cough with frothy pink sputum.

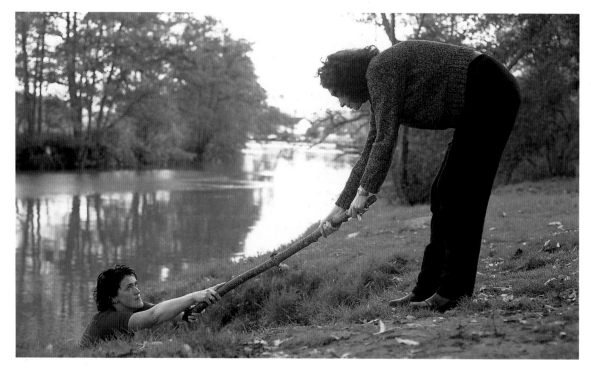

◁ Never jump in the water when dealing with a potential drowning. Hand the person something to hold on to. If nothing is available, lie down and extend your arms so that they can haul themselves up to the safety of the bank.

FIRST AID FOR DROWNING

Remember that the casualty may have swallowed a lot of water, as well as inhaling it. If they vomit, they may inhale the swallowed water into their lungs. To avoid this occurring, try to keep their head lower than the rest of their body when you take them out of the water.

Once the person has been rescued from the water, check their breathing. If they are not breathing, give 5 initial rescue breaths if trained or willing to do so.

Follow DRABC until help arrives. If you are on your own, do two minutes CPR before calling for help.

Do not try to empty their lungs and stomach of water.

Keep them warm, as they may be suffering from hypothermia. Take off the wet clothes – but only if you have dry ones to use in their place. Cover the ground under them, as heat is lost via this route.

If they start breathing; place in the recovery position, protecting their neck and spine. As there is a risk of secondary drowning, they must go to hospital, even if they appear to have completely recovered. Symptoms may appear up to 72 hours later.

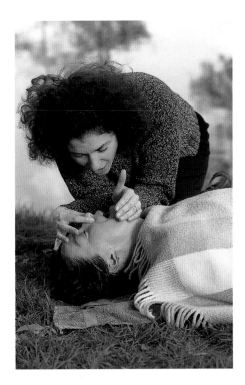

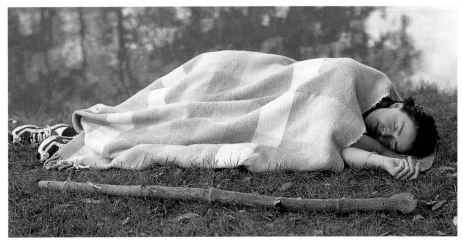

RESCUE SAFETY TIPS

➤ Do not enter the water if you can avoid it (never dive in). Water rescue is a skilled operation for which you need training.

➤ Throw the person a rope attached to a buoyancy aid and tow them ashore, or use a pole such as an oar from a rowing boat to get them ashore.

➤ Remember that, in cold water, hypothermia may make it difficult to detect signs of a circulation.

◁ Lose no time in resuscitating. If you are alone, act as you would when resuscitating a child and perform CPR for 2 minutes before calling for help.

▽ If breathing, place the casualty in the recovery position, keeping them warm and well covered until the emergency services arrive.

PREVENTION OF DROWNING

To minimize the chances of an accidental drowning, follow these guidelines:

➤ Children should be supervised whenever they are near water – at the beach, by a lake, river, pond or paddling pool. Even competent swimmers should be watched. Toddlers have drowned in minute amounts of water. Any water in the home should be kept covered – even fish tanks and toilets.

➤ Avoid alcohol if going for a swim. Many drownings are linked with excessive alcohol intake, especially in teenagers.

➤ Fence off swimming pools and ponds. Make sure the gate is self-shutting and the catch too high for a child to reach.

➤ Keep away from unfamiliar rivers, lakes or ponds, and never dive into unexplored or shallow waters.

➤ Ask the lifeguard on the beach about swimming conditions such as hidden currents or other hazards.

➤ Never swim outdoors if there is a storm brewing, as the risk of lightning striking the water is high and lethal.

Hanging and strangling: what to do

SEE ALSO
➤ What is first aid?, p12
➤ Responsiveness and the airway, p28
➤ The recovery position, 36

Both hanging and strangling involve compression of the windpipe and major blood vessels in the neck, which eventually causes death. In hanging, when the body is suspended by a noose around the neck, the neck is often broken. Strangling is constriction around the neck. Babies and young children are very vulnerable to strangulation by items such as blind cords, cot rails, banisters or railings. Such accidents also occur with adults, for example if clothing is caught in machinery. Deliberate hanging as a form of suicide is also a possibility.

Although most cases of strangling in babies and children are accidents, hanging is the second most common method of suicide (after firearms), and strangulation is often the method used in homicide. Death occurs because constriction of blood vessels in the neck stops oxygen reaching the brain, rather than because the airway is blocked. In hangings, the situation can be complicated because the neck is often broken.

It is essential to remove the constricting item and give first aid as quickly as possible to give the best chance of restoring breathing. If you are dealing with a hanging casualty you must handle them very carefully to avoid aggravating a spinal injury.

△ Before you release a victim of hanging to lay them on the ground, try to support them in some way. This is in order to prevent a heavy fall and further injury – you will find this much easier if you have a helper.

SIGNS OF HANGING OR STRANGLING

➤ Numerous tiny haemorrhages above the constriction line, including the whites of the eyes.

➤ Bruising, scratches and swelling around the neck – even finger marks may be obvious.

➤ Blue-grey discolouration of the skin.

➤ Very noisy breathing, due to the swelling around the airway, as well as a muffled voice and cough.

REDUCING THE RISKS

Babies under three months old are vulnerable to accidental strangling in crib bars or railings as they are not strong enough to physically push themselves out of trouble. Toddlers may lie with their neck over an object, and their body weight is enough to cause strangulation. Never leave babies and children alone in the house and be vigilant for hazards from ropes and cords. Never hang a pacifier on a string around their necks. Make sure looped blind cords are fitted with an approved safety device.

Older children may take great risks when they are playing, and rope swings of any kind are especially treacherous sources of potential danger. Children should be taught never to wrap anything around their neck and should be supervised at all times when climbing or near any equipment with moving parts, such as a treadmill or an escalator in a shopping mall, in case loose cords get trapped.

Automatic doors in shops and public buildings, and electric car windows, are responsible for significant numbers of accidental stranglings. Getting dangling clothing caught in escalators is another potential hazard. Always watch children very carefully whenever they are around such devices.

FIRST AID FOR HANGING

You need to act swiftly in an incident of hanging or strangling as the combination of a compressed airway and a possible neck injury can lead to a very rapid death. Your aim is to remove the constriction, restore breathing and summon the emergency services.

If the casualty is still hanging, try to support their body as you lift them down (call for help with this if you can).

Cut off the rope or constricting object as quickly as you can.

Lay them flat and assess their ABC. Be aware that there may be spinal injury at the neck, and so you must not over-flex the neck during any resuscitation efforts.

If they are breathing, place them in the recovery position while protecting their spine. You can then go for help.

DEALING WITH A HANGING

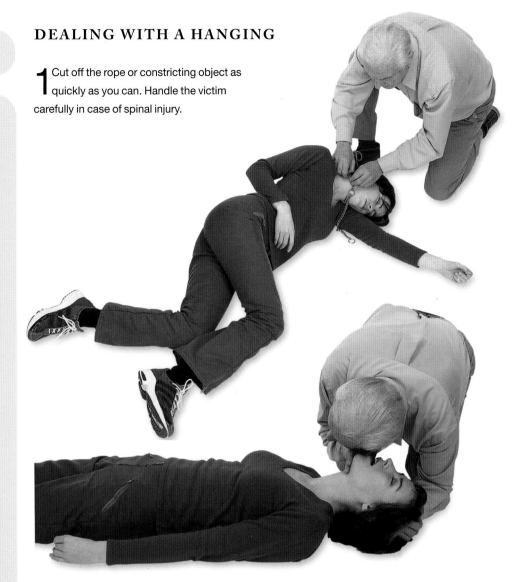

1 Cut off the rope or constricting object as quickly as you can. Handle the victim carefully in case of spinal injury.

2 Check for responsiveness and, if necessary, start resuscitation without delay.

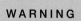

3 If breathing, place the casualty in the recovery position and call the emergency services.

WARNING
The incident may have to be investigated by the police. In this event, it is vital that any potential evidence, for example the rope or piece of clothing found around the casualty's neck, is not destroyed or tampered with in any way.

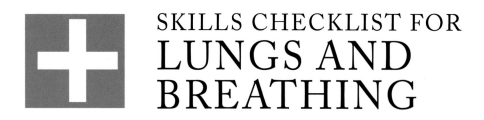

SKILLS CHECKLIST FOR
LUNGS AND BREATHING

KEY POINTS

- Always take any breathing difficulty seriously, and watch closely for deterioration ☐

- Swiftly follow basic guidelines for dealing with breathing difficulties, even if you don't know the root cause of the problem ☐

- Never put yourself at risk when dealing with noxious fume or drowning scenarios ☐

- Use common sense vigilance to prevent all kinds of strangling and hanging accidents ☐

SKILLS LEARNED

- Recognizing the signs and symptoms of breathing problems ☐

- How to help an asthma sufferer during an attack ☐

- Recognizing the severity of an asthma attack ☐

- How to treat hyperventilation ☐

- How to help casualties who have inhaled toxic fumes ☐

- Preventing and dealing with drowning ☐

- Dealing with hanging and strangulation ☐

5

HEART AND CIRCULATION

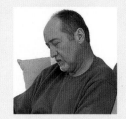

The heart and circulation are together responsible for providing every single cell in the body with blood – without blood there is no life. When things go wrong with this system, the outcome can quickly be catastrophic, so it is important to be prepared. This chapter describes the first aid to be given in conditions that affect the circulation, such as shock and anaphylaxis. Appropriate first-aid techniques are also given for heart attack and other abnormal heart conditions, including angina, heart failure and cardiac arrest. Knowing how to deal with such conditions can be life-saving.

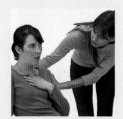

CONTENTS

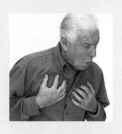

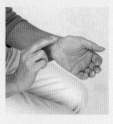

Understanding the cardiovascular system

SEE ALSO

➤ What is first aid?, p12

➤ Chest compressions, p30

➤ Full resuscitation sequence, p33

The cardiovascular system is made up of the heart ("cardio") and the blood vessels ("vascular"). The heart – which is essentially a large, powerful muscle about the size of your clenched fist – pumps blood at an average rate of 60–80 times a minute for a person's entire lifespan. The heart and the circulatory system can develop a range of disorders, due to the great demands placed on them. A number of these problems call for prompt emergency first-aid techniques in order to save the casualty's life.

THE HEART

Situated between the lungs, the heart is slightly to the left side of the body. The hollow area inside the heart muscle is made up of four separate compartments: two on the left and two on the right.

In healthy people, the two sides of the heart have no communication with each other. However, some babies are born with a communication between the two – a condition known as having a "hole in the heart".

Each side of the heart has two chambers, an upper atrium and a lower ventricle, giving four chambers in total: the left ventricle and atrium, and the right ventricle and atrium.

THE CIRCULATION

The left ventricle sends oxygenated blood through the main vessel leaving the heart, the aorta, to all parts of the body. Blood travels through arteries, which branch out into smaller vessels called arterioles. These then become minute vessels called capillaries, which form a network that bathes all body tissues allowing easy delivery of oxygen and nutrients and collection of carbon dioxide and other waste products. The capillaries then join with tiny vessels called venules, which form larger and larger veins, until the two vena cavae carrying deoxygenated blood arrive back at the right side of the heart. The superior vena cava returns blood from the head and arms and the inferior vena cava brings blood from the lower body and legs.

Deoxygenated venous blood arrives in the right atrium, moves down into the right ventricle, and is then pumped out of the heart through the pulmonary artery to

STRUCTURE OF THE HEART

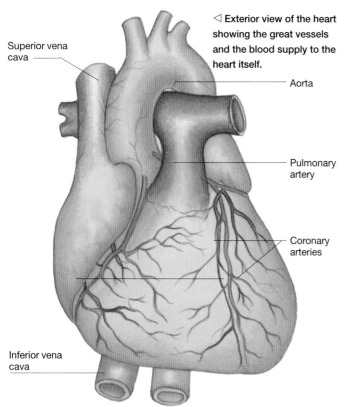

◁ Exterior view of the heart showing the great vessels and the blood supply to the heart itself.

Superior vena cava

Aorta

Pulmonary artery

Coronary arteries

Inferior vena cava

▽ Cross-section through the heart showing the four chambers surrounded by a thick muscular layer around the outside.

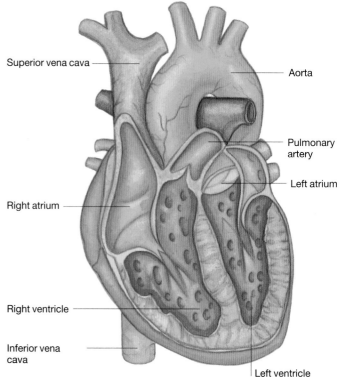

Superior vena cava

Aorta

Pulmonary artery

Left atrium

Right atrium

Right ventricle

Inferior vena cava

Left ventricle

CIRCULATING OXYGEN IN THE BLOOD

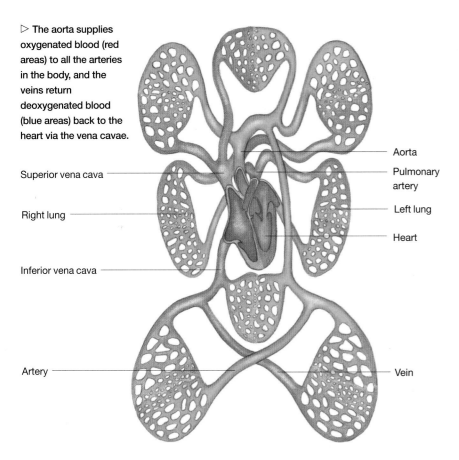

▷ The aorta supplies oxygenated blood (red areas) to all the arteries in the body, and the veins return deoxygenated blood (blue areas) back to the heart via the vena cavae.

Superior vena cava

Right lung

Inferior vena cava

Artery

Aorta

Pulmonary artery

Left lung

Heart

Vein

ARTERIES AND VEINS

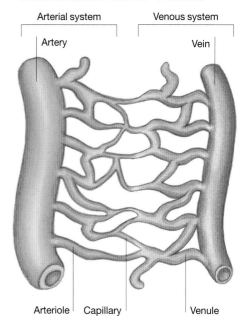

Arterial system | Venous system

Artery

Vein

Arteriole | Capillary | Venule

△ Close-up of a section of the circulatory system. The arterial system, which carries oxygenated blood (red), runs into smaller and smaller arteries until it reaches the tiny veins in the venous system, which carries deoxygenated blood (blue). The veins gradually enlarge until the blood reaches the vena cavae.

the lungs to be re-oxygenated. From the lungs it travels back to the heart, entering the left atrium and passing into the left ventricle. It then exits the heart via the aorta (the body's biggest vessel), starting its journey round the body again. The entire blood volume circulates around the body about once per minute, with the heart beating on average about 70 times per minute at rest.

Oxygenated blood pumped out into arteries from the left side of the heart is bright red, whereas the deoxygenated blood arriving back at the right side of the heart from the veins is a dark red colour.

THE BLOOD
Blood delivers nutrients around the body, as well as carrying oxygen from, and carbon dioxide to, the lungs. It protects against blood loss through its clotting ability, and infection through its white blood cells.

Fifty-five per cent of blood is made up of a straw-coloured clear fluid called plasma, which is rich in proteins. Within the plasma float red and white blood cells, plus components (such as platelets) that are needed for clot-forming. White cells are mainly involved in fighting infection, while red cells carry oxygen.

WHAT IS THE PULSE?
Each beat of the heart causes a pressure wave to travel through the arterial system.

▽ The "carotid" pulse in the neck is often a good one to find. Use two fingers to feel in the groove on either side of the windpipe.

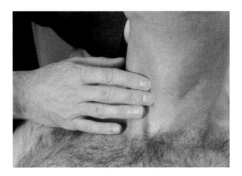

This can be felt as a pulse at various points where arteries are close to the body surface, including the neck, wrist and groin.

It can be much trickier than most people imagine to determine whether someone has a pulse, so this check is often best left to those with medical experience. Remember that vital signs such as coughing, gasping, twitching or blinking also indicate a circulation, and anyone can check for those.

▽ Practise feeling for a pulse. Try on an adult and also on a child.

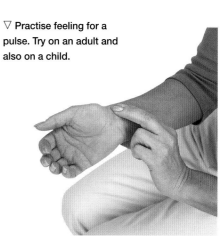

Dealing with shock

SEE ALSO

➤ What is first aid?, p12
➤ Full resuscitation sequence, p33
➤ Managing anaphylactic shock, p70

Shock is a serious condition caused by a sudden and dramatic drop in blood pressure. Without swift medical attention, shock can be life-threatening. It can be caused by any illness or injury that causes too little blood to circulate around the body, such as a heart attack or serious bleeding. This deprives the body of oxygen, leading to the pale, cold, collapsed state that typifies shock. This so-called physiological or circulatory shock must not be confused with the psychological or emotional shock that often occurs after a traumatic event.

Normally, the circulation provides a perfect balance between delivering oxygen and other nutrients to all cells in the body and removing toxic waste products. If this system fails and the amount of blood circulating around the body drops, the combined effect of a lack of oxygen reaching vital organs and a build-up of toxins leads to circulatory shock. If untreated or not attended to quickly enough, shock can be fatal.

WHAT CAUSES SHOCK?

Any trauma or illness that reduces blood circulation is capable of causing shock. If the heart is unable to pump effectively, after a heart attack for example, shock may follow. Abnormal heart rhythm can lead to shock. Electrocution can cause the heart to stop pumping blood.

Another common cause of shock is excessive loss of body fluids, which may be due to blood loss after a serious accident or fluid loss caused by extensive burns or prolonged diarrhoea and vomiting. A person can lose up to 0.5 litre (1 pint) of blood without any effect; after a loss of 2 litres (3.5 pints), symptoms of shock become apparent; and after losing 3 litres (5 pints) of blood, which is half the body's normal capacity, the end stages of shock, including loss of consciousness and heart failure, appear.

A severe head or spinal injury might affect control of the body's blood flow. The blood vessels may widen abnormally in severe infections and some types of poisoning. A severe allergic reaction in susceptible people may lead to the same symptoms – a very specific and rapidly life-threatening condition known as anaphylactic shock.

SIGNS AND SYMPTOMS OF CIRCULATORY SHOCK

➤ Pale or grey skin that feels cold and clammy.

➤ Fast, weak pulse.

➤ Profuse sweating.

➤ Fast, shallow breathing.

➤ Dizziness and faintness.

➤ Nausea and vomiting.

➤ Blurred vision.

➤ Thirst.

➤ Yawning, sighing, and gasping for air.

➤ Restlessness.

➤ Anxiety and/or confusion.

➤ Loss of consciousness.

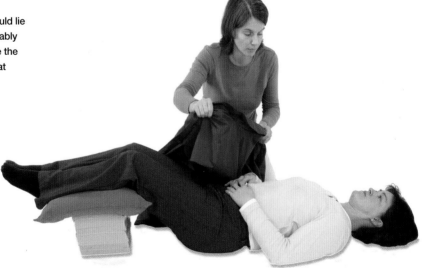

▷ If the casualty is conscious, they should lie down with their legs supported comfortably on an object that raises their legs above the level of their heart. (Do not raise legs that may be fractured, however.) The knees should be bent, as shown, to prevent straining the hamstring tendon at the back of the knee. You might want to pad the object with a folded blanket, garment or cushion. Do not raise their head up on cushions, as this restricts the airway – place on a blanket or similar if needed. Once in position, cover the casualty to keep them warm.

FIRST AID FOR CIRCULATORY SHOCK

If the casualty is unconscious, check DRABC.

Call the emergency services, if you have not already done so.

Start resuscitation, if necessary. Get someone to control any heavy bleeding, if possible.

If the casualty is unconscious but breathing, put them in the recovery position. Stop any heavy bleeding.

If the casualty is conscious, lie them down and reassure them. Staunch any heavy bleeding.

Check the body for fractures, wounds, and burns. Deal with these as necessary; make sure any heavy bleeding is controlled.

Unless you think their legs may be fractured, place their legs on a low, padded support (with legs higher than heart).

Cover the casualty with a blanket, and try to keep them calm and monitor their condition until help arrives.

Do not give the casualty anything to eat or drink. Moisten an uncomfortably dry mouth with a wet flannel or towel.

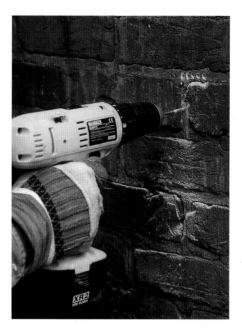

△ Electrocution is one of the traumas that can lead to circulatory shock. A common cause of electrocution around the home is using electrical DIY or gardening equipment.

SYMPTOMS OF SHOCK

In reaction to the reduced circulation of blood, the body directs blood to vital areas such as the heart and lungs, and away from the skin. This makes the skin cold and pale. The body releases adrenaline as an emergency response and this causes a rapid pulse and sweating. As the blood flow weakens further, the brain begins to suffer from lack of oxygen, leading to nausea, dizziness, blurred vision, and confusion. If blood circulation is not restored rapidly, the casualty will start gasping for breath and will soon lose consciousness.

WHAT YOU CAN DO TO HELP

If you think you have come across a casualty in shock, it is crucial to call the emergency services because medical help is always necessary. First-aid measures can help maintain the limited blood circulation to the brain, heart and lungs while waiting for expert help. Should the casualty slip into unconsciousness, you must assess them (ABC) and then administer life-saving techniques as necessary, for as long as you are able or until help arrives at the scene.

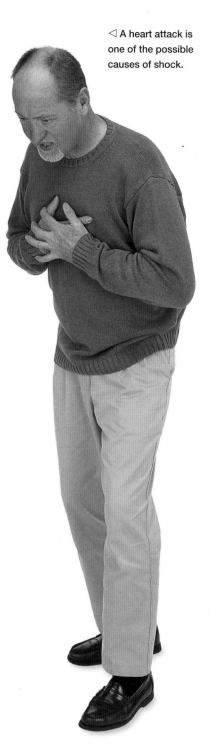

◁ A heart attack is one of the possible causes of shock.

WARNING

Do not try to warm the casualty by any means other than by covering with a blanket. Avoid hot water bottles, electric blankets, fan heaters or any other form of direct heat, as overheating the body will increase the danger.

Managing anaphylactic shock

SEE ALSO

➤ What is first aid?, p12

➤ Full resuscitation sequence, p33

➤ Dealing with bites and stings, p104

Anaphylactic shock is a massive allergic reaction that can develop after contact with a trigger substance. This is a potentially fatal condition caused by the body's response to a substance that usually has no serious effect on other people: a food, a drug or an insect sting, for example. It is a form of circulatory shock, but the effects usually develop suddenly and worsen rapidly. A susceptible person may need to carry an injection of adrenaline in case of accidental exposure. Once the condition has developed, the risk of anaphylaxis usually lasts for life.

What causes anaphylactic shock? The body's immune system overreacts to what it sees as a foreign body, even though, in most people it would not cause any reaction. People become sensitized to a substance, often at an early age, and may not initially have any reaction to the substance – it is often the second and subsequent exposures that can cause an allergic reaction and may lead to anaphylaxis. From that time on, such people will remain at risk for the rest of their lives.

Even a tiny amount of the substance can set off a reaction – a trace of peanut oil in a sandwich might be enough for a person sensitive to nuts. Their body releases a massive amount of histamine; this makes their blood vessels dilate and leak fluid, and the lungs go into spasm, causing symptoms similar to asthma. The victim may feel faint, confused or anxious, with a rapid heartbeat and clammy skin. They may have an itchy, raised rash (hives), facial or tongue swelling, abdominal pain or nausea and vomiting. If swelling involves the airway consequences are potentially fatal. The most common causes of anaphylaxis are peanuts, sesame seeds and oil, fish, shellfish, dairy products, eggs, wasp or bee stings, latex, antibiotics and other drugs.

People known to be allergic to peanuts, for example, must be very vigilant when buying processed foods, ensuring that they check the ingredients label to check for nut traces. They must also take great care when ordering food in restaurants and even more so if buying food from street markets and stalls.

RECOGNIZING ANAPHYLAXIS

Anyone who has had an anaphylactic reaction should be referred to an allergy specialist, because subsequent reactions can be sudden and severe. The specialist

SIGNS AND SYMPTOMS OF ANAPHYLACTIC SHOCK

➤ Intensely itchy rash, often with red raised areas (hives).

➤ A sudden drop in blood pressure (difficult to determine and not visible).

➤ Extreme anxiety, including a sense of imminent doom.

➤ Swollen face, lips, tongue and throat.

➤ Rapid pulse.

➤ Puffy eyes.

➤ Difficulty speaking or swallowing.

➤ Wheezing, tight chest and breathing difficulty.

➤ Abdominal pain, feelings of nausea and vomiting.

➤ Faintness.

➤ Loss of consciousness.

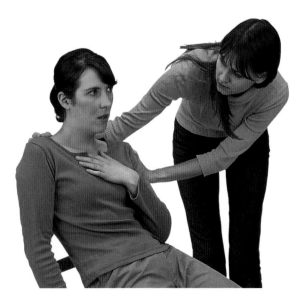

◁ Check through the ABC of resuscitation if necessary. Look for signs of shock, including breathing difficulty, swelling of the mouth, tongue or throat and pale skin.

cannot always identify exactly what has caused the reaction, but skin prick and blood tests may be useful. In some cases of food allergy, a challenge test may be carried out in which minute quantities of the suspect allergen are ingested. This is the only certain way to confirm the allergen. Such a test is done only in a clinic or hospital setting with facilities to deal with a severe reaction should one develop.

In some countries, desensitizing treatment, either as injections or drops under the tongue, are given to try to reduce a person's sensitivity to a substance. However, this can induce anaphylaxis, and many people feel the risk is too great.

FIRST AID FOR ANAPHYLAXIS

People with a history of anaphylaxis who have been prescribed an epinephrine auto-injector should carry it with them at all times. Search in their bag for one if they are too ill to do so themselves. Ideally they should inject themselves, but this is a life-threatening situation and you may need to administer it if they are unable. Full instructions are given on the tube containing the injector pen (also called Epipens). If the person continues to suffer severe symptoms, or they recur, give a second injection after 5–15 minutes if there is a second injector available.

Dial the emergency services.

Remove any trigger if possible, such as a bee sting still stuck in the skin.

Lie the casualty down flat unless they have breathing difficulties or are pregnant. Keep them comfortable until the ambulance arrives.

Insist that the sufferer go to hospital, even if they feel better. Anaphylaxis can recur up to several hours after contact with the agent and it may be more serious next time around.

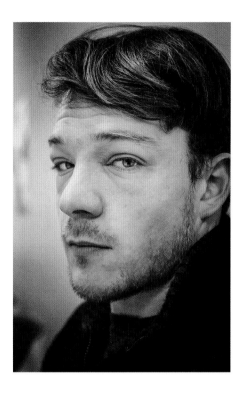

△ This young man's puffy eyes and red raised areas of skin are some of the signs of an allergic reaction to some food or substance he has come into contact with.

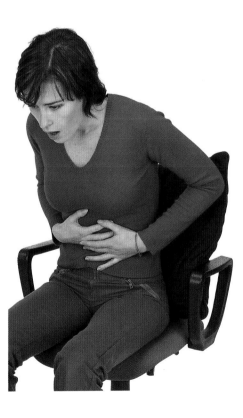

◁ Abdominal pain, nausea and vomiting are among the common symptoms of anaphylactic shock.

TIPS FOR ANAPHYLAXIS SUFFERERS

➤ Always carry your adrenaline auto-injector with you. If you have been prescribed two, carry both in case you needed a second injection. If you have to use your injector, replace it straightaway.

➤ If you are allergic to a food, be extra careful when eating out. Do not rely on menu descriptions: tell the waiting staff what you are allergic to and ask them to check with the chef that your chosen dish doesn't contain it.

➤ Always read food ingredients labels when shopping. You may miss something vital otherwise. If in doubt, avoid the food.

➤ Practise using your adrenaline pen – the manufacturer of your auto-injector can supply a trainer device that has no needle or adrenaline. Be comfortable with using it before an emergency occurs.

➤ Tell family, friends and work colleagues what happens when you have an allergic reaction, and ensure that key people around you know that you may need to have adrenaline and where you keep your injector pen. If your child is a sufferer, make sure their teachers and friends' parents know about the allergy and understand the importance of getting adrenaline administered.

➤ Wear a medical ID tag of some kind (often worn as a bracelet).

Coping with a heart attack

SEE ALSO
➤ What is first aid?, p12
➤ Chest compressions, p30
➤ Full resuscitation sequence, p33

Heart attack is one of the leading causes of death in developed countries. For the best chance of survival, immediate hospital admission is necessary. To ensure that this happens you need to recognize when a person is possibly having a heart attack and phone for an ambulance without delay. The cause of a heart attack is nearly always a blockage in one of the major arteries supplying the heart muscle. There may be warning signs, such as angina, or a heart attack may occur suddenly, particularly in people at high risk.

A heart attack is known medically as a myocardial infarction. This literally means the death of an area of heart muscle due to an interrupted blood supply. The coronary arteries, which supply the heart muscle, can become furred up with a fatty substance, plaque, in a condition known as atherosclerosis. Reduced blood flow through these narrowed arteries causes the pain of angina. Eventually, the plaque may cause a blood clot that entirely blocks the artery and part of the heart muscle dies as a result. This is a heart attack

WHO HAS HEART ATTACKS?

Heart attacks become more common as we get older. However, some people are at greater risk of having a heart attack at an early age. These include:

• People with a family history of heart attacks – a close relative who has had a heart attack under the age of 60.
• Anyone with a high blood level of cholesterol. High levels of this fatty substance are linked to an increased risk of atherosclerosis, leading to heart attack.
• Smokers.
• People who are overweight.
• Anyone with high blood pressure.
• People with diabetes.
• Post-menopausal women, since female

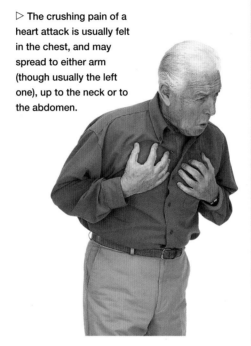

▷ The crushing pain of a heart attack is usually felt in the chest, and may spread to either arm (though usually the left one), up to the neck or to the abdomen.

hormones give pre-menopausal women some protection against heart attacks. After the menopause women are just as much at risk as men.

HOW TO AVOID HEART ATTACKS

If you are in a high-risk group, your doctor may monitor your condition on a regular basis and prescribe drugs. You may also be put on a special diet aimed at reducing the chances of your having a heart attack. For the majority of other people, the risk of heart attack can be reduced by the following guidelines:
• Give up smoking.

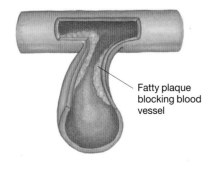

◁ This shows a cross-section of the junction between two arterial blood vessels. A fatty plaque has gathered and is constricting blood flow – atherosclerosis. If this occurs in arteries that supply the heart, a heart attack can occur.

Fatty plaque blocking blood vessel

SIGNS AND SYMPTOMS OF A HEART ATTACK

➤ Chest pain: "crushing" or "tight" pain, usually felt behind the breastbone. The pain may spread to an arm, up to the jaw, neck and teeth, or to the upper or middle part of the abdomen. (Note: some heart attacks are painless, especially in women, older people and those with diabetes.)

➤ Pale/grey colour or blue lips.

➤ Nausea and vomiting.

➤ Sweating and clammy skin.

➤ Feeling restless, often a characteristic sense of impending doom.

➤ Rapid, weak pulse, light headedness.

➤ Breathlessness, cough or wheezing.

➤ Loss of consciousness.

• Keep within the healthy weight range for your height and build.
• Take regular exercise (it is often best to check with a doctor before starting any exercise regime).
• Eat a balanced diet that is low in animal fat, salt and processed/convenience food.
• Learn to manage stress.

WARNING
Beware a persistent pain that is like indigestion, which is not relieved by remedies for indigestion. Many people have died from a heart attack, having put up with what they thought was a bad bout of indigestion for a few days. If in any doubt, go to see a doctor.

FIRST AID FOR SUSPECTED HEART ATTACK

⬇

Call an ambulance.

⬇

Sit the person upright, ideally on the floor and against a wall with their knees bent and their head and shoulders supported.

⬇

Provided they are not allergic to it, give them a standard (300mg) tablet of aspirin and tell them to chew it slowly.

⬇

Do not allow the casualty to eat or drink. Try to keep them calm.

⬇

The casualty's usual angina pills or spray should be administered if required – usually under the tongue.

⬇

Monitor ABC and be prepared to start resuscitation if necessary.

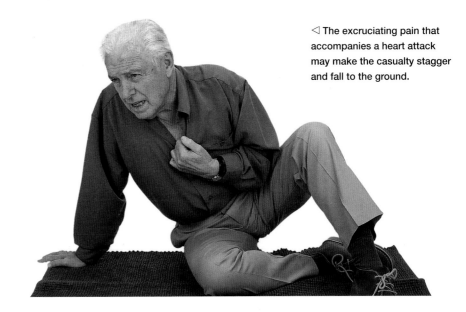

◁ The excruciating pain that accompanies a heart attack may make the casualty stagger and fall to the ground.

ANGINA PECTORIS

Usually shortened to angina, the term angina pectoris literally means pain in the chest. Angina is caused by insufficient blood flow to one or more of the coronary arteries, usually due to obstruction by atherosclerosis but sometimes to spasm of the artery wall. This causes pain that may be relieved by resting or by medication that dilates the arteries, or it may settle spontaneously. Angina may lead on to a full-blown heart attack. People at risk of angina are the same group as those at risk of heart attack.

Those at risk may feel anxious about exercising if this brings on pain, but it is important for them to stay active and exercise in moderation can help to alleviate angina and prevent heart attacks in the long term.

ADVICE FOR DEALING WITH ANGINA

➤ Ensure that the person is sitting down and resting.

➤ If they have had angina before and have an angina spray, let them administer it themselves, or if necessary, help them to use it.

➤ If the pain is worse than normal or lasts for more than 15 minutes despite three doses of medication, or if the sufferer's condition starts to deteriorate, call for an ambulance.

▷ Sit the casualty upright and raise their legs if possible until the emergency services arrive.

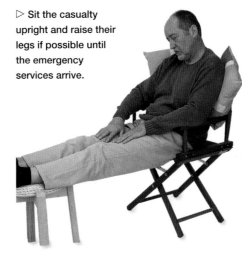

HEART FAILURE

A condition that often develops slowly over months, heart failure does not mean that the heart has stopped working but that it cannot pump efficiently enough to keep up with the body's demands. This results in gradually increasing shortness of breath on exertion, extreme fatigue and fluid building up in the feet and ankles. This is a chronic condition that the person's doctor will aim to manage to reduce symptoms and slow progression.

However, an acute type of heart failure can develop when fluid suddenly builds up in the lungs, causing a severe shortness of breath. This may occur alongside a heart attack or as a result of other heart problems or other conditions such as anaemia or hyperthyroidism. Untreated it may lead to a heart attack. Acute heart failure requires emergency treatment. Sit the person upright, ideally with their legs over the side of a bed. Call the emergency services immediately.

SIGNS AND SYMPTOMS OF HEART FAILURE

➤ Breathing is fast, shallow and laboured.

➤ Skin is cold, clammy and sweaty.

➤ Blue lips, skin and nails.

➤ Sense of confusion and acute anxiety.

Dealing with an abnormal heart rate

Abnormal heart rate or rhythm, known medically as arrhythmia, can cause palpitations and breathlessness. Occasional awareness of one's heartbeat is a normal reaction to fear or excitement, or it may be a sign of too much coffee or alcohol. Frequent palpitations may indicate disease, so this should always be checked by a doctor. Arrhythmias are common after a heart attack, when the heart muscle is in a state of irritability; this is what often causes the heart to stop working altogether, otherwise known as cardiac arrest.

Everyone occasionally feels their heart "leap" – hopefully from love rather than fear, and sometimes for no apparent reason at all. That sudden thump or feeling that the heart has missed a beat is called a palpitation. This is only worrying when it becomes more than an occasional symptom. Frequent palpitations may be an indication of an illness, such as an overactive thyroid or heart disease. However, panic attacks and anxiety may also be the cause of palpitations, as may be over-indulgence in coffee, cigarettes, alcohol or illegal drugs.

WHAT CONTROLS HEART RATE?

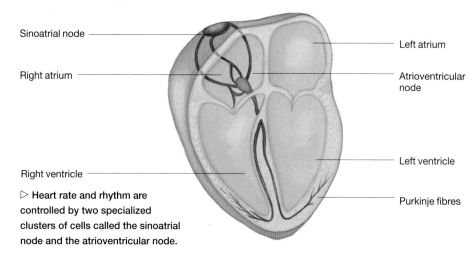

Sinoatrial node

Right atrium

Right ventricle

Left atrium

Atrioventricular node

Left ventricle

Purkinje fibres

▷ Heart rate and rhythm are controlled by two specialized clusters of cells called the sinoatrial node and the atrioventricular node.

HOW THE HEART RATE IS REGULATED

The heart is a muscle that contracts and relaxes continuously and rhythmically between 60 and 80 times a minute, on average, throughout our lives. Heart muscle is unique because it has its own conduction system so it can contract without any outside control. Chemicals such as adrenaline or caffeine can alter the heart rate, as can anxiety, or a drop in blood pressure.

Each contraction of the heart muscle is controlled from within, by the conduction system. This system comprises groups of cells that charge up and fire spontaneously.

One group of cells, called the sinoatrial (S/A) node, sets the rhythm for the rest of the heart – it acts as the heart's internal pacemaker.

An electrical wave spreads from the S/A node through the atria, until it reaches a second node called the atrioventricular node. It is then relayed through branches until it reaches specialized cells called Purkinje fibres in the innermost layer of the ventricles. These form a wiring system that transmits the impulses and synchronizes contraction of the ventricles.

TYPES OF ARRHYTHMIA

Heart rate may be either too high or too low and its rhythm may be irregular. The most serious type of arrhythmia is ventricular fibrillation, which is when the heart muscle "quivers", rather than beating in a coordinated fashion. This is common after a heart attack. The heart cannot pump blood efficiently in this state, and the casualty rapidly loses consciousness and will die as a result of cardiac arrest (when the heart stops) unless the heart can get back into a normal rhythm.

CARDIAC ARREST

A life-threatening emergency situation, cardiac arrest occurs when the heart stops beating. The most common cause is a heart attack, but there are many other causes. After a car accident, cardiac arrest may occur because of massive blood loss, or a collapsed lung. Cardiac arrest may occur in pulmonary embolism, a condition in which a blood clot forms in the lungs. Electrocution or a lightning strike injury may cause a cardiac arrest. Asthmatics may have a cardiac arrest during a severe asthma attack.

Cardiopulmonary resuscitation is not a definitive life-saving treatment for cardiac arrest, and can only keep the blood pumping around the body until specialized help is available. The only effective treatment is defibrillation, in which a high-energy electric shock is applied to the chest wall. The sooner this is done after cardiac arrest, the more likely that the heart will return to a normal rhythm and resume pumping blood around the body.

FIRST AID FOR PALPITATIONS

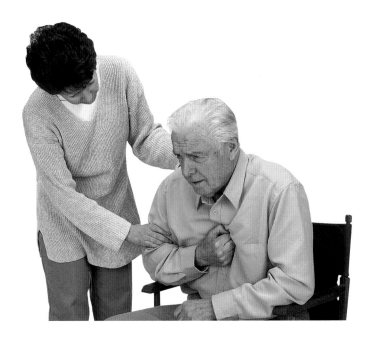

1 If the casualty has chest pains or feels breathless, faint, dizzy or confused, call an ambulance immediately.

2 Sit the casualty down and reassure them if they are anxious. This may be all that is needed to settle the palpitations, most of which are not serious. Talk to them to find out whether they have experienced an abnormal heart rate before and whether they have a diagnosed heart condition.

3 If the casualty has frequent palpitations, advise them to see their doctor in case this is a symptom of a health problem.

Automated external defibrillators (AEDs) are now available in many public places such as shopping malls, factories, sports facilities and doctors' surgeries, for use by bystanders before the ambulance arrives. The emergency operator will be able to direct you to where the closest AED is located, give you the code to open up the device and then instruct you how to use it. The existence of these AEDs has led to a dramatic improvement in survival rates from out-of-hospital cardiac arrest.

▷ Early use of an AED can dramatically improve the survival rate of most heart attack victims.

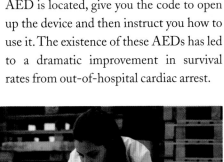

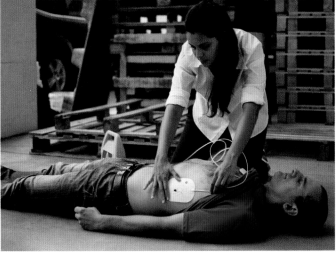

FIRST AID FOR CARDIAC ARREST

The main rule is to assess the casualty according to DRABC procedure, as follows.

Make sure the casualty's airway is clear and open. Check whether the casualty is breathing. If not, call an ambulance and start chest compressions. Keep going until the emergency services arrive.

AUTOMATED EXTERNAL DEFIBRILLATOR (AED)

If someone suffers cardiac arrest in a public place, a defibrillator may be available on site. It is simple to use without training and the emergency operator can talk you through the process if necessary.

➤ If you are already carrying out CPR, only stop when the defibrillator is ready.

➤ Make sure you and any other helpers are not touching the victim while the machine is analysing the heart or administering shocks.

➤ The prompts from the defibrillator should be followed until the paramedics arrive.

SIGNS OF CARDIAC ARREST

➤ Loss of consciousness.

➤ Patient unresponsive.

➤ Breathing is abnormal or absent.

➤ Pale, blue skin.

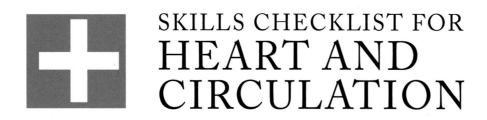

SKILLS CHECKLIST FOR
HEART AND CIRCULATION

KEY POINTS

- Effective blood circulation is essential for an individual to survive ☐

- Always call the emergency services out promptly to shock cases ☐

- Always call the emergency services out promptly if you suspect heart problems – they can quickly become life-threatening ☐

- Frequent heart palpitations must be investigated by a doctor – they are a symptom of various health problems. ☐

SKILLS LEARNED

- An understanding of how the circulatory system works ☐

- Recognizing and dealing with circulatory shock ☐

- Recognizing, treating and avoiding anaphylactic shock ☐

- Recognizing and dealing with a heart attack ☐

- Recognizing and dealing with heart failure and angina ☐

- Dealing with palpitations and cardiac arrest ☐

BRAIN AND NERVOUS SYSTEM

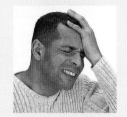

The brain is the control centre of the central nervous system, an extraordinarily complex set of mechanisms that controls the function of the body and mind. Electrical and chemical signals rush around the body causing millions of actions every minute. However, the system is very delicate and easily damaged by injury or disease. Knowing what to do in the event of an accident affecting any part of the nervous system is of prime importance to the outlook for the casualty, and may even save their life. Even something as apparently minor as a headache may warn of a serious condition that must be investigated by a doctor.

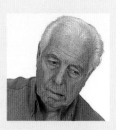

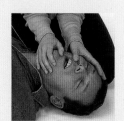

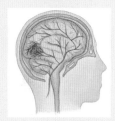

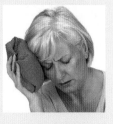

Understanding the nervous system

SEE ALSO
➤ What is first aid?, p12
➤ Dealing with head injury, p80
➤ Coping with headache, p86

The importance of the brain and the central nervous system to the rest of the body cannot be overstated. Every part of the body, and every bodily function, is under its control. For this reason, head and spinal injuries may prove particularly serious and have effects on many parts of the body at some distance from the injury. First aid is of the ultimate importance, particularly maintaining the vital functions of breathing and circulation. Alert the emergency services without delay if you are in any doubt about the casualty's condition.

Human beings have a highly developed and sophisticated nervous system. The brain and nervous system are organized into many parts that serve specific and important functions – together they make up the body's main control centre. All body sensations, muscle contractions, gland secretions and a host of other complex interactions vital to life are relayed through the central nervous system.

HOW THE NERVOUS SYSTEM IS ORGANIZED

The nervous system is divided into two main sections – the central nervous system (CNS), which comprises the brain and the spinal cord, and the peripheral nervous system (PNS), which is made up of all the nerves that branch off the CNS. Nerves from the brain are called cranial nerves and those from the spinal cord are spinal nerves. The PNS is further broken down into nerves under voluntary control, such as those that control the muscles used for conscious movements, and nerves under involuntary control, such as those governing our internal systems – our heart rate and the changing size of our pupil in response to light, for example. The part of the system that regulates actions over which we have no voluntary control is known as the autonomic nervous system (ANS).

We take in information through our five senses – sight, smell, hearing, touch and taste – and the brain can act on this information through the motor system. For example, when a toddler touches a hot oven, the brain receives a message via the senses and acts through the motor system

THE CENTRAL NERVOUS SYSTEM

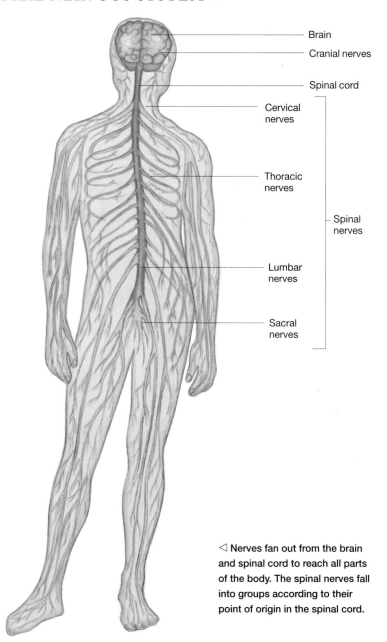

- Brain
- Cranial nerves
- Spinal cord
- Cervical nerves
- Thoracic nerves
- Spinal nerves
- Lumbar nerves
- Sacral nerves

◁ Nerves fan out from the brain and spinal cord to reach all parts of the body. The spinal nerves fall into groups according to their point of origin in the spinal cord.

to make the muscles move. The toddler pulls the hand away from the painful stimulus. Although this is a reflex action, the brain remembers the pain and the toddler will be wary of touching the oven in future.

CROSS-SECTION THROUGH THE BRAIN

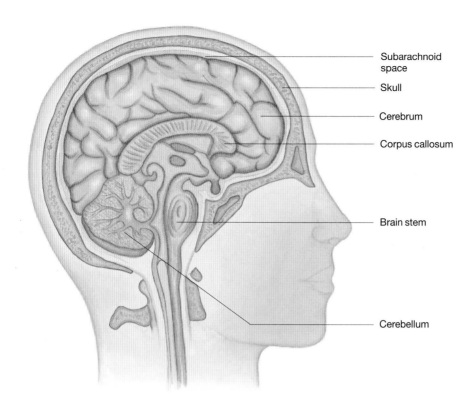

- Subarachnoid space
- Skull
- Cerebrum
- Corpus callosum
- Brain stem
- Cerebellum

MULTIPOLAR NEURONE

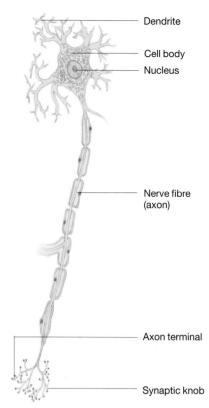

- Dendrite
- Cell body
- Nucleus
- Nerve fibre (axon)
- Axon terminal
- Synaptic knob

THE BRAIN

Our brain controls our thoughts, memories, speech, movements and all the functions of the organs. Divided into three parts, the brain comprises the cerebrum, the cerebellum and the brain stem.

The cerebrum forms the bulk of the brain: it controls sensation, movement, emotion and intellect. The cerebrum is divided into two hemispheres, the left and the right. Many functions are more concentrated in one hemisphere than the other, for example, in right-handed people the brain regions that control speech and language are often in the left hemisphere, which is then called the dominant hemisphere. Left-handed people may have their dominant hemisphere on the right.

The effects of damage to the brain such as after a stroke can be different depending on which areas of the brain are affected. Damage to the left hemisphere may cause speech problems in a right-handed person, but a left-hander's speech will be unaffected.

The cerebellum controls coordination of movement, balance and posture. People with damage to their cerebellum sometimes appear drunk and they may stagger, slur their words and suffer from severe dizziness.

The brain stem regulates the heart rate and breathing, as well as coordinating activities such as coughing, sneezing and swallowing. Brain stem injury can have very severe consequences including leaving people in a coma or vegetative state, and such injuries are often fatal.

NERVES AND NEURONES

The nuts and bolts of the nervous system are cells called neurones and neuroglia. The neurones conduct electrical activity from one part of the body to another, while the neuroglia support and protect the neurones. Billions of these highly specialized cells are joined together to form nerves, which stretch from the brain or spinal cord to every part of the body.

Neurones in the brain are very densely packed and number around 1000 billion. Neurones in the spinal cord and around the body are very long and form an extensive communication system. The cell bodies of neurones are linked together by nerve fibres (axons), and the many projections coming off the cell bodies are called dendrites.

Nerve impulses in the form of electrical signals travel along the neurones at rapid speeds of up to 275 km/h (125 mph). With chemicals called neurotransmitters, signals from the brain are translated into effects at the target cell, for example in a muscle.

NERVOUS SYSTEM PROBLEMS

Although peripheral nerves will regenerate if they are sewn back together fast enough, regeneration is extremely limited in the central nervous system. If the spinal cord is severed, it cannot heal or grow back. If central nervous tissue is damaged, whether due to a stroke or multiple sclerosis, it is likely to cause permanent impairment.

Problems with the nervous system can manifest themselves in many ways, but they are largely determined by the parts of the brain that are affected. Abnormal electrical activity causes epilepsy, degeneration of nervous tissue may cause dementia, and processes that affect neuro-chemicals in the brain can be affected by psychiatric conditions such schizophrenia.

Dealing with head injury

SEE ALSO

➤ What is first aid?, p12

➤ Full resuscitation sequence, p33

➤ Tackling skull and facial fractures, p152

Serious head injury is a medical emergency, particularly if the casualty loses consciousness. The first-aider should protect the casualty's airway, start resuscitation if necessary and alert the emergency services without delay. An obvious cut or bump on the scalp may lead to a suspicion of head injury, but serious internal injury is often not evident from external signs. It is worth remembering also that very young and very old people are especially susceptible to developing delayed reactions to relatively minor head injuries – so may need checking out.

Head injuries are potentially serious because they can damage the brain and surrounding blood vessels. Although the bony skull protects the brain, it also provides an enclosed space in which the brain can be easily shaken and damaged, and where there is little room for any swelling or bleeding following injury.

The main causes of head injuries are road traffic accidents, sporting and recreational activities, falls and assaults.

TYPES OF HEAD INJURY

There are five main types of head injury, and casualties may have several simultaneously:

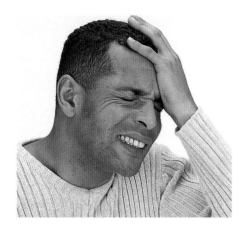

△ A sudden, crushing headache should always be investigated, particularly if it comes on at some point after a blow to the head.

Cuts

Large cuts to the scalp look alarming, and bleed profusely, but are only likely to be serious if caused by a major blow. A large blow may cause brain damage.

Concussion

This is a head injury that temporarily affects brain function. Symptoms may include loss of consciousness, confusion, dizziness, visual disturbances, nausea and vomiting, short-term memory loss, headache and behaviour or personality changes. They may arise immediately following injury nor not for some days or even weeks.

Contusion

Bruising, or contusion, may occur to the brain after an injury, and this causes swelling of the brain tissue. This may lead to prolonged periods of unconsciousness following an accident, and possibly much

SIGNS AND SYMPTOMS OF SERIOUS HEAD INJURY

➤ Deep cuts or tears to the scalp, or goose egg swelling over the scalp.

➤ Nausea and/or vomiting.

➤ Severe headache.

➤ Drowsiness or difficulty being roused.

➤ Unequal sized pupils, or pupils that do not respond to light.

➤ Visual disturbance.

➤ Blood or fluid flowing from ears, nose, eyes and/or mouth.

➤ Paralysis, numbness or loss of function over one half of the body.

➤ Problems with balance.

➤ Behaving as though drunk.

➤ Fits, confusion or unconsciousness.

CONTRA-COUP INJURY

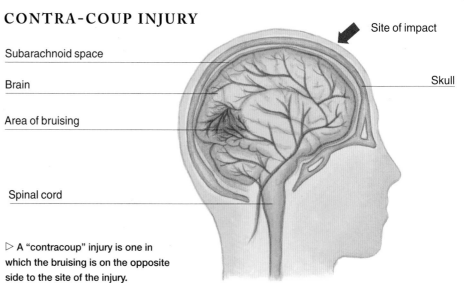

Subarachnoid space

Brain

Area of bruising

Spinal cord

Site of impact

Skull

▷ A "contracoup" injury is one in which the bruising is on the opposite side to the site of the injury.

POSSIBLE SITE OF BRAIN INJURY FOLLOWING BLOW TO BACK OF HEAD

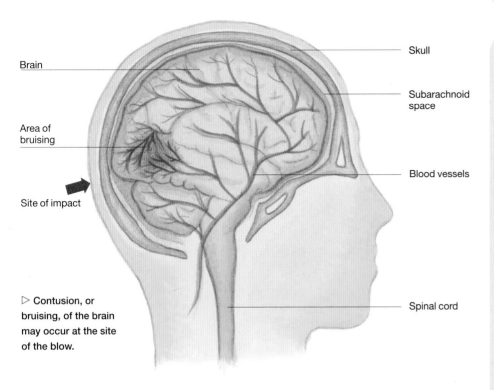

Brain

Area of bruising

Site of impact

Skull

Subarachnoid space

Blood vessels

Spinal cord

▷ Contusion, or bruising, of the brain may occur at the site of the blow.

FIRST AID FOR A HEAD INJURY

Breathing in vomit while unconscious after a head injury may be fatal. The first priority is to protect the victim's airway by tilting back the jaw. Always assume that they may have spinal injuries and protect their neck while trying to keep their airway open: if you can, use the jaw thrust to open the airway. If they are not breathing, start resuscitation.

Carefully apply direct pressure to any scalp wounds that are bleeding.

Watch for vomiting.

If they are conscious, lay them on the floor with head and shoulders slightly raised. If unconscious, place them in the recovery position while protecting their neck.

Call the emergency services.

See how alert they are using AVPU. Reassure them if they are alert.

Continue to watch their breathing, circulation and level of consciousness until help arrives and be prepared to resuscitate if necessary. Even if they regain consciousness, insist that they go to hospital to be checked out.

---

longer periods of amnesia after regaining consciousness. In addition there may be signs of brain injury in other parts of the body, such as paralysis, numbness or changes in breathing.

The bruising may be directly at the site of the injury, or it may be on the opposite side of the skull as the brain bounces away – this is called a contracoup brain injury.

Haemorrhage

Bleeding within the skull, or intracranial haemorrhage, is a common consequence of head injury. The tough sheath (dura mater) attached to the inside of the skull is well supplied with blood vessels. These may be damaged and cause bleeding; sometimes the effects are delayed for several weeks after the injury.

Compression

The skull is an enclosed space, and if there is any swelling or bleeding within it, a point is reached when there is no more room for expansion. Compression of the

SIGNS AND SYMPTOMS OF RISING PRESSURE WITHIN THE SKULL

➤ Intense headache, worse when lying flat and/or with physical exertion.

➤ Vomiting.

➤ Unequal or dilated pupils.

➤ Weakness on one side of the body.

➤ Noisy, irregular breathing.

➤ Irritable or aggressive behaviour.

brain can lead to quite severe damage and a wide range of symptoms. In extreme cases, it can cause brain tissue to squeeze out of the base of the skull – a condition known as coning. This is fatal so it is absolutely vital that any rise in pressure within the skull is recognized before this happens.

Even after seemingly minor head injuries, always be very vigilant for signs of increased cerebral pressure and get help promptly if you spot any.

Coping with epilepsy

SEE ALSO
➤ Responsiveness and the airway, p28
➤ The recovery position, p36
➤ Recognizing a stroke, p84

Epileptic fits, or "seizures", are caused by an instability of electrical activity in the brain. Such fits can be alarming, but there is usually no physical damage to the brain itself. There are over 40 types of seizure, which may be partial (affecting part of the brain) or generalized (affecting the whole brain). These many types range from an "absence" seizure (once called *petit mal*), where the sufferer simply seems to be daydreaming briefly, to a full-blown "tonic-clonic" fit (once called *grand mal*), where the sufferer writhes uncontrollably.

The nature of epileptic seizures depends on which part of the brain is affected. At one end of the scale, there is a brief "absence" of attention; at the other, the major jerking and total unconsciousness (tonic-clonic fit) traditionally associated with epilepsy. Partial seizures may develop into generalized ones. So, for example, someone might start off with one hand affected by jerky movements and progress to a complete tonic-clonic fit. It is reassuring to know that many people only ever have one fit during their lifetime.

WHAT CAUSES SEIZURES?
All kinds of things can cause a seizure:
• Brain damage caused by:
   – Head injury;
   – Difficulties at birth;
   – Reduced brain oxygen (for example, suffocation);
   – Brain problems (tumours, bleeding, swelling).
• Certain diseases (diabetes, liver failure).
• Certain poisons (such as pesticides).
• An inherited low "seizure threshold".
• A large intake of alcohol. Also, alcoholics may have seizures if they suddenly stop drinking alcohol.

• A high temperature (in children). Children up to the age of five years may have convulsions, typically as part of a feverish illness. They usually grow out of these in middle childhood. Feverish convulsions do not indicate that a child may develop epilepsy later on.
• The cause often remains unknown.

CHARACTERISTICS OF SEIZURES
In an absence seizure, the person typically stops what they are doing and stares into space for 10–15 seconds. They have actually lost consciousness briefly and are unaware of their surroundings. They will then continue as if nothing had happened, and will have no memory of the event.

In a tonic-clonic seizure, the person is fully unconscious for up to 10 minutes and may be very sleepy for an hour or two after the seizure. The main features include:
• A change in mood/behaviour several hours or days before a fit – known as a prodrome.
• Immediately before the fit an imaginary smell or vision may be apparent, or a sense of déjà vu – called an aura.
• Sudden unconsciousness, followed by stiffening of the arms and legs – the tonic phase. Then jerky movements of the limbs and face – the clonic phase.
• There may be loss of bladder control and the sufferer may bite their tongue.

HOW TO RECOGNIZE EPILEPSY
Someone who has fainted may jerk slightly – this is not epilepsy. There are many other non-epileptic causes of "funny turns".

A person who has had an epileptic seizure will come to in a confused state. It will help them to hear from a witness what has happened, particularly on the first occasion, as this can then be reported to the emergency services or the hospital.

Epilepsy is diagnosed by neurological tests. These include electroencephalography (EEG), in which brain activity is measured by attaching electrodes to the scalp, and a computerized tomography (CT) scan to exclude brain tumour and stroke. A person recently diagnosed with epilepsy needs reassurance and support to build up their confidence for leading a normal life.

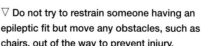

▽ Do not try to restrain someone having an epileptic fit but move any obstacles, such as chairs, out of the way to prevent injury.

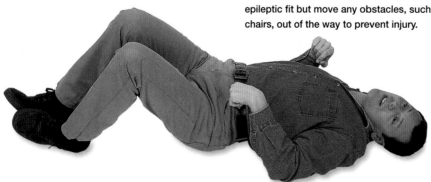

COMMON TRIGGERS

➤ Excess alcohol.
➤ Tiredness.
➤ Emotion (stress/excitement).
➤ Failure to take medication regularly.
➤ Certain foods/not eating properly.
➤ Illness.
➤ Hormonal changes.
➤ Flashing lights.

FIRST AID FOR AN EPILEPTIC FIT

You may want to look quickly to see if the casualty is wearing a medical ID tag, or is carrying a card that says they suffer from epilepsy and tells you what to do.

During the seizure: prevent any avoidable injury. Remove obstacles that might hurt the sufferer and protect their head by placing cushions or rolled up clothing around it. Never restrain them or put anything in their mouth.

After the seizure: put them into the recovery position and make sure that they have a clear airway. Note the duration of the seizure.

CALLING THE EMERGENCY SERVICES

There is usually no need to call an ambulance for a routine seizure suffered by a diagnosed epileptic. However, you should call an ambulance if:
- They do not stop fitting after 5 minutes.
- The fit is worse than usual: more prolonged or violent.
- They suffer a series of fits with short gaps.
- Serious injury has occurred.
- The person remains unconscious for more than 2–3 minutes.

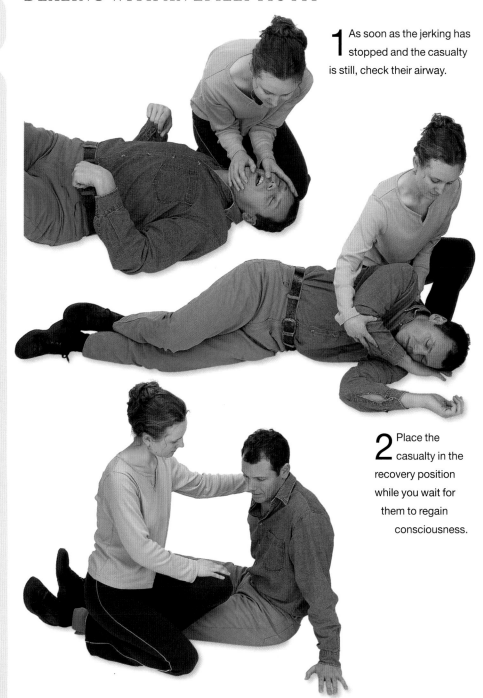

1 As soon as the jerking has stopped and the casualty is still, check their airway.

2 Place the casualty in the recovery position while you wait for them to regain consciousness.

3 Explain to the casualty what happened. Find out whether this has occurred before, and if not they should see a doctor for assessment as soon as possible. Ask whether they would like you to contact anyone.

HOW IS EPILEPSY TREATED?

Epilepsy is usually controlled with anticonvulsant drugs, taken until the sufferer has been seizure-free for 2–3 years. Women with epilepsy considering pregnancy should speak to their doctor first as they may have to be put on a different anticonvulsant drug.

WARNING

For their own safety, people with epilepsy should not swim alone under any circumstances or cycle in traffic-dense areas. Driving is not allowed for six months to a year or even longer after diagnosis, depending on the individual case.

The situation is reviewed regularly, and driving may be permitted again if the epilepsy is well controlled and there is no risk of a seizure.

Recognizing a stroke

SEE ALSO

➤ Dealing with an abnormal heart rate, p74
➤ Coping with headache, p86
➤ Managing dizziness and fainting, p88

Strokes are caused by a sudden stoppage of the blood supply to part of the brain. They are usually the result of a blood clot or a ruptured artery, and vary in severity: some leave no lasting effects, others cause paralysis on one side of the body, and some prove instantly fatal. Although more common in older people, people who smoke, have high blood pressure, or take the combined oral contraceptive pill are at increased risk of having a stroke. First-aid treatment aims to maintain breathing and circulation until the emergency services arrive.

A stroke occurs when the blood supply to a part of the brain is cut off. This may be caused by a blood clot in a vessel in the brain or by bleeding into the brain. A stroke's short- and long-term effects depend on which part of the brain is affected.

A stroke may occur very suddenly with very little warning, or may follow a series of 'mini-strokes' called transient ischaemic attacks. If you find yourself having to administer first aid to a probable stroke victim, it is important to act swiftly and call the emergency services without delay.

WHAT CAUSES A STROKE?
Generally, strokes tend to affect older people, and people with high blood pressure or a circulatory problem.

There are also a number of other factors that can increase a person's risk of having a stroke. These include taking the combined oral contraceptive pill, having a high blood cholesterol, being diabetic, smoking, and being overweight.

Atherosclerosis
Atheroma is a thick, fatty substance that builds up in the arteries over the years, gradually narrowing them and eventually blocking them altogether. This condition, known as atherosclerosis, slows the flow of blood around the body and encourages the formation of blood clots. If a blood clot occurs in one of the cerebral arteries, it will cause a stroke.

Embolism
A fragment of material travelling through the bloodstream, often a piece of blood

CROSS-SECTION OF BRAIN AFTER A STROKE

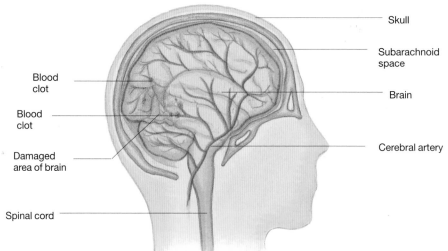

△ A common cause of stroke is a blood clot in a cerebral artery, which supplies blood to the brain. This will starve nearby tissue of oxygen and other nutrients, which will cause temporary or permanent loss of function.

clot, is called an embolus. An embolus may arise in the heart, travel to the brain and cause a stroke. Anyone with a heart valve abnormality or an abnormal heart rhythm is more likely to develop an embolus.

Aneurysm
Some people are born with a weakness in one of the arteries at the base of the brain; this is called an aneurysm. It may leak, causing warning headaches, but often it will suddenly burst, causing a severe and often fatal stroke.

HOW TO RECOGNIZE A STROKE
Minutes matter in a stroke as early treatment in hospital can make all the difference between full recovery and permanent disability. Use the FAST test to check if the casualty has suffered a stroke.
Face – Ask the casualty to smile. Is one side of the face drooping?
Arms – Ask the casualty to raise both arms. Does one flop down?
Speech – Is the casualty's speech slurred or strange?
Time – to call an ambulance if the answer to any of those questions is yes. Note what time the symptoms appears.

Symptoms may include numbness or weakness on one side of the face or body, confusion, dizziness, balance problems, visual disturbance, difficulty speaking or a sudden very severe 'thunderclap' headache. Even if you're not sure the person is having a stroke, call an ambulance right away.

Usually, the part of the body affected by a stroke is on the opposite side to the side of the brain affected. For example, if the person is right-handed then a left-sided stroke will usually affect their speech.

Occasionally a person may be totally unaware that they have a right or left side at all. For example, they might only eat food on the side of the plate that they are aware of.

CAN STROKE BE PREVENTED?

Although none of us can escape the increased risk of having a stroke that comes with growing older, there are a number of measures we can take to reduce the risk.

Smoking increases the risk of a stroke occurring by several hundredfold, and high blood pressure is also closely linked to a higher chance of having a stroke. People with high levels of cholesterol and other fats in their blood may develop atherosclerosis; this is a build-up of a fatty substance that can block arteries and may cause a stroke, amongst other conditions. The risk can be reduced by a healthy diet, exercise, abstention from smoking and, if necessary, appropriate drugs.

F-A-S-T: SIGNS AND SYMPTOMS OF A STROKE

Stroke charities have developed a quick and easy acronym to help people to remember, recognize and diagnose the signs and symptoms of a stroke. This is known as the FAST (Face-Arms-Speech-Time) guide:

➤**F** – Face: the person's face may have dropped on one side, they may not be able to smile, or the mouth or eye may have drooped.

➤**A** – Arms: the person may not be able to lift both arms or keep them in the air, because of weakness in one arm.

➤**S** – Speech: they may not be able to speak, or their speech may be garbled or slurred.

➤**T** – Time: if you see any of the above symptoms, call for the emergency services right away. Note the time that the symptoms began, as this is important for treatment.

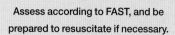

FIRST AID FOR STROKE

Assess according to FAST, and be prepared to resuscitate if necessary.

Call 911 even if you're not sure whether it's a stroke or not – prompt assessment and treatment in hospital is vital to prevent brain damage and possibly permanent disability.

If unconscious (or unable to keep upright), but breathing, put in the recovery position. This is so that, if they vomit, they do not inhale it into their lungs, which can be fatal (stroke victims often lose their gag reflex).

If conscious, lay them on their back with head and shoulders comfortably raised.

Look for a medical ID tag. The casualty may be suffering from another condition, such as diabetic hypoglycaemia.

Do not give food or water at any stage.

▷ In many stroke casualties, the side of the face droops and they may be unable to speak, smile or swallow without dribbling. There may be loss of sensation in one arm. These symptoms may not appear straightaway.

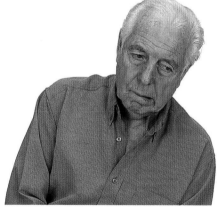

◁ Stroke casualties may vomit copiously. Make sure they are not in a position where they might inhale their vomit, as this can prove fatal.

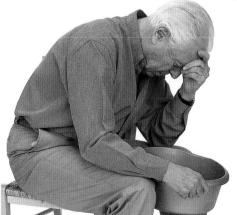

TRANSIENT ISCHEMIC ATTACKS

A transient ischemic attack (TIA) is like a mini-stroke. Symptoms last briefly and totally disappear within 24 hours. TIAs are often a warning sign of a full-blown stroke, there being about a 10 per cent risk that a stroke will happen within a year. The sufferer should be investigated urgently for the cause of the TIA in order to prevent either a recurrence or a full stroke. They may be put on aspirin or an anticoagulant by their doctor, to thin the blood and make clotting less likely.

Coping with headache

SEE ALSO
➤ Dealing with head injury, p80
➤ Recognizing a stroke, p84
➤ Tackling skull and facial fractures, p152

Headaches are such a common complaint that very few people will go through life without experiencing one. Usually a headache is associated with stress, tension, overwork or too much alcohol; it quickly passes with self-help remedies and there is no need for concern.

However, it is important to be aware that severe, persistent or recurrent headaches may have a more serious underlying cause and should be investigated by a doctor. A person experiencing a migraine attack for the first time should also seek the advice of a doctor.

Everybody suffers from headaches at some time in their life and their cause is usually obvious. Persistent headaches that do not ease with simple painkillers, or severe ones that start suddenly, may mean you should see a doctor. Headaches have many different causes, including alcohol, caffeine-withdrawal, lack of fresh air, dehydration (a very common cause, often arising from excess alcohol), stress, menstruation and sinusitis, but very few causes are in any way life-threatening.

Headache following head injury is common and may last for months and even years after the accident. Seek medical attention if there are other symptoms, such as fever, fainting, fits or any discharge from the ears or nose.

TYPES OF HEADACHE

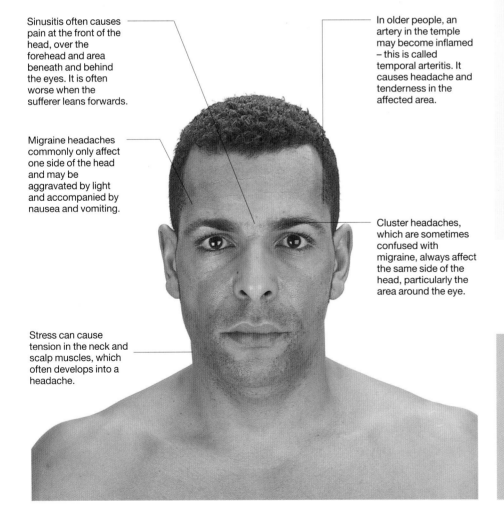

Sinusitis often causes pain at the front of the head, over the forehead and area beneath and behind the eyes. It is often worse when the sufferer leans forwards.

Migraine headaches commonly only affect one side of the head and may be aggravated by light and accompanied by nausea and vomiting.

Stress can cause tension in the neck and scalp muscles, which often develops into a headache.

In older people, an artery in the temple may become inflamed – this is called temporal arteritis. It causes headache and tenderness in the affected area.

Cluster headaches, which are sometimes confused with migraine, always affect the same side of the head, particularly the area around the eye.

WHEN TO SEE A DOCTOR

A person with any of the following types of headache should be seen by a doctor:

➤ Sudden onset.

➤ Persistent headaches.

➤ Associated with a fever and neck stiffness.

➤ Accompanied by a rash.

➤ Following head injury.

➤ Feels like "the worst headache ever".

➤ Accompanied by persistent or severe vomiting.

➤ Worse when lying flat or straining.

➤ Accompanied by confusion, drowsiness or loss of consciousness.

➤ Accompanied by numbness, tingling of the limbs or any other neurological problem.

➤ Regular headaches starting after the age of 50.

WARNING

Any severe headache that persists for several days should be investigated promptly by a doctor. There may be a serious underlying cause, although in most dangerous conditions, such as a brain tumour or stroke, additional symptoms usually accompany the headache.

MIGRAINE

Migraines are a problem often passed down through generations of a family. Migraine is believed to be caused by abnormal brain activity temporarily affecting nerve signals, chemicals and blood vessels in the brain. This causes severe, throbbing pain, vomiting, and visual or sensory problems. The root of these changes is as yet unknown, although the neurotransmitter serotonin may play a big role, as does the chemical, tyramine, found in various foods (see "Triggers" box).

Recognizing migraine

Migraines are usually felt on one side of the head, and they might last up to three days. In some people, a migraine attack is preceded by a warning called an aura. This is primarily visual, such as seeing zigzag lines or spots in the field of vision. There may be other symptoms present such as dizziness, tingling, temporary speech difficulties and blurred vision. Since visual problems often accompany migraine it is not advisable to attempt to drive during an attack.

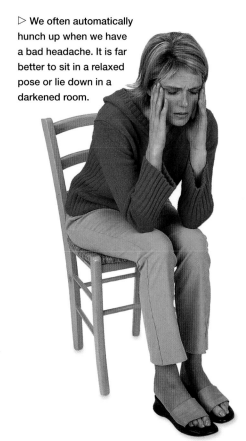

▷ We often automatically hunch up when we have a bad headache. It is far better to sit in a relaxed pose or lie down in a darkened room.

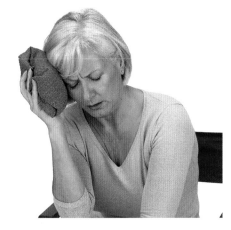

△ Wrapping a bag of frozen vegetables in a cloth and placing it against the headache site may ease the pain a little. Heat applied in the same way may also work.

Treating migraine

A large selection of drugs is available to prevent and treat migraine. Both over-the-counter and prescription drugs are available, and it is best to discuss the options with your doctor. You need to consider the frequency of attacks, how long each attack lasts and the extent to which the debility affects everyday life. There are over-the-counter drugs that combine paracetamol with an anti-sickness treatment, and some people find that ibuprofen helps.

MIGRAINE TRIGGERS

➤ Stress, or relaxing after stress.

➤ Tiredness, sleep disturbances, shift work, jet lag

➤ Strong smells, loud noises, flickering screens.

➤ Hormone changes around the time of a woman's period.

➤ Contraceptive pill.

➤ Missing meals, leading to low blood sugar.

➤ Foods, such as: chocolate, ripe cheese, pickled foods, citrus fruit, monosodium glutamate, yeast extract, cola drinks, red/fortified wine, caffeine. (Some of these contain the amino acid tyramine.)

HOME REMEDIES FOR ROUTINE HEADACHES

➤ Over-the-counter painkillers.

➤ An ice pack or heating pad over the site of the headache.

➤ Bed rest, preferably in the dark.

➤ Relaxation techniques.

➤ Complementary remedies, including herbal remedies such as feverfew, valerian, lavender and betony. Never take feverfew with any blood-thinning drugs and always check the safety of a herbal preparation in case you have a condition that makes its use unsafe.

➤ Massage and acupressure.

Some people find acupuncture effective to help prevent migraine attacks. Transcranial magnetic stimulation (TMS), which involves using a small device held near the head that delivers magnetic pulses through the skin, has been used for both treatment and prevention of migraines.

▽ Nausea and vomiting are very common in migraine – try taking an anti-sickness drug.

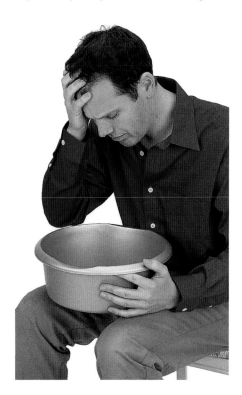

Managing dizziness and fainting

SEE ALSO
➤ What is first aid?, p12
➤ Dealing with head injury, p80
➤ Coping with headache, p86

Dizziness, or a feeling of unsteadiness, is a common complaint and is usually a momentary sensation of no consequence. Dizziness may lead to fainting, which is a short-lived loss of consciousness with a drop to the floor that usually resolves the giddiness. A brief dizzy spell, with or without fainting, can be caused by a hot, stuffy atmosphere, fatigue, anxiety, emotional shock, lack of food, blood loss, or standing still for too long. Vertigo, or the sensation that your surroundings are spinning for no apparent reason, may have a more serious cause.

The main issue with dizziness is whether or not it is caused by a balance disorder.

CAUSES OF DIZZINESS

Non-vertigo dizziness might be felt as wooziness or light-headedness and may be due to anything from low blood sugar (not eating regularly) to high blood pressure, anaemia, or wax in the ears. If this type of dizziness occurs regularly, you should see your doctor, who will determine whether an underlying condition is to blame. The dizziness will have to be controlled, so that activities such as driving can be continued.

One common trigger for dizziness is standing up suddenly. This is often caused by your blood vessels not adjusting fast enough to accommodate a changed body position. It can also happen if you bend down or turn around very quickly. If this persists, see a doctor.

CAUSES OF VERTIGO

Balance is controlled by a part of the inner ear called the labyrinth, and also centrally in the brain. A problem with any part of this system might cause dizziness. The dizzy sensation in this case is more dramatic and is known as vertigo – the person feels their surroundings spinning around them alarmingly (for example after drinking too much alcohol or going on a fairground ride).

Vertigo is often due to a viral infection of the labyrinth, known medically as labyrinthitis, which may last a few weeks but from which complete recovery is usual. It responds well to medication that controls the dizziness and nausea that often accompany true vertigo.

Another reasonably common illness that causes dizziness is Ménière's disease. In this instance, typical symptoms that accompany the vertigo include intermittent deafness and tinnitus (ringing, hissing or other noises in the ear, without an external cause). This condition usually develops in middle age and is treated with drugs. It may go into remission after a few years.

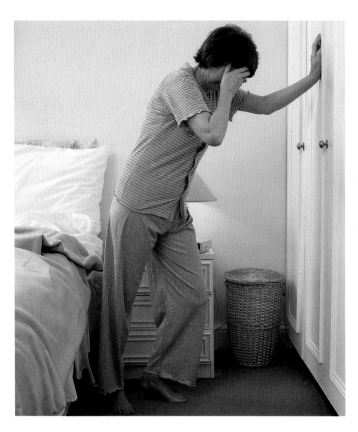

▷ If you get dizzy on standing up suddenly, for example when you first get up in the morning, lean against the wall in case you faint and then kneel or sit down till the dizziness clears. When you get up again, do so more slowly than you did first time round.

WHEN TO SEE A DOCTOR

Most types of dizziness are short-lived but you should see your doctor if any of the following apply:

➤ Dizziness happens regularly.

➤ You have vertigo rather than light-headedness.

➤ Other symptoms, such as deafness, earache, ear popping, tinnitus, nausea or vomiting accompany the dizziness.

➤ There is a family history of Ménière's disease.

➤ You are taking any medication that could be causing the dizziness.

FIRST AID FOR DIZZINESS

Your main concern should be to stop the sufferer from hurting themselves or others, for example if they are driving a car when dizziness strikes.

Sit the sufferer down. If the dizziness continues, lie them flat so that if they faint they won't hurt themselves.

Unless they have sustained a head injury, raise their legs higher than their head.

Ask whether this has happened before, and whether they have any anti-dizziness medication that you could give them.

FAINTING

This occurs when there is a temporary lack of oxygen to the brain. It may happen for many reasons, including hunger, a sudden change of atmosphere from cold to warm, or standing still for a long time. If a person stands still without regularly clenching their calf muscles, the blood pools in their legs and they may faint as the brain does not receive enough oxygen. By fainting, the body is able to get blood and oxygen back up to the brain again – and so the person "comes to" as the brain recovers its function.

Fainting can often cause a lot of worry about more serious complaints such as brain tumours or epilepsy. The following features may distinguish simple fainting from other causes of brief unconsciousness:

- There may be certain brief sensations that warn of a fainting episode: a sense of narrowed vision or of voices becoming distant, for example.
- The victim's skin looks very pale and feels clammy to the touch.
- The victim's pulse becomes slow.
- When they recover, there is no prolonged drowsiness (as there is with epilepsy).
- They may jerk slightly after they pass out, but there is no epileptic-type fit.

FIRST AID FOR FAINTING

Make sure the casualty is breathing If so, lie them flat on their back and raise their legs higher than their head (unless they have a head injury/pains).

Loosen their clothing – especially around the neck – and if the atmosphere is hot and stuffy, open doors and windows.

If they don't wake up after a few minutes, re-check their ABC, place in the recovery position, and call the emergency services. Monitor their airways and breathing until help arrives.

Tell the casualty exactly what happened when they fainted; this witness information may be vital in distinguishing a simple faint from something more alarming. The casualty should see their doctor if there were any unusual signs, such as loss of bladder control or drowsiness, after the faint.

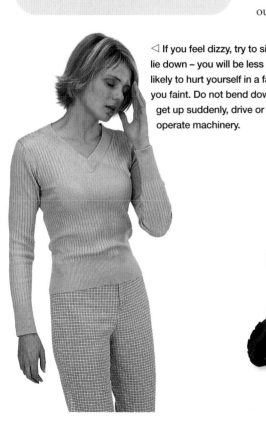

◁ If you feel dizzy, try to sit or lie down – you will be less likely to hurt yourself in a fall if you faint. Do not bend down, get up suddenly, drive or operate machinery.

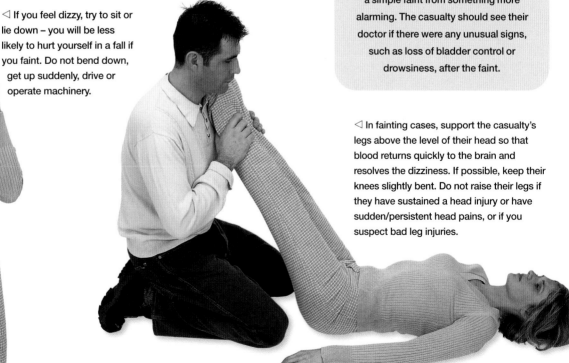

◁ In fainting cases, support the casualty's legs above the level of their head so that blood returns quickly to the brain and resolves the dizziness. If possible, keep their knees slightly bent. Do not raise their legs if they have sustained a head injury or have sudden/persistent head pains, or if you suspect bad leg injuries.

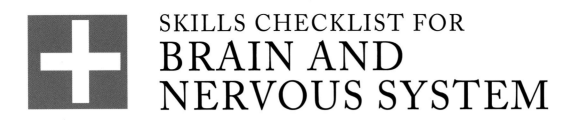

SKILLS CHECKLIST FOR
BRAIN AND NERVOUS SYSTEM

KEY POINTS

- After someone has sustained any blow to the head, be very vigilant for further problems ☐

- Never try to restrain someone who is having an epileptic fit ☐

- Get emergency aid to a stroke casualty as fast as possible ☐

- Persistent or unusual headaches or dizziness should be investigated by a doctor ☐

SKILLS LEARNED

- Recognizing the signs of a serious head injury ☐

- Dealing with a head injury ☐

- What to do if someone has an epileptic fit ☐

- Recognizing and dealing with a stroke ☐

- Knowing when to consult a doctor about headaches ☐

- Giving first aid for dizziness and fainting ☐

- Knowing when to consult a doctor about dizziness and fainting ☐

OTHER MEDICAL EMERGENCIES

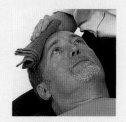

This chapter describes what to do in the event of a range of potentially critical situations. In some of them, including antenatal emergencies, emergency childbirth and diabetic crisis, the emergency services are needed, but there is action you can take to minimize risk before the ambulance arrives. Others are conditions that can usually be dealt with by home first-aid action but that might develop into more serious conditions requiring expert help; these include allergies, bites and stings, and heat and cold disorders. More common symptoms, such as abdominal pain, nausea and vomiting, and fever, are also covered.

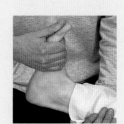

CONTENTS

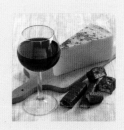

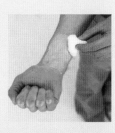

Coping with antenatal emergencies

Situations sometimes arise in pregnancy that call for immediate action. These include bleeding, severe abdominal pain, some types of headache, continuous vomiting, early breaking of the waters, and a reduction in or lack of foetal movements. The first priority is to call for the emergency services and explain what has happened as clearly as you can. While waiting for assistance to arrive, keep the mother calm and reassure her that help is on the way. Monitor her condition and take appropriate action if necessary.

Problems in pregnancy may occur that require getting to hospital quickly, and occasionally rapid action is needed prior to reaching hospital. In addition to antenatal problems, pregnant women are liable to have ordinary accidents and illnesses just like everyone else. It's important that you always make medical and emergency personnel aware that the victim is pregnant, as this may affect their actions. Always seek medical advice if you are in any doubt at all about a pregnant woman's symptoms.

COLLAPSE IN PREGNANCY

Any woman of fertile age who suddenly collapses should be considered possibly to be pregnant. The main concern is that the collapse may be due to a tubal or ectopic pregnancy, in which an embryo implants outside the uterus, most often in one of the Fallopian tubes. This can be life-threatening and requires emergency surgery.

A heavily pregnant woman should not be laid on her back if she collapses. Keep her tilted slightly towards her left side at about a 30-degree angle, for example by putting a wedge such as a pillow or rolled jacket under her right hip. This helps to stop the uterus compressing important vessels returning blood to the heart. For the same reason, if you need to put a pregnant woman into the recovery position, place her onto her left side.

However, if chest compressions become necessary, proceed as for normal CPR with the woman lying flat – it is most important that compressions are effective. If you have help, get the second rescuer gently to press the side of the bump to tilt the uterus towards the left while you do compressions.

BLEEDING IN EARLY PREGNANCY

Any vaginal bleeding during the first eight weeks of pregnancy could be due to an ectopic pregnancy. There is often, but not always, low pelvic pain before the bleeding starts. The combination of pain and bleeding should prompt any woman to see her physician or obstetrician urgently, even if the bleeding is very light. This also applies if she feels unwell, is pale, dizzy or prone to fainting.

Another possible cause of bleeding in early pregnancy (up to 20 weeks) is miscarriage (sometimes called spontaneous abortion),

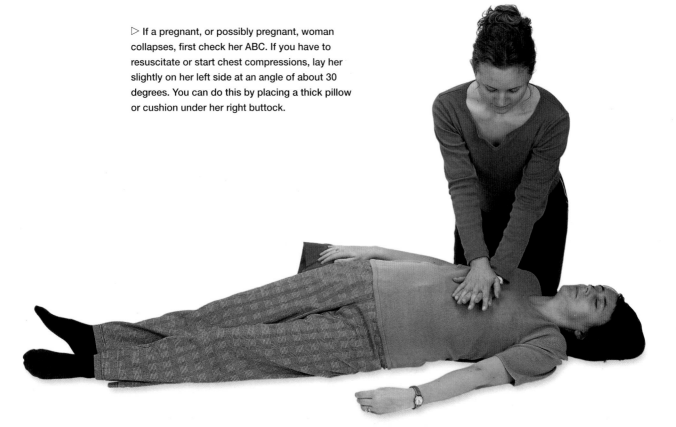

▷ If a pregnant, or possibly pregnant, woman collapses, first check her ABC. If you have to resuscitate or start chest compressions, lay her slightly on her left side at an angle of about 30 degrees. You can do this by placing a thick pillow or cushion under her right buttock.

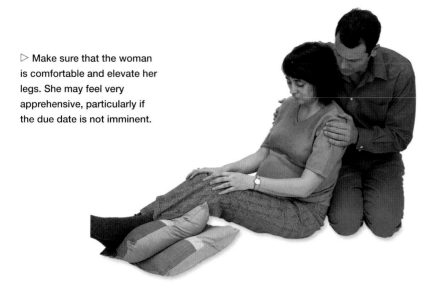

▷ Make sure that the woman is comfortable and elevate her legs. She may feel very apprehensive, particularly if the due date is not imminent.

and the woman should see her obstetrician urgently or go to hospital, depending on the severity of symptoms. Sometimes there is only a very small amount of blood and very little abdominal pain. This may be a threatened miscarriage, which is very common, and bed rest and avoidance of sex may be the only advice from the doctor.

In other cases, the bleeding from a miscarriage may be extremely heavy and accompanied by clots and cramp-like pains in the lower abdomen. There may even be signs and symptoms of shock when the miscarriage has become inevitable, and there may also be visible parts of the placenta and fetus in the blood. Such severe symptoms require admission to hospital, where it is likely that an operation will be performed under anaesthetic to ensure that the entire contents of the uterus are removed to prevent further hemorrhage or infection.

BLEEDING IN LATE PREGNANCY

Any bleeding after 20 weeks should be taken very seriously, and the woman should be taken to a doctor or emergency department immediately. It may only be a harmless "mucus plug", which sits in the cervix until near the end of pregnancy. However, it may also be a sign that the placenta is situated low in the uterus and is bleeding, or that it has started to rupture away from the wall of the uterus. These placental conditions are known as placenta previa (in which bleeding is usually painless) and placental abruption (in which there is severe pain). Both conditions can threaten the baby's life and is a medical emergency.

BREAKING OF THE WATERS

The membranes surrounding the baby in the uterus normally rupture during labor, although sometimes the waters breaking is the first sign that labor is imminent. This may release a gush of amniotic fluid or a more gentle leakage. Sometimes, however, the waters can break before the baby is ready to be born. The woman should contact her obstetrician for advice. She may need to be checked over and may be offered an induction or monitoring in case of infection.

▽ In case a pregnant woman passes out, put her in the recovery position, with her left side down while waiting for the emergency services to arrive.

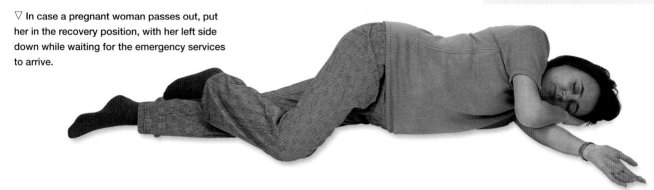

Helping with emergency childbirth

SEE ALSO

➤ Full resuscitation sequence, p33

➤ CHILDREN'S LIFE SUPPORT, p43

➤ Coping with antenatal emergencies, p92

It is not usually first-time mothers who deliver on the kitchen floor but the more experienced second- and third-timers, whose labours are less predictable and occur at a faster pace. Knowing what to do if a woman goes into labour is essential first-aid knowledge.

Although the mother does most of the work during labour and birth, there are a number of things you can do to help. Newborn babies sometimes struggle to breathe, and you might have to provide crucial help. Bringing a new life into the world is an unforgettable experience.

LABOUR

There are three stages of labour. The first stage starts with contractions and ends when the cervix is fully dilated. The second stage begins as the baby descends through the birth canal and ends when the baby is born. The third stage is when the placenta or afterbirth is delivered.

First stage

During this stage the cervix dilates to allow the baby's head through at the second stage. The first labour signs come on at this stage – the contractions. These are regular pains that start like a much more intense version of period-type cramps, usually felt across the lower abdomen. They come and go initially every 5-20 minutes, lasting up to 30 seconds. The mother may also feel the "waters breaking", as the amniotic fluid around the baby gushes out. If the fluid is brownish, rather than clear yellow, the baby may be in distress, and you should seek urgent medical advice.

Second stage

Signs that birth is imminent include regular contractions coming at one to two minute intervals, an overwhelming urge to push or bear down with each contraction, and the baby's head becoming visible at the vaginal entrance ('crowning') during contractions. The mother may involuntarily open her bowels. Try to clear away the faeces without contaminating the vulval area and risking infecting the baby.

Encourage the mother to get into whatever position feels comfortable for her. The baby is ready to be born when you can see the head sitting behind the vulva at the vaginal entrance all the time. Do not try to control the baby's descent, simply allow the head to come down with each contraction.

As the baby's head arrives, it will normally be facing the floor. Support the head with your hand beneath it – the head naturally turns 90 degrees at this stage. Let it come naturally and do not pull. As soon as the baby's head is out, check to see if the umbilical cord is around the neck. If it is, then slip it carefully over the baby's head. The shoulders should appear next.

The rest of the body arrives quickly after this. The emerging baby will be slippery, so be careful not to drop it. Wipe

FIRST AND SECOND STAGES OF LABOUR

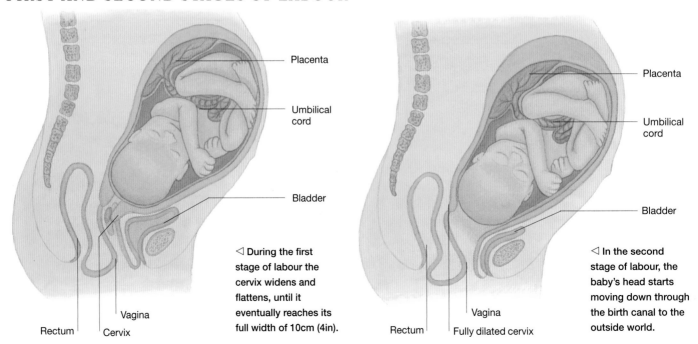

Placenta

Umbilical cord

Bladder

◁ During the first stage of labour the cervix widens and flattens, until it eventually reaches its full width of 10cm (4in).

Rectum   Vagina
Cervix

Placenta

Umbilical cord

Bladder

◁ In the second stage of labour, the baby's head starts moving down through the birth canal to the outside world.

Rectum   Vagina
Fully dilated cervix

any fluid or mucus away from the baby's nose and mouth. It will probably begin to breathe and cry almost at once. If not, drying the baby with a warm clean towel should encourage it.

If there are no signs of breathing, flick the baby's toes with your fingers. If there is still no breathing, remove obvious obstructions or mucous plugs from the mouth and give 2 rescue breaths with your mouth over the baby's mouth and nose. Continue as per the standard basic life support routine for a baby.

Once it is breathing, wrap the baby in clean sheets and a warm blanket, if available, and place it gently on the mother's abdomen. Encourage the mother to breastfeed the baby - this will also promote

DELIVERY OF THE BABY

delivery of the placenta and reduce bleeding. Remember to note the time of birth and congratulate the mother.

Third stage

The placenta may arrive within a few minutes of the baby, but may not be delivered until several hours later. It should arrive naturally without any action by you. Under no circumstances should you pull on the cord. Do not cut the cord. Keep the placenta in a container for the midwife or obstetrician to inspect. If bleeding continues after the placenta has come out, gently massage the top of uterus, which feels like a firm mass just below the navel, and encourage the baby to breast feed as this promotes contraction of the womb bleeding.

Stay with the mother until a midwife or other healthcare professional arrives.

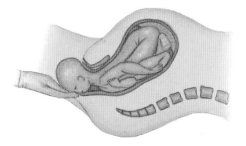

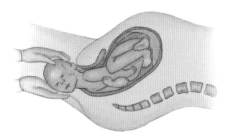

1 Most babies come out with the back of their heads facing towards the mother's front and their faces pointing towards her back.

2 Gently cushion the head rather than pulling on it, to avoid causing any damage.

3 When most of the body has emerged, keep it at the same level as the mother. Make sure you hold the baby carefully as it will be covered in blood and amniotic fluid and will be very slippery.

4 Place the baby on the mother's chest or abdomen in a tilted position with its head slightly lower than the rest of its body in case it vomits. Cover them both to keep warm.

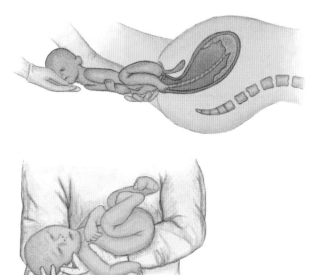

HOW TO PREPARE FOR AN EMERGENCY DELIVERY

If a pregnant woman is having almost continuous contractions, or is feeling the urge to push, there may be no time to get her to hospital and you must prepare for an emergency delivery. First, call for an ambulance. The ambulance controller can give you step-by-step instructions while the paramedics are on their way. Listen carefully. What they say may well contain the following advice, but always stick to their instructions.

Cleanliness is vital. Mother and baby are vulnerable to infection, so take all possible precautions to prevent its spread.

Use a large plastic sheet to cover the lowest and firmest bed in the house, or clear a space on the floor. Find two or three clean sheets.

Find a nappy or something you can use as one for the baby. Arrange towels, flannel and warm water for the mother.

Wash your hands thoroughly with soap and water, wear medical gloves if available, and ideally change them whenever you have been in contact with potentially contaminated material, such as blood or faeces.

Managing diabetic conditions

SEE ALSO
➤ Responsiveness and the airway, p28
➤ The recovery position, p36

Diabetes is a condition in which the body cannot control sugar levels in the blood. This can create all kinds of symptoms, from excessive thirst to loss of consciousness, and complications ranging from blindness to kidney disease to amputations. It is estimated that almost one in 16 of the UK population has diabetes, which has more than doubled since the 1980s. Since a diabetic crisis can be life-threatening it is important to recognize the signs of an impending episode and to take appropriate first-aid action.

People with diabetes mellitus (DM) have a problem with control of blood glucose. The body obtains glucose mainly from sweet and starchy foods such as biscuits, bread and potatoes. The carbohydrates in these foods are broken down into glucose, which is absorbed into the blood through the gut and provides fuel for all our body cells.

In people without diabetes, blood glucose levels are regulated by insulin, a hormone produced by the pancreas. Diabetes means the pancreas produces too little or no insulin, or that the body does not fully respond to it. A diabetes sufferer's blood sugar levels are not controlled properly, which may cause symptoms that can develop into a crisis.

WHAT ARE THE TYPES?

There are two main types of diabetes mellitus –Type 1 DM, which accounts for about 10 per cent of cases, is where the body cannot make insulin. It is a lifelong condition that usually needs insulin treatment. Type 2 DM, the majority of cases, happens when the body either doesn't make enough insulin or doesn't use it efficiently, a problem known as insulin resistance. It can often be managed by lifestyle changes or tablets and is potentially reversible. Type 1 DM is the form usually seen in children, though it can develop later in life. Type 2 DM tends to begin later in life, though is now being seen in children too. It is typically seen in people who are overweight, and its incidence has increased dramatically in many countries in recent years.

CAUSES OF DIABETES

Type 1 diabetes is believed to occur when the immune system mistakenly attacks the cells of the pancreas that make insulin. The attack may be triggered by an infection in someone who has a genetic vulnerability to diabetes.

Type 2 diabetes may also run in

SIGNS AND SYMPTOMS OF DIABETES

People with Type 1 diabetes can become ill quite quickly over several weeks. Type 2 diabetics may be symptom-free for many months or years before the condition is discovered. Symptoms include:

➤ Passing urine often, in large amounts.

➤ Exceptional thirst.

➤ Tiredness.

➤ Blurred vision.

➤ Weight loss, despite healthy appetite.

➤ Recurrent boils or abscesses.

➤ Numbness or tingling in the hands and feet.

➤ Genital thrush (yeast) infection.

▷ The pancreas is an elongated gland that secretes insulin. It actually lies just behind the stomach, but has been shown in front here so that it can be seen clearly.

LOCATION OF THE PANCREAS

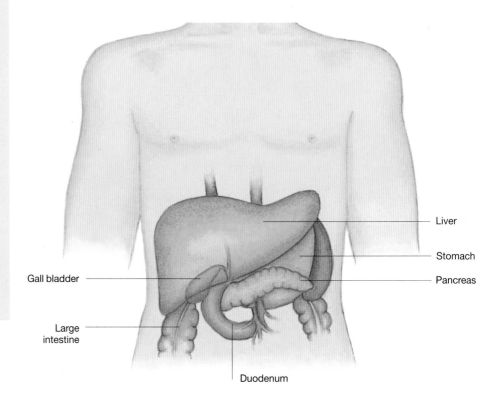

Liver

Stomach

Pancreas

Gall bladder

Large intestine

Duodenum

FIRST AID FOR HYPOGLYCAEMIA AND HYPERGLYCAEMIA

IF UNCONSCIOUS:

Follow DRABC and call an ambulance. Do not try to give them anything to eat or drink. If breathing, place in the recovery position and monitor breathing while waiting for the ambulance.

IF CONSCIOUS:

Loosen tight clothing. In hypoglycaemia, give a sugar-sweetened drink such as cola, lemonade, fruit juice, or some squares of chocolate. Do not give "diet"/diabetic drinks of any kind. Call emergency services if the person's condition seems at all worrying or does not improve. If the person has blood sugar testing equipment, help them to use it.

In hyperglycaemia, call emergency services straightaway. Do not administer insulin, even if you find it on the casualty. If properly alert, they will know to take it themselves. Look for clues about their condition so you can inform emergency services: medical ID tags/cards, an insulin "pen", glucose tablets, medication or a blood-testing kit.

If you're not sure if the person has hypoglycaemia or hyperglycaemia, give them something sweet anyway. It will help a 'hypo' and won't do any harm in the case of hyperglycaemia.

families and has very strong links with obesity and other lifestyle factors such as lack of exercise. Type 2 DM usually begins with insulin resistance, in which the body becomes less and less responsive to the effects of insulin.

HOW IS DIABETES TREATED?

The aim of diabetes treatment is to keep blood sugar levels stable and as close to normal as possible. In type 1 DM, insulin is needed, usually by injection; the person will have to test their blood glucose regularly and adapt insulin dose and dietary intake accordingly.

Diet is also crucial in type 2 DM, which may be manageable without insulin, either with diet and lifestyle changes alone or diet plus tablets. Recent evidence suggests that in some cases successful weight loss may be able to reverse the condition.

WHAT CAN GO WRONG?

There are some long-term health risks associated with diabetes, but the only likely emergencies are hypoglycaemia or, less commonly, hyperglycaemia.

Hypoglycaemia

This crisis, often called a "hypo" or "low", results from too little blood sugar. It can be caused by lack of food, delayed meals, insufficient carbohydrate, too much insulin, taking exercise without adjusting insulin dose or carbohydrate intake, shock or stress, and can be so sudden that the person is unable to take the necessary action, (generally, eating some form of sugar). See Signs and Symptoms box.

Hyperglycaemia

This results from too high a level of blood sugar, sometimes caused by too much food, insufficient insulin or missed tablets, or by a virus. It develops more slowly than hypoglycaemia, except in children or with viruses, but is more difficult to treat and likely to need medical attention. A viral illness unsettles the blood sugar balance, making a person with diabetes dehydrated,

with abnormal levels of sodium and potassium and acid in the blood. This makes them very ill and may even lead to a coma. See Signs and Symptoms box.

▽ Cola or lemonade, a few squares of chocolate or a milky sweetened drink are good first-aid choices for hypoglycaemia.

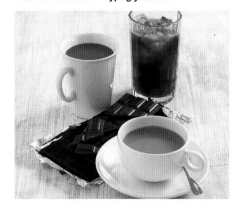

Dealing with nausea and vomiting

SEE ALSO

➤ Dealing with head injury, p80

➤ Coping with headache, p86

➤ ACTION ON POISONING, p185

Nausea and vomiting are common symptoms that are usually short-lived with no serious consequences. They arise from all kinds of causes, notably food poisoning, travel sickness, migraine, viral infection, allergic reaction, a drug side-effect or pregnancy. Nausea and vomiting may also have more serious causes, such as a heart attack, which will need to be investigated at your nearest hospital accident and emergency department. Prolonged vomiting can lead to dehydration, which can quickly become a medical emergency.

There are many causes of nausea and vomiting. Most of them are "self-limiting", which means they will settle without the need for further treatment or investigation. However, nausea and vomiting may be the beginning of a serious illness, and if they persist or dehydration sets in, the patient should seek medical advice.

CAUSES OF NAUSEA

Common reasons for nausea and vomiting include:

• Motion sickness.
• Migraine.
• Food poisoning.
• Viral gastroenteritis.
• Pregnancy.
• Drug side-effect.

More serious causes of nausea and vomiting, such as head injury, appendicitis, heart attack, hepatitis, urinary tract infection and bowel obstruction, will usually be accompanied by other symptoms such as headache, abdominal pain, chest pain, yellow conjunctiva (whites of eyes), fever, frequent and burning urine or abnormal bowel movements, which may range from loose and frequent to entirely absent for a few days.

TREATMENT FOR VOMITING

Urge the patient to drink small sips of iced fluid, every 30 minutes or so, and to refrain from eating for 12 hours. When vomiting stops and the appetite returns, stick to bland foods, such as rice. If there are signs of dehydration, seek medical advice.

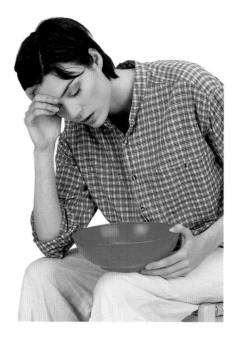

△ Seek immediate medical assistance if vomiting is accompanied by a headache that might be due to head injury.

SIGNS AND SYMPTOMS OF DEHYDRATION

Mild

➤ Headaches.

➤ Thirst.

➤ Dark urine.

➤ Dry, scaly-looking lips and tongue.

Moderate

➤ No urine passed in over 24 hours.

➤ Breath smells of nail-varnish remover.

➤ Sunken eyes.

Severe

➤ The skin remains in folds even after letting go of a pinch.

➤ Drowsiness.

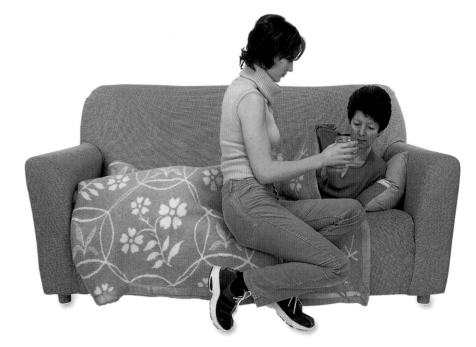

▷ Encourage the patient to drink a little plain water every half an hour in order to prevent any danger of dehydration.

Tackling diarrhoea, fever and cramp

SEE ALSO
➤ Dealing with nausea and vomiting, p98
➤ Dealing with abdominal pain, p100

Diarrhoea is a common complaint that usually clears up on its own, although persistent cases or those occurring after travel abroad should be investigated. Fever is usually a symptom of infectious illness. If the temperature is very high or persists, see a doctor. With fever and diarrhoea, replacing fluid is all-important. Cramp may be exacerbated by fever (or any other factor that raises body temperature). Cramp spasms occur when muscle fibres over-contract. This often happens after exercise, due mostly to a build-up of lactic acid in the muscles.

DIARRHOEA

Characterized by loose, frequent bowel movements, diarrhoea usually gets better without treatment. It may be accompanied by vomiting, and is commonly caused by gastroenteritis, which may be viral or caused by contaminated foods – especially shellfish, meat, milk or egg products – that have not been cooked or stored properly. Diarrhoea may occur in many other gut conditions, from irritable bowel syndrome to bowel cancer, or with certain medicines. Even constipation can lead to diarrhoea, as loose stools start to overflow the blocked-up bowel. Seek medical advice if:

• Diarrhoea is not improving after 2 days in adults or 24 hours in babies or young children.
• The stools are black and tarry or blood-stained.
• There is accompanying vomiting such that the casualty cannot keep down any fluids.
• Dehydration is developing.

• There is fever more than 102°F (39°C).
• The person recently returned from a trip abroad.
• There is persistent abdominal pain or cramps.

FEVER

A raised temperature is a sign that the body is fighting infection or illness. It makes people tired and shivery, and they may have cold-like symptoms, feel sick or even vomit. Other symptoms that may accompany fever and give a clue as to its cause include diarrhoea or a burning sensation when passing urine.

It is useful to have a thermometer in your medicine cabinet, particularly if you have children. Modern digital thermometers are very easy to use and are mercury-free.

It's best not to try to bring down a temperature with medicines, unless the person is very uncomfortable. Increase fluid intake to make up that lost in sweating and to protect against possible dehydration.

TAKING TEMPERATURE
Normal body temperature varies slightly depending on where, and at what time of day, it is taken:

Method	°C	°F
Under arm	36.5	97.7
Oral	37.0	98.6

CRAMP

Cramp is usually felt at night, and it happens most commonly in the calf muscles. Getting out of bed and walking around is the best way of relieving cramp, or try massaging the affected muscle or pulling the toes towards you as far as they will go.

Cramp may also occur with exercise, dehydration, vitamin deficiencies, some medications or during pregnancy. Occasionally cramp-like symptoms when exercising, relieved by rest, may be a sign of serious circulation problems, particularly in older smokers. The person should seek medical advice.

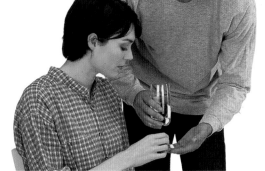

◁ Ibuprofen or paracetamol tablets, capsules or syrup are best avoided unless the casualty is very distressed by the raised temperature.

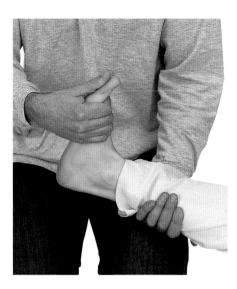

▷ In order to relieve calf muscle cramp, extend the leg through the pain and the cramp will disappear.

Dealing with abdominal pain

SEE ALSO

➤ Coping with antenatal emergencies, p92

➤ Dealing with nausea and vomiting, p98

Abdominal pain is one of the most common symptoms, with causes ranging from menstruation to appendicitis or even occasionally pneumonia. In helping a casualty with abdominal pain, you need first to ascertain how serious is the likely cause. When the pain started, where it is sited, how severe it is and any accompanying symptoms, such as vomiting or vaginal bleeding, will help your assessment. Call a doctor or an ambulance if the pain is severe and prolonged, or if there is unexpected vaginal blood, or blood in the motions, vomit or urine.

Of all the areas in the body, apart from the chest, the painful abdomen probably causes the most worry. Abdominal pain is very common in all age groups, and even recurrent pain may be due to completely benign and treatable causes.

In attending a person with abdominal pain, it is important to be able to make a distinction between a minor episode that will pass without any problems and a serious, possibly life-threatening, condition such as an ectopic pregnancy.

WHERE AND WHY ABDOMINAL PAIN ARISES

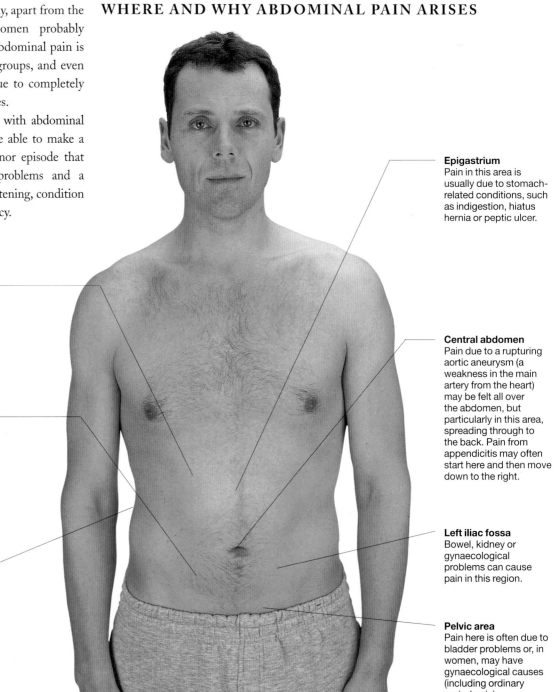

Epigastrium
Pain in this area is usually due to stomach-related conditions, such as indigestion, hiatus hernia or peptic ulcer.

Right upper quadrant
The gall bladder, liver and pancreas lie in this area. Pain here is often due to gallstones or pancreatitis.

Right iliac fossa
This is typically where the pain of appendicitis is felt, although bowel, kidney and gynaecological problems can cause pain here.

Right and left loin
This is where the kidneys lie, and pain from them is often felt here, spreading down to the lower pelvic areas.

Central abdomen
Pain due to a rupturing aortic aneurysm (a weakness in the main artery from the heart) may be felt all over the abdomen, but particularly in this area, spreading through to the back. Pain from appendicitis may often start here and then move down to the right.

Left iliac fossa
Bowel, kidney or gynaecological problems can cause pain in this region.

Pelvic area
Pain here is often due to bladder problems or, in women, may have gynaecological causes (including ordinary period pain).

ASSESSING ABDOMINAL PAIN

Before you start to consider what might be causing the abdominal pain, you should bear in mind the following considerations:

• Remember that the pain may not just be over a specific organ as it can be "referred" to other areas. This is especially true in appendicitis.

• Any woman of childbearing age with abdominal pain might be pregnant.

• Very ill or old people do not necessarily have a high temperature with serious causes of abdominal pain.

• People taking regular anti-inflammatory medication for arthritis or muscular pain can suffer bleeding in their stomach or duodenum with no pain at all until the ulcer perforates or they sustain massive internal bleeding.

CAUSES OF ABDOMINAL PAIN

It is not only the site of the pain that gives clues to its origins. Hollow organs such as the gut and renal tract tend to cause pain that comes and goes rather like labour pains, and this is often called "colicky" pain. Pain due to peritonitis, where the membrane that lines the abdominal cavity becomes inflamed, is a constant, uninterrupted pain. Pains that occur around the time that the bowels open are usually due to a bowel-related problem.

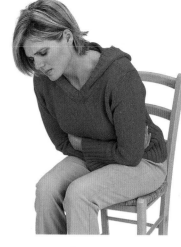

△ Always consider pregnancy as a possible cause of abdominal pain in any woman of childbearing age.

SIGNS OF POTENTIALLY SERIOUS ABDOMINAL PAIN

➤ Profuse nausea and vomiting.

➤ Severe diarrhoea or constipation or an alternation between the two.

➤ Back pain.

➤ Shallow, fast breathing.

➤ Fever.

➤ Signs of developing shock – rapid pulse and sweaty, cold skin.

➤ A bulging or rigid abdominal wall.

➤ Tenderness on pressing the abdomen.

➤ A lump or mass in the abdomen.

➤ Any bleeding from the rectum, in the urine, or non-menstrual vaginal bleeding.

There may be other clues to the origin of the pain, such as symptoms relating to the kidneys (including a burning when passing urine and passing urine often or not at all).

The duration of the pain is important. Regular bouts of pain that settle after a few days may be due to irritable bowel syndrome or diverticulitis. Severe pain of sudden onset is more likely to be a serious condition such as appendicitis.

FIRST AID FOR ABDOMINAL PAIN

Have a vessel nearby in case of vomiting.

GENERAL, NON-ACUTE STOMACH/ABDOMINAL ACHES:
Keep the sufferer comfortable and give them fluids little and often, rather than a glassful that may be vomited straight back. A hot-water bottle or heating pad placed on the painful area may ease the pain. If the pain does not settle with simple paracetamol-based painkillers or medications for heartburn, seek medical advice. Do not give aspirin or anti-inflammatory drugs like ibuprofen as these may irritate the stomach lining.

ACUTE STOMACH/ABDOMINAL PAIN:
If there is severe or sudden acute pain, or pain accompanied by fever, yellow skin or conjunctivae or signs of shock, call the emergency services. Give nothing to eat or drink with acute abdominal pain, and never apply heat if there is fever or acute pain (for example, applying heat to an inflamed appendix would be very dangerous).

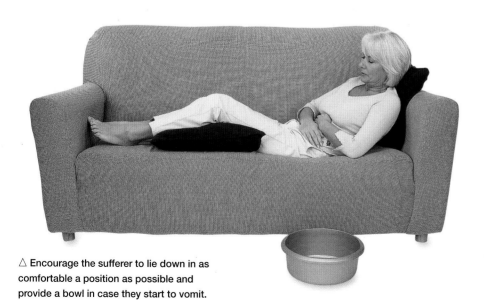

△ Encourage the sufferer to lie down in as comfortable a position as possible and provide a bowl in case they start to vomit.

Coping with allergy

SEE ALSO
➤ LUNGS AND BREATHING, p53
➤ Managing anaphylactic shock, p70
➤ Dealing with bites and stings, p104

Allergic responses may be minor or they may be severe. At worst, an allergen can cause anaphylactic shock, which demands immediate action to prevent serious illness and even death. People with allergic illnesses, such as asthma and eczema, are likely to develop other allergic responses. A relatively minor response on the first exposure to an allergen may be followed by a much more dramatic response the next time. You should be familiar with the first aid necessary to assist the casualty and know how to prevent exposure in future.

The immune system is designed to protect us, but in allergy it works against us. Normally harmless substances, such as pollen or cat fur, are called allergens, because they can cause an allergic reaction if they come into contact with the immune system of a susceptible person. The immune cells act as if the allergens are dangerous invaders and the cells release damaging chemicals, such as histamine, in order to eradicate the invader. This causes allergic symptoms in the sufferer.

Once sensitized to a particular allergen, the immune system will react to it in every future contact. This may cause a wide variety of symptoms from wheezing and running eyes to vomiting or hives. The

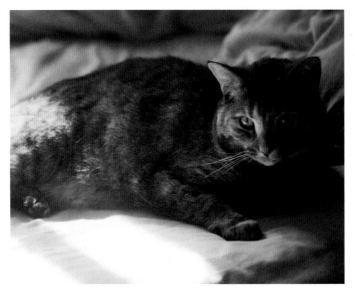

◁ Cats are well-recognized causes of allergic reaction, often causing the sufferer to wheeze and sneeze within minutes of entering the same room.

respiratory allergens such as pollen, dust and animal hairs tend to lead to fairly mild reactions, while reactions to allergens such as antibiotics or bee stings may be more severe.

At its worst, an allergic reaction can cause anaphylactic shock, with the risk of serious illness and death.

HOW TO SPOT AN ALLERGY

Allergic reactions vary depending on which part of the body is reacting. Respiratory allergies tend to cause hay fever or asthma. Intestinal allergies cause diarrhoea and vomiting as well as stomach pain. Skin allergies may cause a rash called hives or urticaria that looks like a nettle sting but is often more widespread. Severe allergies may cause shock and impaired breathing.

You may start to recognize a seasonal pattern to certain symptoms, or that they only happen when there is a cat in the house or when mowing the lawn. Blood,

skin prick or patch tests can help identify if a reaction is allergic or not, and may be able to identify a specific allergen.

FOOD ALLERGY OR INTOLERANCE?

Many people believe they have allergies to foods when, in fact, they have a food intolerance. A food intolerance is due to a lack of a digestive enzyme, such as lactase, that breaks down lactose in milk, or to susceptibility to a chemical such as tyramine in cheese, histamine in poorly-stored fish or salicylates in food, such as tomatoes.

A true food allergy should be suspected if the person has repeated symptoms, such as abdominal pain, diarrhoea, vomiting, hives or breathing difficulties every time after eating a particular food.

If symptoms develop slowly it may be difficult to identify which food is causing them. Seek medical advice before following an exclusion diet that cuts out major food groups.

COMMON ALLERGENS

Almost any substance can be an allergen but these are the most common culprits:

➤ Foods, including fish, shellfish, milk, nuts, eggs, chocolate, wheat and soya.

➤ Antibiotics, such as penicillin or tetracycline.

➤ Other drugs, such as insulin and contrast agents used in certain X-rays and scans.

➤ Venoms – wasp, bee, snake, scorpion, jellyfish.

➤ Dust mites, animals, plants, pollens and moulds.

➤ Chemicals – latex, dyes, base metals, such as nickel.

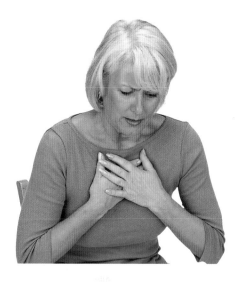

△ Coughing, a tight chest and breathing difficulty may be potentially worrying signs of an allergy that is affecting the respiratory system.

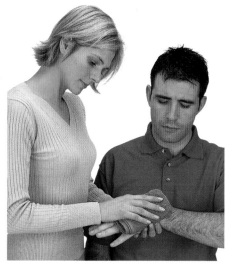

△ Try using a wrapped ice pack or bag of frozen vegetables to reduce the pain and inflammation of an insect sting or bite.

WHEN TO CALL 999

Call 999 or your local emergency number if the person experiences:

➤ Any breathing difficulty or trouble swallowing.

➤ Swelling of the lips or eyes.

➤ Hives around the mouth or elsewhere on the face.

➤ Collapse, dizziness, faintness or confusion.

➤ Palpitations, rapid heartbeat.

➤ Severe nausea, abdominal cramps or vomiting.

KEEPING HOUSE-DUST MITES UNDER CONTROL

➤ Avoid carpets – floorboards, tiles, vinyl flooring or linoleum are healthier.

➤ Keep the house well ventilated and damp-dust regularly.

➤ Buy dust-resistant pillows and mattresses or mattress covers, or vacuum the mattress daily.

➤ Put soft toys and pillows into the freezer every few months to kill house-dust mites.

➤ Avoid sheepskin underlays, as they attract house-dust mite.

➤ Use damp cloths rather than dusters for cleaning around the house.

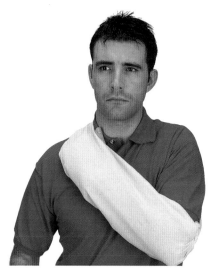

△ If you are dealing with an insect sting, elevate the affected part of the body in a sling if this is possible.

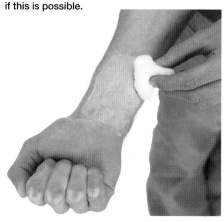

△ Calamine lotion is a cooling first-aid remedy for itchy rashes and insect bites.

FIRST AID FOR ALLERGIC REACTION

If there is any swelling around the face or neck, any difficulty breathing or symptoms threatening loss of consciousness, such as dizziness, get medical aid urgently. With any severe reaction, follow DRABC and look for any allergy information or medication that the sufferer may carry. If conscious, help them into a position that eases breathing. If unconscious, check ABC; be prepared to resuscitate if necessary.

Try ice on swellings due to insect bites; scrape off the stinger and elevate the affected part in a high sling if possible.

Antihistamines can be bought over the counter and may help with many allergies, including a nettle-type rash common in skin allergies.

Calamine lotion and ice are useful for itchy rashes or insect bite reactions.

Anti-allergy nose drops can be bought over the counter and can be useful for hayfever-type reactions.

In the long term, avoiding the allergen is the best option if you can, for example by not having pets or mowing the lawn in the middle of the day when pollen is most troublesome.

Dealing with bites and stings

SEE ALSO
➤ What is first aid?, p12
➤ Dealing with breathing difficulties, p56
➤ Coping with allergy, p102

When travelling abroad, animals, insects, snakes, and sea creatures may all present a hazard and any bite or sting is potentially dangerous due to allergy or infection, as well as the wound itself and the possible effects of venom. There are very many venomous snakes around the world. Alligators are endemic in southeastern states of America. Dogs can inflict very nasty wounds, and occasionally may be carrying rabies; jellyfish and other sea creatures may inject poison; even cats can cause unpleasant wounds; and some people are allergic to bee and wasp stings.

Many countries are home to a variety of dangerous animals, poisonous snakes and insects, and knowledge of how to treat any problems arising from contact with them will give peace of mind. Even non-venomous bites and stings can cause nasty infections or allergic reactions.

HUMAN AND ANIMAL BITES

Bite injuries are common. Millions of people are attacked by domestic dogs every year and, apart from treating the wound, you should be aware of the high potential for infection. Clean the wound thoroughly, apply antibiotic cream and advise the victim to seek medical attention within 8 hours – they may need antibiotics or measures against rabies or tetanus. Similarly, cat bites and even scratches often become infected, especially if they are on the hand or face. The victim should be alert for symptoms such as redness, heat, swelling, tenderness or pus that may appear up to 2 weeks later and should see a doctor promptly if these develop.

Human bites are the third most common cause, most often sustained "in reverse",

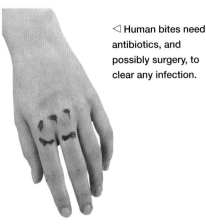
◁ Human bites need antibiotics, and possibly surgery, to clear any infection.

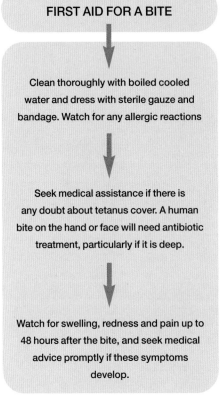

FIRST AID FOR A BITE

Clean thoroughly with boiled cooled water and dress with sterile gauze and bandage. Watch for any allergic reactions

Seek medical assistance if there is any doubt about tetanus cover. A human bite on the hand or face will need antibiotic treatment, particularly if it is deep.

Watch for swelling, redness and pain up to 48 hours after the bite, and seek medical advice promptly if these symptoms develop.

when someone punches someone else in the mouth and teeth break the skin of their knuckle. The underlying joint frequently becomes infected, requiring antibiotics or specialist treatment. Again clean the wound thoroughly and always seek urgent medical attention.

Horse, squirrel, rabbit, skunk, monkey, rodent and ferret bites may also cause serious infections. Although rare, attacks by wolves, bears, mountain lions and wild boar can cause infection as well as serious injury. Alligator attacks are becoming more common, especially in Florida, USA, and have obvious deadly potential. Although the majority of encounters result in survivable

injuries, even seemingly superficial bites can become very seriously infected and you should always call for emergency help. Bites and scratches often lead to infection, especially on the hand and face.

SNAKE BITES

Poisonous snakes release venom when they bite, which can cause pain and swelling, abdominal pain, vomiting and diarrhea. Shock may develop and in extreme cases a bite may be fatal. Copperheads inflict the greatest number of bites, but their venom is the least toxic; most fatal bites are due to rattlesnakes.

If someone is bitten by a snake, call the emergency services immediately, wash the affected area and try to keep it below the level of the heart. Keep the victim calm and still, and wrap a bandage around a bitten limb above the bite, tightly enough to impede the spread of venom but not so tight as to cut off circulation. Monitor the victim constantly and institute DRABC procedures if necessary.

SYMPTOMS AND SIGNS OF A VENOMOUS BITE

➤ Puncture marks in the skin.

➤ Feeling generally unwell.

➤ Lack of appetite.

➤ Abdominal pains.

➤ Rash, headache or fever.

➤ Muscle spasms.

➤ Joint pains.

SPIDER BITES

Most spider bites do not cause serious harm, but black widows and brown recluse spiders can be very dangerous, so in any case where you are not completely sure of the type of spider, call an ambulance. Symptoms such as swelling, pain, cramps, fever or chills, sweating or vomiting may not develop until later.

SEA CREATURES

Some marine animals can inflict damage, either by puncturing the skin with spines, or by injecting venom. Some, such as weever fish or stonefish, are effectively invisible as they blend with sand and rocks. Sea urchins may be visible, but if you step on one, the spines can break off and remain embedded in the foot. Remove any spines if you can, clean the wounds and seek medical attention urgently.

Most jellyfish stings are painful but not dangerous. Rinse the area with vinegar and extract the tentacles – warm water may help. A few jellyfish inject a neurotoxin that can stop muscles working and lead swiftly to respiratory arrest and suffocation. If any breathing difficulties arise, call an ambulance and be prepared to start CPR if necessary.

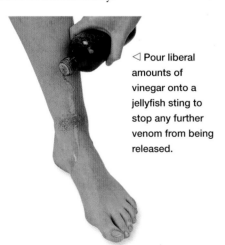

◁ Pour liberal amounts of vinegar onto a jellyfish sting to stop any further venom from being released.

Shark attacks are rare but if not fatal can cause deep puncture wounds and severe lacerations as well as broken bones and sometimes amputations. Call an ambulance immediately, put pressure on checks if necessary and treat for bleeding and shock while waiting for help to arrive.

WASP, BEE, YELLOW JACKET AND HORNET STINGS

Most reactions to insect stings are mild, causing short-lived pain, redness, itching or swelling, though they can cause an allergic reaction in a susceptible person. Suspect an allergy if there is severe swelling, dizziness, fainting, difficulty breathing, nausea or vomiting, hives or a tight throat or chest. If an allergic reaction develops, call an ambulance immediately. Administer adrenaline if the victim carries an auto-injector.

A bee may leave behind a sting attached to a venomous sac. If you squeeze it, more venom will be released. Instead, scrape it out carefully with a fingernail or the edge of a credit card, and wash the area with soap and water. Place ice over the sting to reduce swelling and pain. Taking an oral antihistamine may be advised, in case an allergic reaction develops.

TICK BITES

Most tick bites cause only minor soreness and swelling, but some can transmit infections such as Lyme disease or Rocky Mountain spotted fever. Prompt tick removal reduces the risk of Lyme disease. Grip the tick with fine-tipped tweezers to as close to the skin as possible and gently pull with a steady upward motion. Don't squeeze or twist the tick; don't use petroleum jelly, nail polish or a hot match, and don't touch it with your bare hands. If the head remains buried in the skin, take the victim to a doctor. Even after complete removal, the person should seek prompt medical attention if a spreading red ring like a bulls-eye, or flu-like symptoms, develop over the subsequent 2 weeks.

FIRST AID FOR SNAKE, SCORPION AND SPIDER BITES

Institute the DRABC procedures and be prepared to resuscitate if necessary. Do not bite, cut, squeeze, suck or apply ice or a tourniquet to the bite.

⬇

Calm the casualty and keep them as still as possible, so the poison does not spread.

⬇

Call the emergency services or get the sufferer to medical help quickly so that anti-venom can be given if necessary. Follow any instructions given over the phone by the emergency services.

⬇

If you cannot get medical help or advice within 30 minutes, bandage the bitten part firmly, but not so tightly that it stops blood reaching or leaving the affected part. Splint the bitten part to keep it immobile.

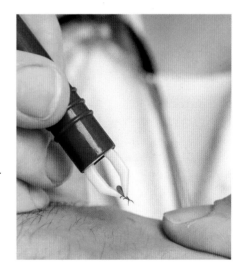

△ Use a fine-tipped pair of tweezers to remove a tick. Grab as close to the head as you can and gently pull upwards.

Managing heat and cold disorders

SEE ALSO

➤ Dealing with breathing difficulties, p56

➤ Dealing with shock, p68

➤ Dealing with nausea and vomiting, p98

It takes time for our bodies to get used to a different temperature. The brain controls our response to hot and cold conditions mainly by altering sweat production and the amount of blood circulating near the surface of our body. If it is not given sufficient time to adapt to extreme temperature change, we may become ill – sometimes dangerously so. Temperature disorders in which the sufferer overheats include heat stroke, heat exhaustion (which may lead to heat stroke) and heat cramps; extremes of cold can cause frostbite and hypothermia.

HYPOTHERMIA

Caused by cold conditions, hypothermia occurs when the body's core temperature drops below 35°C (95°F).

It most commonly occurs:

• In a poorly heated home, particularly with older or undernourished people of any age.

• In cold outdoor conditions, such as moors and mountains and at some road traffic accidents. Temperatures do not have to be freezing. It is more likely in wet and windy conditions.

• During or after immersion in cold water, even for short periods of time.

In cold and temperate climates, older people are particularly vulnerable to hypothermia in the winter: they may sit still for long periods, they may not eat properly or be unable to heat their home sufficiently, and their metabolism is slower than that of a younger person.

Diagnosis can be difficult, and unconscious hypothermia sufferers may be mistaken for dead. However, due to the body's reduced need for oxygen when very cold, even prolonged resuscitation efforts have been successful.

HEAT EXHAUSTION

Due to excessive loss of water and salt from profuse sweating, heat exhaustion often occurs after heavy exercise and prolonged other recreational activities on hot days. Heat exhaustion is not usually serious if you can cool down the casualty within 30 minutes, but if not treated promptly, it may develop into heat stroke, which is an emergency.

FIRST AID FOR HYPOTHERMIA

BASIC PRINCIPLES:
• Prevent further heat loss • Get urgent help • Rewarm the casualty – gradually
• Follow DRABC and be prepared to start resuscitation if needed.

Keep movement of the casualty to a minimum, and very gentle. Sudden movement can cause heart problems.

IF OUTDOORS
Get the casualty to shelter if possible. Replace wet clothing with dry, ideally warmed (e.g. from dry, warm bystanders). Cover the casualty's head and insulate them against cold from the ground. Wrap them in something warm such as a sleeping bag or foil blanket, or ideally a survival bag. If you can't get them to a safe indoor place within a short time, call the emergency services for help.

IF INDOORS
Rewarm gradually in a generally warm room. Replace any cold, damp clothing. If alert enough to eat/drink, give hot fluids like soup (no alcohol) and a little high-calorie food. Do not: heat up the body too fast, apply direct heat (hot-water bottles, sitting someone against a radiator), massage or rub the skin, get the casualty to exercise.

SIGNS AND SYMPTOMS OF HYPOTHERMIA

Mild – body temp. 35°C (95°F) or less

➤ Casualty feels very cold, with pale, dry skin.

➤ Uncontrollable shivering.

➤ Stumbling, poor coordination, slurred speech, mild confusion, odd behaviour.

Deep – body temp. 33°C (91.4°F) or less

➤ Casualty has no sensation of cold.

➤ Shivering stops.

➤ Drowsy, becoming unconscious.

➤ Breathing slows.

➤ There may be no detectable pulse.

HEAT STROKE

A very serious condition, heat stroke may be fatal. It may start as heat exhaustion, but if the body does not cool down, its heat-regulating mechanism fails, and body

SIGNS AND SYMPTOMS OF HEAT EXHAUSTION

➤ Occurs gradually over several hours.

➤ Body temperature may be normal, but may rise to 38–40°C (100.4–104°F).

➤ Headache, dizziness, confusion, tiredness, nausea, shallow breathing.

➤ Cold, pale, clammy skin and sweating.

➤ Arm, leg and stomach cramps.

➤ Feeling faint or actually fainting.

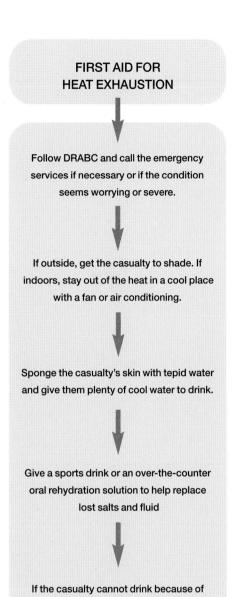

FIRST AID FOR HEAT EXHAUSTION

Follow DRABC and call the emergency services if necessary or if the condition seems worrying or severe.

↓

If outside, get the casualty to shade. If indoors, stay out of the heat in a cool place with a fan or air conditioning.

↓

Sponge the casualty's skin with tepid water and give them plenty of cool water to drink.

↓

Give a sports drink or an over-the-counter oral rehydration solution to help replace lost salts and fluid

↓

If the casualty cannot drink because of nausea or vomiting, or there is no improvement after 30 minutes, call an ambulance.

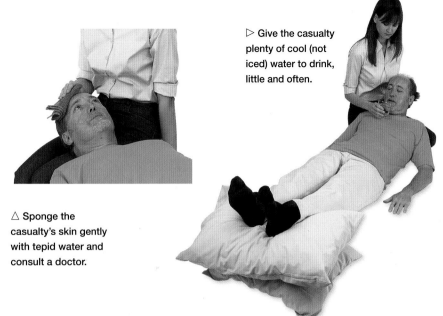

△ Sponge the casualty's skin gently with tepid water and consult a doctor.

▷ Give the casualty plenty of cool (not iced) water to drink, little and often.

tissues start to heat up dangerously. Muscles and major organs begin to break down. Heat stroke tends to happen mainly in a very hot environment or with a fever.

Older people and those who are disabled or infirm, obese, alcoholic or have diabetes are more vulnerable to heat stroke. Some drugs, especially anti-depressants, diuretics and sedatives, can increase susceptibility.

Dealing with heat stroke

A person suffering from heat stroke needs urgent medical attention. Call the emergency services without delay and,

while waiting for them, follow these steps:
• Having followed the DRABC procedures and initiated resuscitation if necessary, move the casualty out of the sun to a shady, cool place, preferably air-conditioned. Remove excessive clothes.
• Lie the casualty flat. If they have heart problems, keep them sitting up.
• Watch for breathing problems or seizures.
• Cool the casualty down but do not immerse them in cold water – this makes blood vessels in the skin close down, increasing core temperature. The best way to cool down a hot person is to spray their skin with water or wrap them in a wet sheet and direct a fan at them.

SIGNS AND SYMPTOMS OF HEAT STROKE

➤ Similar to heat exhaustion but with no sweating.

➤ Throbbing headache, dizziness, rapid shallow breathing.

➤ Temperature is over 40°C (104°F).

➤ Sudden delirium, with confusion and agitation.

➤ Convulsions, coma and death.

➤ Red hot skin.

➤ Muscle cramps and weakness.

Alternatively apply cold, wet cloths or wrapped ice packs to neck, armpits and groin.

HEAT CRAMPS

These may happen after excessive exercise, or exercising in very hot weather. The muscle cramps occur as a result of loss of salt and water from sweating. People may also feel sick and dizzy.

First-aid treatment involves moving the sufferer to a cool place and giving them a sports drink or rehydration fluids to replace lost salts.

PREVENTING HEAT PROBLEMS

Follow these important tips whenever you are in hot conditions:
• Stay in the shade and use air conditioning when it is available.
• Drink 5–6 litres (9–10½ pints) of fluid per day if sweating a lot in a hot climate or because of exercise or fever, and avoid excessive alcohol. (Normal daily fluid intake is 2–3 litres/3½–5 pints; dark urine is a clear sign that you must drink more fluids.)
• Avoid over-exertion and take frequent cool showers.
• Ensure adequate ventilation indoors.
• Wear a wide-brimmed hat outdoors.
• Avoid going out when the sun is at its hottest – between 11 a.m. and 3 p.m.

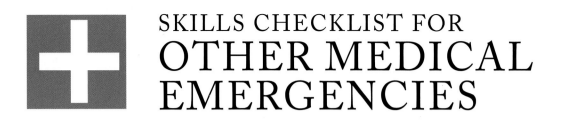

SKILLS CHECKLIST FOR
OTHER MEDICAL EMERGENCIES

KEY POINTS

- Unusual symptoms in pregnancy should always be dealt with urgently ☐

- Always consider blood-sugar problems when the cause of collapse is unknown ☐

- Although usually self-limiting, nausea and vomiting can point to serious conditions ☐

- Consult a doctor for persistent or severe abdominal pain ☐

- Always seek rapid medical help in the event of a serious allergic reaction or snake bite ☐

SKILLS LEARNED

- What to do for collapse and bleeding in pregnancy ☐

- Assisting at the birth of a baby ☐

- Coping with a diabetic crisis ☐

- Dealing with sickness, diarrhoea, fever, cramp and dehydration ☐

- Recognizing severe abdominal pain ☐

- Coping with allergic reactions and bites and stings ☐

- Dealing with temperature-related conditions: hypothermia and heat stroke ☐

CHILDHOOD PROBLEMS

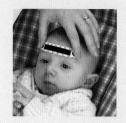

Babies and young children can deteriorate alarmingly quickly when they are ill. It is therefore wise to take seriously any symptoms they may have. Symptoms such as fever, vomiting, diarrhoea, breathing difficulties, coughs, abdominal pain and headache may be signs of routine, non-threatening childhood complaints, but they could signal something more serious. As a preventative measure, you should leave your child only with trusted and experienced childminders or at registered nursery schools where you can be sure that your child will receive good care in the event of developing an illness.

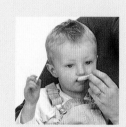

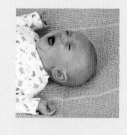

CONTENTS

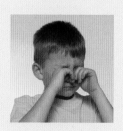

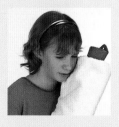

Recognizing childhood illness

SEE ALSO

➤ CHILDREN'S LIFE SUPPORT, p43

➤ Dealing with problems in babies, p112

Babies and young children can become seriously ill within a very short space of time. It is vital that the parents and any other carers are familiar with what is normal for that particular child and, therefore, know when something is wrong. Very often children are unable to articulate exactly what the problem is and so you have to be prepared to make an informed guess about the cause. Whenever you are in any doubt about the health of a child you should consult a doctor or go to hospital immediately, no matter what time of day, or night, it is.

Children are not simply miniature adults – their bodies are different and respond differently to illness and trauma. The responses of a baby will differ to those of a toddler, and the responses of a 7-year-old or a teenager will differ too. Children may not be physically or emotionally able to articulate how or why they feel ill, or where it hurts. This is why it is always important to listen to their parents. Parents may not be certain of what the problem is either, but they know that "something is not right" with their child.

Doctors always find time to see children, as they know how difficult it can be to judge childhood illness, and that problems may develop rapidly. At the same time, being able to deal with the common, short-lived childhood illnesses and with minor accidents yourself may allow you to avoid seeking unnecessary medical help or to improve matters until further medical help is available.

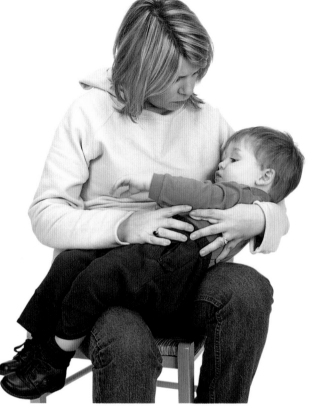

◁ The young sick child will probably be clingy and tearful. Look closely for any signs of illness.

▽ The sick child is usually unhappy and subdued, although they may be unable to explain exactly what is wrong.

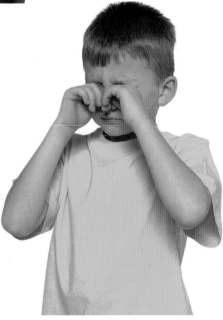

ASSESSING AN ILL CHILD

Children react differently to illness at different ages. So, since babies tend to breathe through their noses, their small nasal passages make a cold a very distressing experience that affects sleep and feeding, whereas an older child tolerates the symptoms more easily. There are, however, a few pointers to illness that apply more generally:

➤ How alert is the child? If they show interest in their toys and in people around them, this is a good sign. If they are slumped, silent and inert in their parent's lap, you should be concerned.

➤ Look for rashes or abnormal skin colour, for example a greyish pallor may indicate a very sick child.

➤ Identify any areas of pain. You can ask an older child where the pain is, but in babies and younger children you may have to use your intuition.

➤ Is there any restricted movement in the arms or legs? The child may be protecting an injured limb.

➤ Babies' cries can offer clues – a high-pitched cry is often a sign of illness.

RECOGNIZING A SERIOUSLY ILL CHILD

Children can get seriously ill very quickly, and often recover just as suddenly. Potentially worrying signs include:

➤ Altered consciousness: not engaging with people, unusually agitated or apathetic, drowsy or unrousable.

➤ Breathing quickly, noisily or not at all.

➤ Grey/white/blue skin colour.

➤ Sunken eyes, caked and dry lips and tongue that suggest dehydration.

➤ Hot trunk and head but cold limbs.

➤ Pupils are unequal/do not react to light.

➤ Aversion to light.

➤ Stiff neck.

➤ Weak, high-pitched cry.

➤ No spontaneous movement.

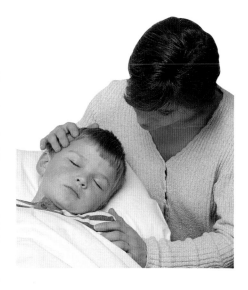

△ If the child is extremely apathetic and drowsy, consult a doctor immediately.

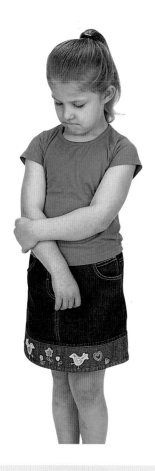

▷ If the child exhibits no sign of illness other than not being her usual self, then she may be unhappy. Childhood depression often goes unrecognized.

A REASSURING MANNER

Always try to calm a sick child – children soak up, and respond to, mood and atmosphere very readily. Being reassuring and friendly lessens their fear, which may, in turn, lessen their pain and distress. If you come across a situation where you are dealing with distraught parents as well as an ill child, unless it's an emergency it's best to put both the parents and the child at ease before attempting to examine the child. Chat calmly to the parents before addressing their child at all, and try to gather as much information about the situation as possible. Then keep the child occupied by playing and chatting quietly with them.

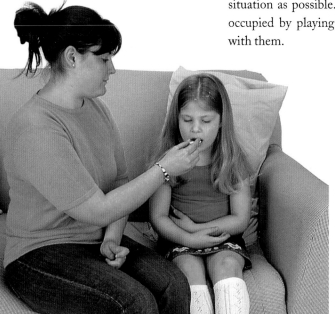

 Avoid giving your child paracetamol or ibuprofen syrup unless they are in pain or distressed by a fever.

FIRST AID FOR A SERIOUSLY ILL CHILD

Initiate the dRABC procedure and commence resuscitation, if necessary. If the child is unconscious but breathing, put them in the recovery position (for babies under 1 year hold them in the baby recovery position). Call the emergency services straight away.

If the child is conscious but struggling to breathe, you must still call the emergency services at once. Sit the child up and keep them as calm as possible while waiting for the ambulance.

If breathing is adequate but your child is feverish, unwell or has other worrying symptoms seek prompt medical advice.

Dealing with problems in babies

SEE ALSO

➤ CHILDREN'S LIFE
SUPPORT, p43

➤ Recognizing childhood
illness, p110

➤ Coping with fever, p114

Young babies commonly suffer from a number of problems, most of which are perfectly normal. Crying is a baby's main method of communication so a change in the pattern or type of crying may indicate that something is wrong. Parents soon become attuned to their baby's crying. Problems that commonly affect babies include feeding and sleeping difficulty, colic, nappy rash and teething. Symptoms such as fever or diarrhoea should never be attributed to minor baby problems, and you should seek your doctor's advice if such symptoms develop.

New babies arrive after a long and sometimes seemingly endless nine months. It seems that there is ample time to prepare for their arrival, and yet so often these tiny, innocent beings arrive in their expectant households like miniature missiles. This is especially true for first-time parents, who before the birth can rarely see past the labour to the daily care routine beyond.

New babies don't know that they are meant to sleep at night and be more awake during the day. They have no routine – but their parents are often used to rigid schedules that they have stuck to for many years before their child's arrival. In the first few weeks, babies seem to do nothing but sleep, feed and cry, in an entirely random way. It helps to know what to expect.

CRYING

A baby's cry has a remarkably unsettling effect on its parents, especially the mother. Other people may hardly notice the noise but the mother will find it very hard to ignore. There is a good reason for this, rooted in evolution. When a mother is breastfeeding, she is the only person who can feed the baby, and if their cries do not make her run to them, they would starve. Crying is a baby's only means of communication.

Most parents quickly recognize that their baby has different cries. Sometimes it will be the weak, "don't leave me" cry of the tired baby left to fall asleep in their cot; at others, the alarmed and heart-rending cry of the hungry baby. A very sick baby may have a high-pitched cry that sounds odd

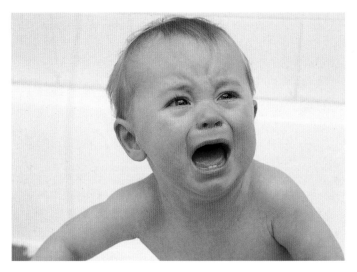

◁ The cry of a sick child is noticeably different to their normal cry. Parents can usually recognize a cry that is simply asking for cuddles or food.

and frightening, or may be too weak to cry at all. Some babies hardly seem to cry while others never seem to stop.

Babies cry for many reasons including hunger, tiredness, pain, colic and dirty nappies. Babies differ in their tolerance of discomfort: some can have a filthy nappy and not fret at all, while others cannot bear even to be just a little wet.

COLIC

Characterized by very sudden attacks of crying and obvious distress, colic may cause the baby to draw up their legs and

cry inconsolably for several hours, day after day. No one knows what causes colic, which makes it rather difficult to treat. Colic often follows a definite pattern: it occurs at specific times of the day, usually in the evening, and it peaks at two to three

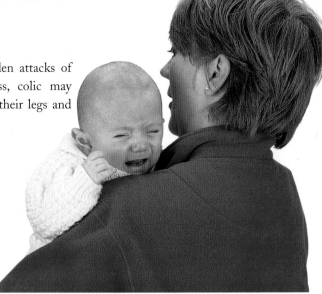

▷ A colicky baby may cry inconsolably for many hours, but is not ill and feeds well.

SIMPLE WAYS OF DEALING WITH COLIC

➤ Rock your baby gently or walk around with your baby either in your arms or in a baby sling.

➤ Put your baby into the pram or buggy and wheel it to and fro inside the house, or, if convenient, go out for a walk with the baby.

➤ Gently rub or massage your baby's abdomen in a clockwise direction, following the path of the digestive system.➤

➤ Dill, fennel and chamomile are age-old traditional herbal remedies for colic – but check with your doctor before giving any remedies to a small baby.

➤ If you are breast-feeding, then you should try to rest during the day if at all possible – this will help to replenish your supply of milk, ready for the evening feeds.

➤ Making sure that you always drink plenty of fluids, and eat good, nutritionally balanced meals, will help to keep your milk supply going well.

▽ Nappy rash can be alleviated by regularly leaving the baby on a towel with no nappy, allowing the circulation of air.

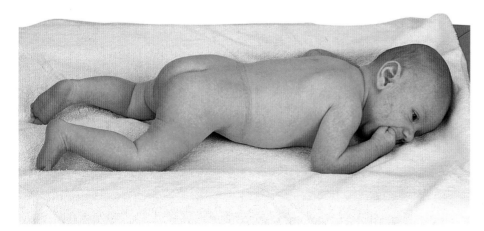

months of age, usually improving or disappearing altogether by around six months.

Parents of colicky babies need to be reassured that there is nothing at all wrong with their baby; and they will often need emotional support, or someone else to look after the baby for a while.

RASHES

Babies often have blotchy skin when they arrive, and for a few weeks out of the womb, their skin often becomes dry and spotty.

Milia

These little white "milk spots" appear round the nose of a newborn baby's face. They usually disappear after a few weeks.

Nappy or diaper rash

Babies have very sensitive skin, and so it is not surprising that their bottoms become sore from contact with urine and feces. To reduce the likelihood of nappy rash occurring, always change your baby if the nappy is dirtied or wet. Using a liberal application of a barrier cream at each change helps protect the skin. Avoid harsh soaps, detergents, talc and bubble bath. Give your baby as much time as possible without a nappy during the day.

When a baby is teething or ill, especially with diarrhoea or fever, they are much more susceptible to nappy rash. Be aware of this and make sure you do not delay changing their nappy.

PREVENTING NAPPY RASH

➤ Use a barrier cream on their bottoms all the time – zinc and paraffin oil creams are best.

➤ Try to use only water and cotton wool in the early weeks, as they may react to wipes or lotions.

➤ Change their nappies regularly, rather than wait for them to start leaking through clothes.

➤ If a baby's bottom is beginning to look a little red, try leaving them on a towel without a nappy for a while. This will allow some air to circulate around their bottom.

If there are little red and white spots either within or outside the general rash area, then the baby may have a yeast infection. Over-the-counter creams are available for this condition but if there is no improvement within 48 hours, or if open sores or blisters develop, see your doctor.

TEETHING

Some babies cut their teeth with very little fuss, whereas others seem to have a lot of trouble. The incisors at the front of the mouth usually arrive fairly painlessly around 6 months, but the bigger teeth at the back (molars), which arrive later, can cause a lot of upset.

Rubbing the gums with special teething gel may help, but avoid those containing benzocaine, which is no longer recommended for infants under two. For babies older than three months, liquid ibuprofen or paracetamol may be given if the baby is clearly distressed.

For babies between three and six months, seek advice from your pediatrician first. Do not give these medications to babies under three months. For some babies, biting on a hard or cool object, such as a special teething ring can help to relieve the pain.

Coping with fever

SEE ALSO
➤ Recognizing childhood illness, p110
➤ Dealing with problems in babies, p112

Fever is usually a sign of infection – although it can be caused by immunization or by being overdressed or in an overheated room. A raised temperature is a natural response that helps the body to fight infection. However it can be more serious in very young babies. Seek an urgent medical appointment if you think a baby has a fever, especially if they are under six months old. Keep a look-out for signs of dehydration and for other symptoms that might give a clue as to the cause of a fever, and always call a doctor if you are concerned.

A child's temperature often rises for up to 24 hours or even longer with no other obvious signs of infection, such as an earache, a sore throat or a common or garden cold. In many ways, it is reassuring when the first signs of a runny nose and cough appear as the cause of the temperature is then obvious.

NORMAL TEMPERATURE

Under arm/forehead	36.5°C (97.7°F)
Oral	37.0°C (98.6°F)

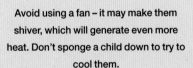

FIRST AID FOR A CHILD WITH A FEVER

If the room is warm, turn down the central heating or any other source of direct heat, and avoid too many bed covers or clothes.

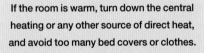

Avoid using a fan – it may make them shiver, which will generate even more heat. Don't sponge a child down to try to cool them.

Fever is a natural response to help the body fight infection, but if the child is very distressed, think about giving ibuprofen or paracetamol syrup (never aspirin) at the correct dose for their age. Babies should not have paracetamol under two months or ibuprofen under three months unless a doctor advises it.

DANGER SIGNS AND SYMPTOMS – CALL YOUR PEDIATRICIAN

➤ Baby under three months old.

➤ Fever over 38°C (100.4°F) in a baby under three months, or over 39°C (102.2°F) in a baby from three to six months old.

➤ Baby refusing feeds or has a seizure.

➤ Signs of dehydration such as producing less urine than normal, or very dark urine, sunken eyes, crying with little or no tear flow, or the soft spot on a baby's head (fontanelle) appearing sunken.

➤ Other signs of illness, such as a rash.

➤ Fever persists for more than 48 hours without any obvious source of infection, or that has lasted for more than five days in total.

Call an ambulance if:

➤ A rash that does not disappear when a glass is pressed on it.

➤ Cold or mottled hands or feet, blue lips or skin.

➤ A child who is drowsy or difficult to rouse.

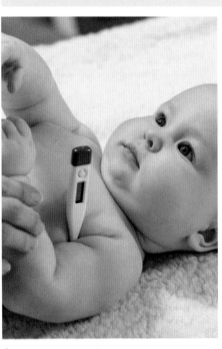

△ You can take a child's temperature using a digital pen thermometer under the arm.

SEPSIS

Small children, particularly premature babies and infants, are vulnerable to infection spreading in the bloodstream (septicemia), which may lead to a life-threatening response called sepsis or septic shock. It may develop after any infection, including wounds, pneumonia, meningitis, ear or urinary tract infection and even influenza. Symptoms include a high fever, shortness of breath, confusion, drowsiness, a drop in urine output and, in babies, seizures, a swollen abdomen and vomiting. More children in the UK die of sepsis than of pediatric cancers, and many survivors are left with long-term disability. Early detection and treatment in hospital, most likely in the intensive care unit, is vital. If you suspect sepsis, call an ambulance immediately.

Dealing with vomiting and diarrhoea

SEE ALSO
➤ Recognizing childhood illness p110
➤ Dealing with problems in babies p112

Extremely common symptoms in babies and children, diarrhoea and vomiting usually clear up quickly without any special treatment. Viral gastroenteritis (an infection of the gut) and food intolerance are common causes. If diarrhoea and/or vomiting is profuse and persistent there is a danger of dehydration, particularly in babies and very young children. It is important to make sure the child drinks plenty of clear fluids for the duration of the illness. If other symptoms develop or there is no improvement after 48 hours, you should seek a doctor's advice.

DEHYDRATION DANGER

What cannot be stressed enough with these childhood complaints is that babies and children are more prone to dehydration than adults because they are less able to replace fluid losses.

BABIES

Vomiting and diarrhoea without a serious cause occur quite often in babies because their digestive systems are still immature.

A little vomiting after feeding is normal and is called "posseting". Some babies are prone to bringing up a lot of their feeds, which is worrying only if the baby is not gaining weight. Babies may vomit as a sign of a general infection.

You should ask for medical advice with:
• Repeated vomiting such that a child cannot keep down fluids.
• Unwell baby with a fever.
• Green-stained vomit or vomit containing blood.
• Projectile vomiting.
• Signs of dehydration.
Breast-fed babies have runny, bright yellow stools that smell like cottage cheese; babies on formula often have dark green, liquid bowel motions. Diarrhoea is different – watery, frequent, and often foul-smelling stools.

OLDER CHILDREN

There are many causes of vomiting and diarrhoea in children, but the most common is viral gastroenteritis. Although this gets better without treatment, dehydration may develop if the child does not drink enough. Encourage your child to drink clear, diluted fluids and avoid fizzy and milk-based drinks. An alternative is oral rehydration salts that can be bought from the pharmacist.

▽ A child who is vomiting may be drowsy and listless. Take the child's temperature and consult your doctor if you are worried.

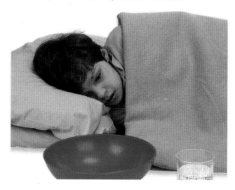

FIRST AID FOR A BABY WITH VOMITING AND/OR DIARRHOEA

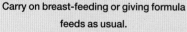

Carry on breast-feeding or giving formula feeds as usual.

Ask your doctor or pharmacist if the baby needs rehydration fluids as well. These are special powders that you make into a drink containing the sugars and salts lost through diarrhoea or vomiting.

Seek medical advice if the baby cannot keep down rehydration fluids, if the problem persists for more than 48 hours or if you are worried.

FIRST AID FOR A VOMITING CHILD

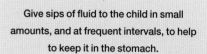
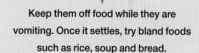

Give sips of fluid to the child in small amounts, and at frequent intervals, to help to keep it in the stomach.

Keep them off food while they are vomiting. Once it settles, try bland foods such as rice, soup and bread.

Keep a child with diarrhoea and vomiting away from other children until 48 hours after the last time they had symptoms.

DANGER

If a child is vomiting and has a rash, stiff neck or headache, call for an ambulance or take the child to the emergency department immediately.

SIGNS AND SYMPTOMS OF DEHYDRATION

➤ The soft spot on top of a baby's head becomes sunken.

➤ The eyes become sunken and hollow looking.

➤ The lips are parched and the tongue is dry.

➤ Urine production falls. A baby's nappy may remain dry all day.

➤ They may be drowsy and listless.

Managing abdominal pain

SEE ALSO
➤ Coping with fever, p114
➤ Dealing with vomiting and diarrhoea, p115

Abdominal pain is a very common symptom in young children, and it is usually short-lived. It can occur for a wide range of reasons, which may or may not affect the digestive tract. Children tend not to suffer from indigestion, but anxiety and even migraine can cause stomachache. However, there are a few serious conditions that require immediate medical attention, and you should be alert for other symptoms that might signal such a situation. If you have any doubts, you should always consult a doctor immediately.

Children often complain of tummy ache, but the pain will usually disappear spontaneously without any intervention. Even children admitted to hospital with stomach pain are often sent home with no definite diagnosis. Children sometimes experience this kind of physical symptom as a result of unhappiness or anxiety. For example, a child who complains of recurring stomach pain may have problems at school or at home.

CAUSES OF ABDOMINAL PAIN

In children, abdominal pain is often not connected with the digestive system and may have causes such as a twisted testicle or abdominal migraine (recurrent episodes of pain often with similar triggers to migraine headaches in adults). Urinary tract infections, which are more common in girls, can cause abdominal pain. Even a general infection, such as a cold or flu, might give a child a stomachache – this is due to the glands swelling in their abdominal cavity as well as the head and neck area.

The type of pain and its location often give valuable clues to what might be causing it, but it is often difficult for a child to describe the pain accurately or to tell you exactly where it is situated. Accompanying symptoms, such as fever, diarrhoea or vomiting, can help to narrow down the possible causes but you should never hesitate to contact your doctor if you are at all concerned.

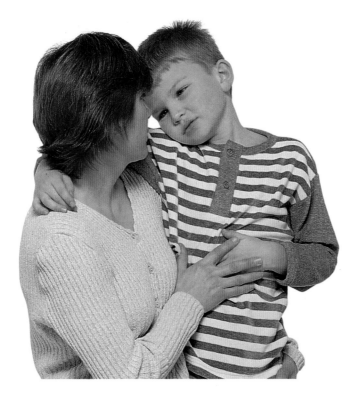

FIRST AID FOR A CHILD WITH ABDOMINAL PAIN

Try to find out exactly where the pain is and when it occurs. Is the pain there all of the time or does it relate to opening the bowels or urinating?

Encourage the child to eat bland foods such as dry toast or rice, and avoid fatty or spiced foods.

Don't give your child painkillers except on medical advice, as they could mask a possible serious cause for the pain.

A wrapped hot-water bottle placed on their stomach can be extremely comforting.

If the child is also vomiting or is suffering from diarrhoea, then they should avoid solid foods for 12–24 hours. Give them little amounts of fluid often.

◁ Talk to your child to try to assess whether the abdominal pain has an emotional rather than a physical cause.

PAINFUL CONSTIPATION

If you have never seen the distress that constipation – passing infrequent hard stools – causes in a baby, this may seem an odd condition to discuss in a first-aid book. However, it is one of the commonest causes of abdominal pain in children, and it is very useful to be aware of this fact.

A baby who screams and strains at the same time, while drawing up their knees, may be constipated. They may pass very hard, pellet-like stools or not have any bowel movements for a few days. It often happens briefly when bottle-fed babies change from the "first milks" to the more filling "second milks". A baby who has had bowel difficulties from birth may have a problem with the nerves that supply the gut – this is known as Hirschsprung's disease. It is a rare but serious condition that always requires surgical treatment.

Constipation may begin to be a problem during potty training. Parents should be aware that this can impede the learning process, as it is obviously unpleasant for the child – a situation to look out for and handle carefully. A child might also pass one large, hard motion that tears their anus. If they then start holding on to their stools to avoid pain, this could set up a vicious cycle which may eventually lead to the child being unable to control their bowel motions and soiling themselves. Plenty of fluids and high-fibre foods are needed to stop this scenario from developing – the earlier the better. Seek medical advice if the problem persists.

◁ A wrapped hot-water bottle placed on the child's stomach can be comforting and may also relieve the pain.

WHEN TO CALL THE DOCTOR

Call the doctor if a child's abdominal pain is accompanied by any of these symptoms:

➤ Sudden, severe pain, particularly if it is confined to one area of the abdomen.

➤ If the abdomen is swollen or painful when gently pressed.

➤ Vomiting, diarrhoea or fever.

➤ Blood in vomit or stools, or from the back passage.

➤ If there are signs of dehydration, for example dry lips and mouth, no urine passed for several hours or noticeably sunken eyes.

➤ If there is pain in the groin or a swelling of a testicle.

➤ If the pain has lasted intermittently for 24 hours and is getting worse.

APPENDICITIS

The appendix is a tiny tube of gut attached to the intestine that may become blocked and inflamed. Children of all ages can develop appendicitis. Pain often starts around the navel, and after a few hours shifts to the lower right-hand side of the abdomen, where the appendix is sited. The child may vomit, lack appetite, or have a fever and bad breath. There is a danger of perforation, so if you think appendicitis is a possibility you should go seek a doctor's advice and go to hospital without delay.

FIRST AID FOR A BABY WITH CONSTIPATION

⬇

Try giving them plain water in a bottle or on a spoon between milk feeds.

⬇

Try a teaspoon or syringe of prune juice or orange juice diluted 50/50 with water.

⬇

A small amount of petroleum jelly applied around the anus can help move a hard stool that may have formed.

⬇

Your health visitor is a good source of advice but you must see the doctor if the baby passes blood, starts to vomit or fails to gain weight.

INTUSSUSCEPTION

A condition that typically occurs between the ages of 3 months and 2 years, intussusception must be treated as an emergency. The cause is often unknown, but the result is that a section of intestine folds into itself, rather like the sleeve of a jersey. The child will be in severe pain and highly distressed. Vomiting may occur and a red, jelly-like stool may also be passed. If any of these symptoms occur, you must call an ambulance straight away.

WARNING

Call an ambulance if your child has any of the following symptoms:

➤ Pain that has lasted continuously for over 6 hours.

➤ Pain in the groin or testes.

➤ Greenish-yellow vomit.

➤ Red material in the faeces.

Coughs and breathing difficulty

SEE ALSO

➤ CHILDREN'S LIFE SUPPORT, p43
➤ Choking in babies and children, p50
➤ Dealing with breathing difficulties, p56
➤ Recognizing childhood illness, p110

Colds and coughs are very common in young children. They are not usually a cause for concern, and home remedies can generally provide relief. Occasionally, however, a child may experience severe difficulty in breathing: this constitutes an emergency and you should call an ambulance immediately. Causes of breathing difficulty range from asthma to choking, and some childhood infections, such as bronchiolitis. Breathing difficulty can be life-threatening and is alarming for both parent and child; never hesitate to call for help.

Children's air passages are smaller than adults', and so they are more likely to become blocked. A child can be unwell with a cough and a runny nose, but this on its own is seldom something that is likely to lead to any serious breathing problems. However, some conditions can lead to sudden breathing problems that may require first aid or emergency medical treatment.

COUGH

Coughs and colds are all too common in childhood, but rarely serious. Sometimes the type of cough may give clues to what is causing it. A barking cough and hoarse voice is characteristic of croup, a viral infection affecting the larynx and vocal chords. The noise can be very alarming, sounding somewhat like a seal barking.

Humidifying the atmosphere with steam can help.

A cough that comes in paroxysms so that at the end of the coughing fit, the child has to take such a deep breath that they make a "whooping" noise, is characteristic of whooping cough. Vomiting with the coughing is common with whooping cough. However, this condition is less common since the advent of the whooping cough vaccine.

NOISY BREATHING

Children may make all sorts of noises when they breathe, but noisy breathing does not necessarily indicate difficulties with breathing. The type of noise they make may help to pinpoint what the problem is likely to be.

Wheezing

Usually heard when a child breathes out, wheezing is a rather musical noise. Most people associate wheezing with asthma, but wheezing can also be due to viral infections, principally bronchiolitis. This is mostly seen in infants under 1 year and may require hospital admission if they have feeding problems, but is usually self-limiting. It is possible they may go on to develop asthma.

Noisy in-breaths

A harsh noise made as a child breathes in ("stridor") comes from the upper airways. It is caused by the airways being blocked or narrowed. Croup causes this type of noise, but it may also be due to inhaling a foreign body or very rarely due to a bacterial infection called epiglottitis.

TIPS FOR TACKLING CHILDREN'S COUGHS

➤ Use a humidifier or boil some pans of water to create a steamy atmosphere. Do this twice an hour if necessary.

➤ Place a wet towel on a warm radiator to moisten the air.

➤ Run the shower or a bath and sit the child in a steamy bathroom.

➤ Menthol and eucalyptus oil added to a bowl of warm water, or on the pillow or sheets, can help to ease a cough caused by an infection.

➤ Never smoke in the house.

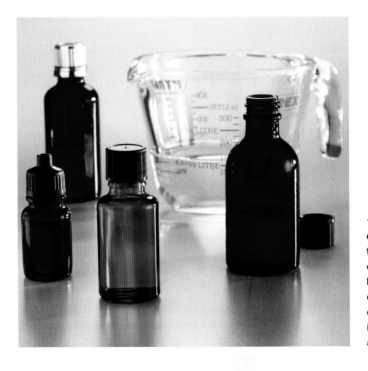

◁ Menthol or eucalyptus oils added to a bowl of hot water or onto a pillow can help ease a child's cough. A few drops of oil mixed with water in a room spray may also help.

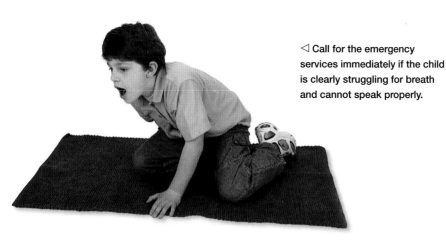

◁ Call for the emergency services immediately if the child is clearly struggling for breath and cannot speak properly.

FIRST AID FOR SEVERE BREATHING DIFFICULTY

↓

Sit the child upright. Try not to panic – this could make the child worse.

↓

Known asthmatics should take several puffs of a reliever inhaler (usually blue) through a spacer device, if available.

↓

Call a doctor/emergency services, depending on the severity of the problem.

Grunting

This noise can indicate serious breathing difficulties in a baby, and often pneumonia in an older child.

Snuffling

Babies will often snuffle when they have a cold. They then find it difficult to sleep and feed, which disturbs both them and their parents. However, most babies manage to find a way over this temporary problem without too much difficulty.

▽ If your child is on asthma medication, and they start to cough or wheeze, they must take some of the "reliever" drug (often in a blue case), preferably using a "spacer device", which assists uptake. You may need to help them take the drug.

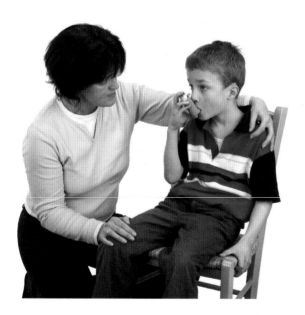

ASTHMA

Childhood asthma can be hard to recognize – for example, it often shows itself as sudden coughing fits or night-time coughing rather than wheezing. Children with asthma may cough, wheeze and, in severe attacks, have extreme breathing problems that require hospitalization. As asthma is potentially life-threatening it is essential to recognize the symptoms that need hospital treatment.

A child who has been diagnosed with asthma will have one or more inhalers, which normally keep the condition well controlled. Occasionally, maybe in the summer when the pollen count is high or if the child has a bad cold, the asthma does not respond to the normal treatment and breathing difficulties develop. This may mean that it is necessary to make a reassessment of the medication that the child is taking.

An asthmatic child who is having breathing problems can become seriously ill very rapidly, so never hesitate to call for an ambulance or take them to a hospital.

WARNING

Call an ambulance immediately if:

➤ Breathlessness and noisy breathing start suddenly, especially after choking.

➤ Breathing is so laboured that a baby or child is unable to feed/eat or drink.

➤ The child cannot speak in proper sentences or even utter sounds.

➤ The child is drowsy or confused.

➤ There is a visible "sucking in" of the ribcage as they breathe in and out.

➤ The child stops breathing altogether for more than a few seconds.

➤ The lips turn blue.

Specific asthma danger signs:

➤ Too breathless to speak or feed/eat.

➤ Breathing rate over 50 breaths/minute.

➤ Pulse over 140/minute.

➤ Blue lips.

➤ Very wheezy chest turning into no wheezing – no air is getting through.

➤ Fatigue/exhaustion.

➤ Drowsiness/agitation.

Tackling headaches

SEE ALSO
➤ Recognizing childhood illness, p110
➤ Coping with fever, p114

Headaches are a very common complaint in childhood. Usually, the headache passes quickly without the need to consult a doctor. Often a headache can signal the beginning of a childhood infectious illness, so look out for other symptoms. Occasionally, a headache can be a sign of a serious condition, such as meningitis, that requires urgent medical help. On the other hand, a headache may have its root in something as simple as a child having stayed out a little too long in the sun or not having drunk enough fluid.

Because children often complain of having a headache, the difficulty is knowing when to worry about it and seek help, and when to assume it has a self-limiting cause and will settle down by itself. Younger children obviously may not be able to articulate that they have a headache, but their actions may suggest it, for example they may dislike having their head moved, or be very irritable when moved at all, or they may be very sensitive to bright light or noise.

COMMON TYPES AND CAUSES OF HEADACHES

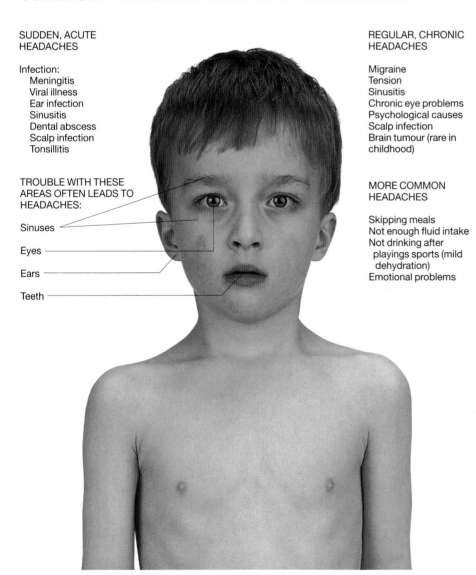

SUDDEN, ACUTE
HEADACHES

Infection:
   Meningitis
   Viral illness
   Ear infection
   Sinusitis
   Dental abscess
   Scalp infection
   Tonsillitis

TROUBLE WITH THESE
AREAS OFTEN LEADS TO
HEADACHES:

Sinuses

Eyes

Ears

Teeth

REGULAR, CHRONIC
HEADACHES

Migraine
Tension
Sinusitis
Chronic eye problems
Psychological causes
Scalp infection
Brain tumour (rare in childhood)

MORE COMMON
HEADACHES

Skipping meals
Not enough fluid intake
Not drinking after playings sports (mild dehydration)
Emotional problems

FIRST AID FOR A CHILD'S HEADACHE

Remove your child from any noisy, bright or disturbing environment and encourage them to rest in a quiet, dark room and to sleep if they can.

⬇

Make sure they drink plenty of clear liquids but avoid caffeine-containing drinks.

⬇

Try placing a cooled, damp flannel on their forehead to soothe the pain.

⬇

If the headache persists you could offer ibuprofen or paracetamol in a dose appropriate for their age. Children under 16 should never be given aspirin except on the advice of a doctor.

⬇

Look all over the body for a rash – this might signify a childhood infectious disease.

⬇

If they vomit, are drowsy, are very sensitive to light, have neck stiffness or any other worrying symptoms, or if the headache does not shift, call a doctor immediately.

WHEN IS A HEADACHE SERIOUS?

Your child's behaviour and distress level can indicate how serious the headache is, but you should always seek medical advice in the following circumstances:

➤ If it comes on suddenly.

➤ If it is accompanied by vomiting, irritability, fever, drowsiness, rash and/or neck stiffness.

➤ If the headache lasts longer than 24 hours.

➤ If the headaches are recurrent and starts early in the mornings.

➤ If the headaches are becoming increasingly severe and more frequent.

➤ If the headache pain is not relieved by simple, over-the-counter painkillers.

➤ If the headache follows an accident.

➤ If the headache occurs some hours after the child has suffered a bump on the head.

▷ The meningitis rash caused by meningococcal bacteria has a dark red/blue, paint-speckled look. Test for it by pressing a clear glass against the rash to see if it fades. If you can still see the rash through the glass, call for an ambulance.

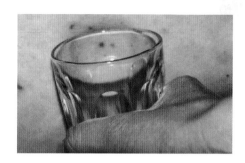

MENINGITIS

A headache can be a sign of meningitis – an infection of the linings covering the brain that is caused by either a bacterium or a virus. It is very worrying for all parents, and difficult to recognize, as it may resemble other, lesser infections.

While a headache is often a principal symptom of meningitis, other signs – such as high fever, drowsiness, cold hands and feet, neck stiffness, light sensitivity and/or profuse vomiting – may be more obvious. A child who has been mildly unwell and then worsens should be examined by a doctor. In bacterial meningitis, there may be a characteristic rash, but this is one of the later symptoms. (In babies with any kind of meningitis, they may just be non-specifically unwell and do not generally have neck stiffness.)

A WORD ON RASHES

Children often develop rashes when they are unwell. As well as meningitis, infections such as chicken pox, measles and German measles have a specific rash that helps diagnose the condition. Many unspecific viral infections cause a child to have a rash, often as their temperature settles and they improve. Drug allergies may cause rashes that resemble nettle stings.

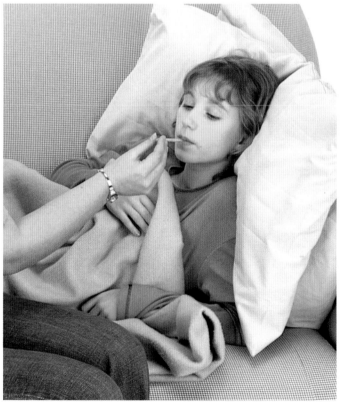

◁ Check your child's temperature and seek medical advice if you are concerned.

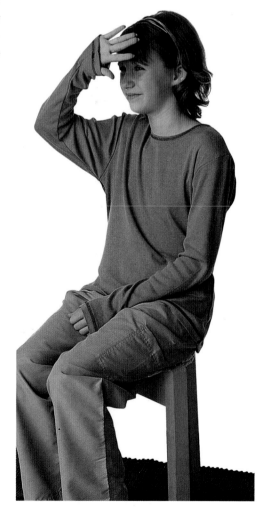

▷ A strong aversion to bright light of any kind can accompany various headaches – from migraines to those caused by meningitis.

Managing other problems

SEE ALSO
➤ Recognizing childhood illness, p110
➤ Coping with fever, p114
➤ Managing abdominal pain, p116

Children's immature immune systems make them very susceptible to a range of minor infections, such as earache and sore throat. It is not uncommon, particularly during the winter, for children to have endless colds and other infections but these are rarely of an emergency nature and can be dealt with safely at home. Toothache tends to affect older children; it is important to look after teeth from babyhood to prevent tooth decay later. If your child is feeling feverish and generally unwell, do not overlook the possibility of a urinary tract infection.

Children are more prone than adults to mild infectious illnesses, probably because their immune systems are still developing and they have countless opportunities to pick up infections from other children. Sometimes these illnesses have serious consequences, such as short-term deafness or lots of time off school, but for the most part, they are minor, self-limiting problems that can be treated at home.

EARACHE

Practically every child has an earache at some stage. It often starts after a cold, the pain from the earache being caused by a build-up of infection behind the eardrum – a condition called otitis media. Pus builds up behind the drum, causing an unbearable increase in pressure that may be relieved when the eardrum finally bursts and lets the pus out. Most children get better in a few days without antibiotics, though these may be prescribed for severe cases. Earache may also be caused by an infection in the outer ear canal, a toothache that is radiating out to the ear or a foreign body in the ear. It can also accompany tonsillitis.

Sometimes a thick, gluey substance remains behind in the ear after otitis media and makes the child temporarily deaf for up to six months; this is called glue ear. Your doctor may examine the ear six weeks after the otitis media, and refer the child to a specialist if glue ear has developed.

FIRST AID FOR A CHILD WITH EARACHE

↓

Give the child a warm flannel or wrapped hot-water bottle to hold against the ear – it is comforting and pain-relieving.

↓

Try giving your child paracetamol syrup to relieve earache pain.

↓

Give frequent small amounts of fluids to stave off any mild dehydration that can worsen the pain.

↓

Prop up the child with pillows or cushions – this may be more comfortable

↓

Avoid getting water in the ear.

WHEN TO SEE A DOCTOR IF YOUR CHILD HAS EARACHE

These are the main pointers for when to seek expert advice:

➤ If the child has a high fever, especially if the fever lasts for longer than about 24 hours.

➤ If there is fluid or blood coming out of the ear.

➤ If there is a foreign body in the ear canal.

➤ If there is any swelling around the ear.

➤ If the child is not drinking, or is generally unwell.

➤ If there is any deafness.

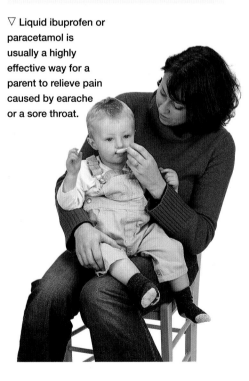

▽ Liquid ibuprofen or paracetamol is usually a highly effective way for a parent to relieve pain caused by earache or a sore throat.

◁ Lying with the affected ear against a wrapped hot-water bottle may help to ease earache pain.

TOOTHACHE

Toothache may be due to an infected tooth, in which case the pain is often throbbing and there may be obvious swelling around the gum area. It may settle by itself, but if it lasts longer than 24 hours the child should see a dentist.

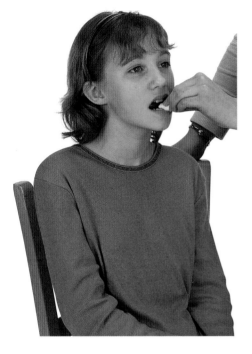

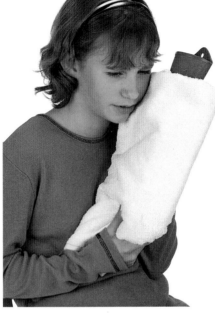

△ Try soaking a small piece of cotton wool in oil of cloves and placing this on the offending tooth – it can be surprisingly effective at relieving pain.

△ Another good way to relieve the pain of toothache is to hold a wrapped hot-water bottle against the offending cheek (but not if an abscess is suspected).

FIRST AID FOR TOOTHACHE

↓

Give your child ibuprofen or paracetamol syrup in the correct dose for the child's age.

↓

Unless an abscess is suspected, try placing a wrapped hot-water bottle against the cheek where the tooth can be felt.

↓

If the child is aged over two, soak a small plug of cotton wool in oil of cloves and hold it against the painful tooth. Oil of cloves is a highly effective pain-reliever and anti-inflammatory.

SORE THROAT

Most sore throats in children are caused by self-limiting viral infections and can be helped simply by giving your child ibuprofen or paracetamol syrup and plentiful fluids. Unless the child cannot swallow fluids or is very hot and unwell, they will usually get better after a few days without needing to see a doctor. However, do keep watch for a high temperature.

URINARY TRACT INFECTIONS

Children can also develop an infection in their urinary tract. This is usually due to bacteria from the gut entering the urinary system, but occasionally it is a sign of other problems within the urinary tract. If infection is not detected and treated, usually with antibiotics, it may damage the kidneys, so always seek medical advice if you suspect a urinary infection.

Symptoms include needing to pass urine more often, and cloudy, bloody or foul-smelling urine. Older children may have pain or a burning sensation when passing urine. Babies and young children may just be unwell with a fever, vomiting, diarrhoea, and feeding difficulties. If a child is hot and unwell for a few days with no other obvious cause for the fever (such as a cold, cough or runny nose), they may have a urinary tract infection. Simple dipstick tests carried out in the GP's surgery can usually tell if there is any infection.

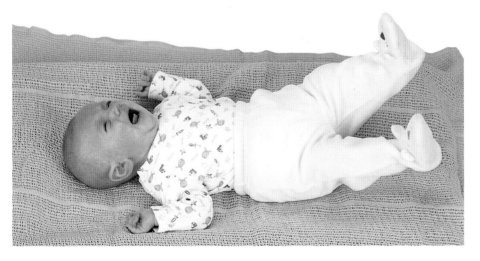

◁ Sore throats can be hard to diagnose in babies. A doctor may be able to tell by shining a light into the back of the throat while the baby is crying.

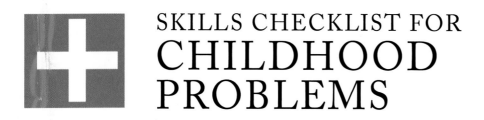

SKILLS CHECKLIST FOR
CHILDHOOD PROBLEMS

KEY POINTS

- Babies' and children's bodies function differently from those of adults ☐

- A baby or child can become seriously ill very rapidly – within the space of a few hours ☐

- Always be on the look-out for dehydration ☐

- If in doubt about a baby's or child's health, consult a doctor immediately ☐

- If abdominal pain, headache or breathing problems in a young child do not resolve quickly, get help; always seek help urgently if you suspect meningitis ☐

SKILLS LEARNED

- Recognizing a seriously ill child ☐

- Managing babies' crying, nappy rash, teething and colic ☐

- Treating fever, vomiting and diarrhoea ☐

- Dealing with abdominal pain and recognizing appendicitis ☐

- When to seek medical assistance for a child with breathing difficulties ☐

- When to seek medical assistance for headaches in a child ☐

- How to recognize meningitis ☐

- Action for earache, toothache, sore throats and possible urinary tract infections ☐

WOUNDS AND BLEEDING

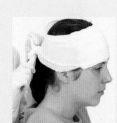

Minor wounds can be carefully cleaned and dressed at home. Any large wound, or a wound that is severely bleeding or contains foreign matter, must be professionally cleaned and treated at a hospital. If you are in any doubt about whether or not a wound needs stitching, take the casualty to hospital – the more promptly this is done, the better the outcome is likely to be. Protecting the first-aider from infection is another important issue when discussing wounds – you will find dealing with blood and other body fluids covered elsewhere.

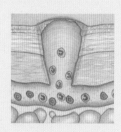

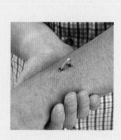

CONTENTS

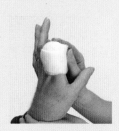

Types of wound

Even minor wounds can become infected and cause real problems with the casualty's health. However, most bites, grazes and cuts heal without too much trouble and can easily be treated at home. It is important that you are aware of the type of wound sustained so that you can carry out the appropriate first aid, described in detail on the following pages. Some wounds, such as puncture wounds, are more likely to cause damage to the underlying tissues and organs, and so they need professional assessment by medical personnel.

There are two main types of wound: closed and open. Closed wounds are usually caused by a blunt object, and vary from a small bruise to serious internal organ damage. A bruise accompanied by significant pain and swelling could signify underlying tissue damage. Open wounds range from surface abrasions to deep puncture wounds. Identifying the wound type helps first-aiders decide whether damage to underlying structures is likely.

ABRASIONS

Abrasions or grazes tend to be caused by a rough object applied at an angle, or by falling on to, or sliding along, a rough surface.

LACERATIONS

A laceration is a wound with jagged edges. These are often seen in car accidents, and may cause heavy bleeding (although some large lacerations show little bleeding). As the object causing the wound may be very dirty, the risk of subsequent infection is high.

INCISIONS

These are clean-edged cuts, such as those caused by a knife or broken glass, and they may be deep. Incision wounds may look relatively harmless, but there can be considerable damage to underlying tendons, nerves, blood vessels and even organs. Deep incisions may be life-threatening, especially if the injury is to the neck or around the chest or abdomen. Bleeding from incisions can take some time to stop. Superficial incisions often heal quickly and well as the edges come together cleanly.

PUNCTURE WOUNDS

Often caused by long, needle-like objects, these can be tricky to assess, as the size of the external wound gives no clue to how deep it goes (and the extent of tissue damage). Professional assessment may be needed.

BITES

All bites carry a high risk of infection, with human bites frequently becoming infected. It is sensible to seek medical advice for a human bite in case antibiotics are needed.

BRUISES

A bruise is discolouration of unbroken skin, caused by blood escaping from blood vessels. This may be minor, as from a small area of broken capillaries after a bump, or may indicate internal bleeding. Most look more alarming than they are, and gradually disappear. A new bruise is usually purple; older ones are brown, yellow or greenish.

SCARRING

The extent of scarring after an injury will vary depending on the individual.

➤ Children's skin is usually flawless and so any scarring will show up more clearly than in an adult. However, children also heal much more quickly and more effectively. A childhood scar will often fade completely over time.

➤ Some people are unlucky and their skin forms what are known as keloid scars. Here, cut or wounded skin heals over-enthusiastically, forming huge, often unsightly, scars.

GRITTY WOUNDS

Dirty or gritty wounds may need to be cleaned by a doctor or nurse to remove foreign bodies and prevent infection.

GUNSHOT WOUNDS

Guns can inflict many types of wound, and bleeding can be external and internal. Handguns, low-calibre rifles and shotguns fire fairly low-velocity projectiles, which usually stay in the body, while high-velocity bullets from military weapons often leave entry and exit wounds. High-velocity bullets create powerful shock waves that can break bones and cause widespread tissue damage.

AMPUTATIONS

The cutting or tearing off of body parts needs urgent help. Keep the severed part dry and cool and take it straight to hospital along with the casualty, as reattachment may be possible.

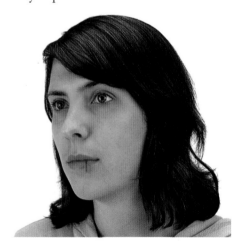

△ A cut that extends beyond the outer edge of the lip should be professionally treated. The cut edges need to be matched up exactly so they heal with minimal scarring.

TYPES OF WOUND

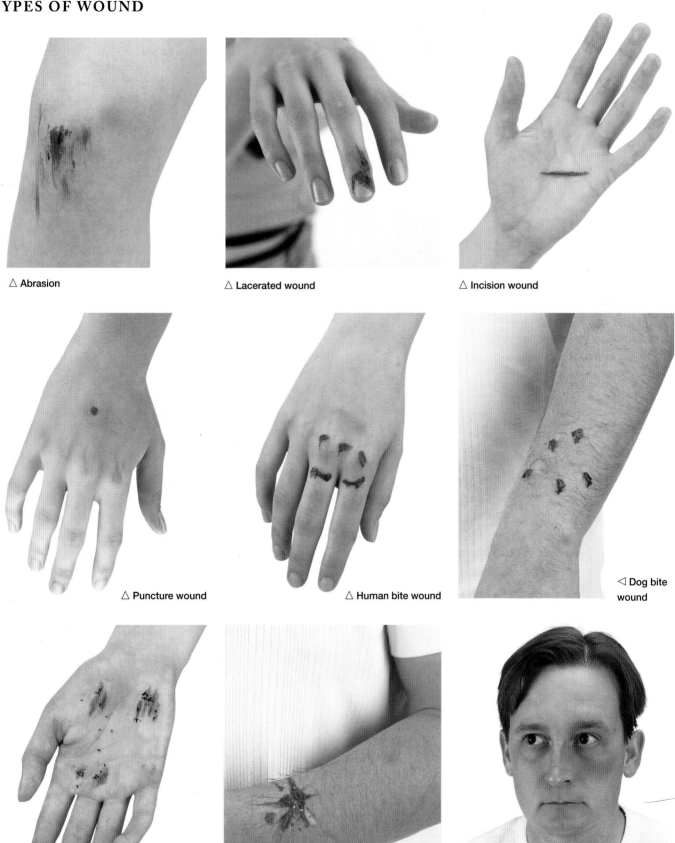

△ Abrasion

△ Lacerated wound

△ Incision wound

△ Puncture wound

△ Human bite wound

◁ Dog bite wound

△ Gritty wound

△ Gunshot wound

△ Bruising

Wounds and wound healing

SEE ALSO

➤ Dealing with major wounds, p134
➤ Controlling severe bleeding, p138
➤ Recognizing internal bleeding, p140

It is very useful for a first-aider to understand both how wounds affect our body as a whole, and how the body heals itself. Remember that any major loss to the body's constantly circulating blood supply is a potential emergency, as it can lead progressively from a drop in blood pressure through to collapse, unconsciousness, loss of breathing and heartbeat, and death. It is also vital to grasp the basic issues of wound care – including stemming blood loss and preventing infection – and also to be able to tell a minor from a major wound.

Our skin has many important functions. Nerves in the skin let us feel temperature, pain, touch and pressure. We get rid of water, salts and toxins through our skin, and changes to the flow of blood to the skin also help us to control our body temperature. The skin produces vitamin D, which helps to keep our bones strong and healthy. Our skin helps to protect the tissues lying beneath it from infection, trauma, dehydration and the harmful rays of the sun. The skin is our first line of defence and is easily damaged.

THE HEALING PROCESS

A superficial wound, such as a surface burn, only involves the topmost layer of skin, called the epidermis. This heals very quickly, in one to two days. A deeper wound takes longer to heal.

As blood rushes into the wound, it clots and effectively seals the wound. The wound then fills with white cells which kill any bugs and absorb foreign matter. However, in a dirty or contaminated wound,

INSIDE A BLOOD VESSEL

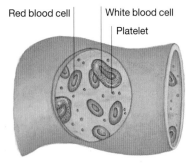

Red blood cell | White blood cell
Platelet

△ Important constituents of wound-healing: white and red blood cells and platelets.

HOW A WOUND HEALS

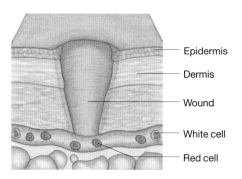

Epidermis
Dermis
Wound
White cell
Red cell

1 A large wound in the skin penetrates both the epidermis and the dermis.

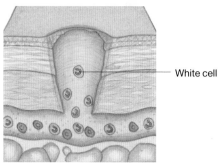

White cell

2 Blood rushing into the wound forms a clot as it exits. White cells fight infection.

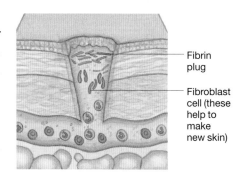

Fibrin plug
Fibroblast cell (these help to make new skin)

3 Strands of fibrin form a plug that slowly shrinks. New tissue forms underneath.

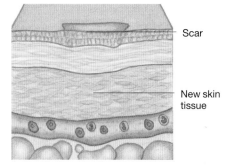

Scar
New skin tissue

4 The plug forms a scab, which eventually drops off. A scar remains.

the white blood cells may be overwhelmed and so infection begins. The wound may also be too big to allow clotting to stop the bleeding, resulting in continual blood loss (and, potentially, shock).

The body does all it can to reduce the bleeding from a wound. Damaged blood vessels within the wound go into spasm, and may stay in spasm for anything up to several hours. At the same time, platelet cells from the blood help to form a "plug" that may be enough to stop bleeding in a small wound. The body also uses a complex series of processes in the blood to produce strands of a substance called fibrin. These stick together to form a substantial protective plug, beneath which new skin tissue forms.

CLOTTING PROBLEMS

When someone's blood clots too easily, a clot may form in an unbroken blood vessel. This condition – "thrombosis" – is more

CLEANING AND DRESSING A WOUND

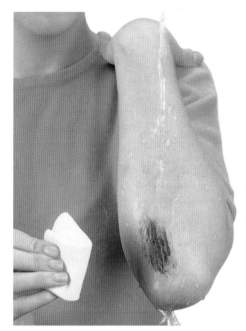

1 Expose the wound and clean it well (grit and dirt can cause infection and slow healing). Staunch any bleeding with direct pressure.

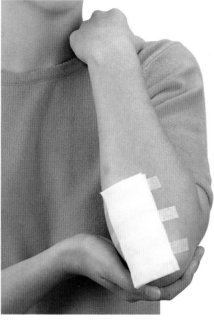

2 Cover small wounds with a plaster. Larger wounds: ideally a non-adhesive dressing and then a sterile dressing and bandage.

likely in people who have had major surgery, in smokers and after immobilisation or long-distance travel. If the blood is slow to clot – as in people taking blood-thinning medication or those who have the inherited condition haemophilia – severe bleeding may occur after relatively minor injuries.

MINOR AND MAJOR WOUNDS

A minor wound is a small wound that stops bleeding easily and is neither too deep nor infected. A brief look at the wound, and finding out how it occurred, will help you to make your assessment and proceed accordingly. You should treat it as a major/serious wound, and seek qualified medical aid, if:

• You can't stop the bleeding.
• The wound looks as if it could be deeper than 1–2mm, as it may need stitching.
• You think that there might be damage to underlying structures such as nerves and tendons – for example, if there seems to be any loss of function or numbness.
• The wound is dirty or contaminated, for example with soil or body fluids.
• There could be a foreign body in the wound.
• The wound may leave ugly scarring, as in facial wounds.
• The wound covers a large area.

   Stitching is needed on some wounds, to stop bleeding or prevent infection. Only use wound closure strips (thin adhesive

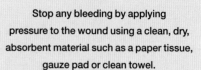

FIRST AID FOR MINOR WOUNDS

⬇

Wash your hands thoroughly. Avoid touching the wound, in order to prevent infection. Wear gloves if you have them.

⬇

Stop any bleeding by applying pressure to the wound using a clean, dry, absorbent material such as a paper tissue, gauze pad or clean towel.

⬇

Take a brief look and find out how and where the wound was caused.

⬇

Wash the wound under running tap water, or bottled drinking water/boiled and cooled water if you are somewhere where the tap water is unsuitable for drinking.

⬇

Dry the wound and apply a sterile adhesive dressing (plaster). For wounds over a larger area, it may be better to use a non-adhesive dressing, sterile dressing and bandage, if you have these to hand.

⬇

The casualty must keep the wound clean and dry for the next few days.

tape designed for smaller wounds) if the wound is shallow, clean, uninfected and there is nothing embedded in it.

KEEPING WOUNDS DRY

A wound must stay fairly dry in order to heal. Wounds kept enclosed and damp are more likely to become infected and can take longer to heal. If the pad of a plaster becomes wet, it should be carefully changed for a dry one. Some small, minor wounds, grazes and open blisters respond well to exposure to the air – provided dirt or dust are unlikely to get into them.

Tackling embedded objects

SEE ALSO
➤ Dealing with major wounds, p134
➤ Miscellaneous foreign bodies, p144

A "foreign body" that has lodged within a wound can cause infection. The object may be relatively easy to remove, as is usually the case with a splinter. However, if you are in any doubt about your ability to remove it safely and cleanly, leave it until you can get professional help. This is essential if the object is large or deeply embedded. A foreign body will frequently lead to infection around the site and impedes wound healing, so needs prompt attention. An embedded object left in the wound could cause an infection of the bloodstream.

Even tiny embedded objects can be very painful, and they may travel and cause further problems – such as pressure on a nerve or an annoying lump. Only remove an embedded body (or any foreign body) if the injury is minor and it is easy to do so; otherwise, get medical help.

Sometimes doctors decide to leave an embedded object in place, because it is more risky to remove it than to leave it where it is.

SMALL SPLINTERS

A small splinter of wood, metal or glass may come out if you gently squeeze the skin on either side. If it is protruding from the skin, it may be easy to remove with a pair of sterile tweezers. Sterilize them in boiling water for a few seconds, or hold them in a gas flame, and allow to cool before using. Pull the splinter out at the angle it went in. (Soft wood may need expert aid, as it falls apart easily.)

Small splinters that are visible just under the skin may be taken out very carefully with sterile tweezers and a sterile needle, but never dig around – you could cause great harm.

WARNING
If you cannot see a splinter, be very wary of poking around trying to remove it. Tiny objects under the skin often work their way out by themselves after a few days. However you should seek medical attention if there are any signs of infection, such as pus or red streaks on the skin.

FISH HOOKS

These can be very sharp and often get stuck in people's fingers. The barb means you may not be able to pull them back out the way they went in.
- Your first priority is to get medical help.
- Ask if the casualty has tetanus cover; if not, medical aid is particularly important.
- If the barb is visible, use pliers to cut the barb off and then pull the hook out.
- If you know that there is a barb, but cannot see it, only try to pull the hook out if no medical help is available. The person may require an anaesthetic before this is done, so it is best to take them to a doctor or nurse. If you do have to remove it, still get them to a doctor as fast as possible to be checked out.

DEALING WITH FISH HOOKS

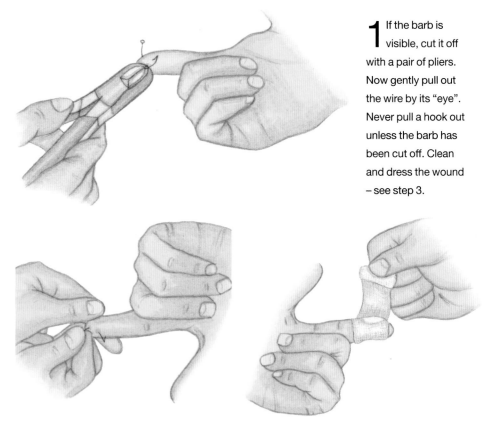

1 If the barb is visible, cut it off with a pair of pliers. Now gently pull out the wire by its "eye". Never pull a hook out unless the barb has been cut off. Clean and dress the wound – see step 3.

2 If the barb is not visible, and no medical help is available, push the hook firmly but carefully through the wound until the barb emerges. Cut the barb off and remove the wire.

3 When the wire is out, clean the wound with tap water, or sterile water (boiled and cooled) where tap water is suspect. Pad the wound with gauze and bandage it up. Seek medical help.

DRESSING ARM WOUNDS WITH EMBEDDED OBJECTS

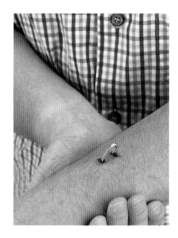

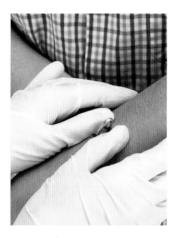

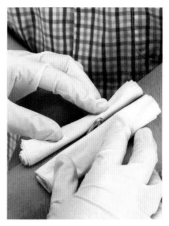

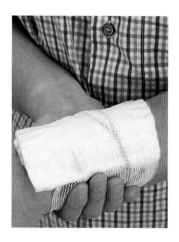

1 Do not try to remove this kind of embedded object as you may cause further damage. Your aim is to deal with bleeding and protect the area from infection, and to get aid promptly.

2 If the wound is bleeding, apply pressure to the surrounding area with your hands. Never apply pressure directly on to an embedded object. Elevating the wounded part will also help.

3 Place padding around the object. If possible, as it would be here, build this padding up until it is as high as the embedded object, ready to bandage over smoothly.

4 Bandage over the padding (or on either side of the object if it is a long one and still protrudes). Apply no direct pressure at all to the object. Now keep the wound elevated until help arrives.

LARGE EMBEDDED OBJECTS

If a large object is embedded in the wound, you should not try to remove it but should seek urgent medical help. This is especially important if the injury is to the chest or abdomen. The object may have cut through large blood vessels or even be embedded in the heart, but while it remains in the wound, it may act as a plug and prevent further bleeding. You could do just as much damage pulling it out as occurred as the object went in.

If someone is impaled, on a railing for example, do not try to get them off it. Only do this is if the person needs to be resuscitated, in which case this takes priority. Instead, help the person to stay still and try to support their weight in as comfortable a position as possible. Cover them with a coat or blanket to keep them warm, and call the emergency services immediately, or ask a helper to do so. Tell the operator that the casualty is impaled, as the fire brigade will be required with cutting equipment. Reassure the casualty that help is on its way, and keep talking to them to keep them calm.

▷ Small children playing with pencils or crayons is one of the many everyday situations that can turn into an embedded object incident – if a child trips they may embed a pencil, pen or other pointed object in their face.

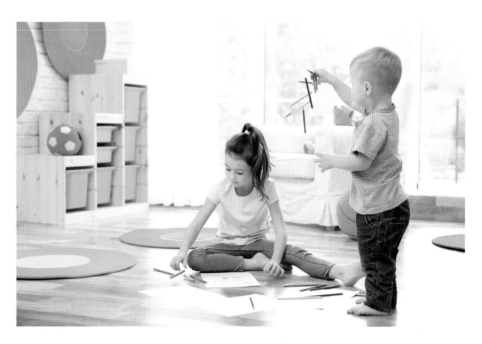

Treating infected wounds

SEE ALSO
➤ Types of wound, p126
➤ Tackling embedded objects, p130

When a wound becomes infected, it will need very careful monitoring and handling. If not treated correctly, the wound may become increasingly infected, spreading to a larger and larger area of the body. An infected wound can also lead to poisoning of the bloodstream, a serious condition known as septicaemia. Bites, whether inflicted by a human or a dog, cat or other animal, are all likely to cause infection unless the site of the wound has been professionally cleaned and treated. The person will often need to take antibiotics.

Sometimes a wound becomes infected despite having been cleaned and dressed correctly, and kept clean and dry. Certain types of wound are more prone to infection – bites, for example, and particularly human or cat bites. If there is a lot of blood under a wound and this is not cleared out and its reappearance prevented, or if a wound is deep and dirty, then infection is more likely. Some people are more vulnerable to infection. These include those with diabetes, those with a compromised immune system (due to drugs or illness), and alcoholics.

There are usually many warning signs that a wound has become infected, giving plenty of time for it to be treated with antibiotics and drainage if necessary.

SIGNS AND SYMPTOMS OF INFECTION

➤ An infection may start to show itself within a few hours of the injury, or may not appear for several days.

➤ Be aware of pain around the site of the wound – this is often an early sign of infection.

➤ Watch for any redness, tenderness or swelling under the wound, red streaks or pus coming from it, or for the start of a fever.

➤ Swollen glands nearby (such as in the neck, armpit or groin).

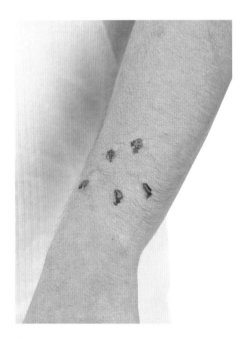

△ This wound, caused by a dog, will need to be assessed by a doctor. Antibiotics may be given as a preventative measure.

FIRST AID FOR INFECTION

↓

Cover the wound with a sterile bandage. Leave the surrounding area visible, so that you can monitor signs of spreading infection – vital information for the doctor.

↓

Elevate and support the infected area if possible. For example, if a forearm is infected, the raised arm could be placed so that its elbow rests on some books topped with a sweater as cushioning.

↓

Get the casualty to a doctor as soon as possible.

WOUNDS THAT ARE PRONE TO INFECTION

Any wound can become infected, but certain kinds are more at risk:

➤ Bite wounds: animal or human.

➤ Wounds/scratches from human nails or the claws of animals.

➤ Stab (penetrating) wounds.

➤ Wounds sustained while working: in soil or manure; in or around waste or excrement; with animals.

➤ Wounds from dirty tools or objects, such as garden injuries or dirty nails in the foot while working on building sites.

➤ Wounds with embedded objects, especially softwood splinters, grit and plant thorns.

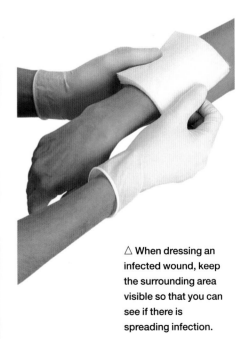

△ When dressing an infected wound, keep the surrounding area visible so that you can see if there is spreading infection.

SIGNS OF INFECTION

You may notice the first signs of infection in and around a wound within hours but it frequently takes longer to manifest itself. The infection may not surface until a day or two after the injury when the casualty may have more or less forgotten the injury.

Pain, redness, tenderness and swelling are all signs of infection. The casualty may also experience fever and notice pus oozing from the wound.

SPREADING INFECTION

Infection may spread under the skin (cellulitis) and/or into the bloodstream (septicemia). Cellulitis may appear even without an obvious wound, and is often from an unsuspected insect bite.

If the wound is near a joint, infection may spread into the joint. This is particularly true of human bites on the knuckles – these may be "self-inflicted", occurring when someone aims a punch at someone's face and sustains a laceration to the knuckles from their victim's teeth. Joint infection can lead to a serious condition called septic arthritis. This may occur with no obvious wound, especially in babies, older people and those with compromised immune systems. Suspect septic arthritis if the joint feels hot or swollen, or if it is exceedingly painful, especially with movement, and the victim develops a fever or chills and fatigue with generalized weakness. Seek rapid medical attention in this case.

You should suspect cellulitis if there is a spreading redness and swelling beyond the wound site. The glands in the armpits, neck or groins may be sore and tender, and there may be a red line going up the limb towards the glands. The wound may leak clear fluid or pus and the person may develop a fever. They should see a doctor urgently – take them to the nearest emergency department if necessary – as they may need antibiotics and possibly further treatment in hospital.

Septicemia means bacteria or other germs are in the bloodstream, which can cause a very serious condition called sepsis. Suspect sepsis if the casualty feels extremely unwell with a fever, thirst, shivering, lethargy, vomiting, rapid breathing or mental confusion.

Sepsis is potentially life-threatening so call an ambulance as they need urgent hospital treatment and possibly admission to the intensive care unit.

TETANUS

A bacterium commonly found in soil and animal feces, tetanus can contaminate the tiniest of wounds. In general, the dirtier the wound, the greater the chance of infection, but some 20 per cent of people with tetanus infection have no obvious wound through which the infection could have entered. It may take three months for signs of the disease to develop, although it is usually obvious within two weeks.

Tetanus is a particularly vicious disease. The tetanus bacterium produces a neurotoxin that causes painful muscle spasms (lockjaw) as well as having a detrimental effect on the heart. People still develop this infection worldwide, and it is a huge killer. However, you can be vaccinated against the disease – both as general preventative and if an injury is sustained that puts you at greater risk of developing it.

Tetanus immunization

Most babies in Western countries are given immunization against tetanus with at least three doses starting at about two or three months, followed by a booster around three or four years old, and again in adolescence. Some countries offer adults further boosters every ten years. If a casualty is not sure whether they are fully immunized, they may be given either the full course or a booster dose. If the wound is very dirty, they may be given tetanus immunoglobulin as a further precaution.

If there is any doubt about tetanus cover, it is best to assume the person is not immune and get them seen by a doctor.

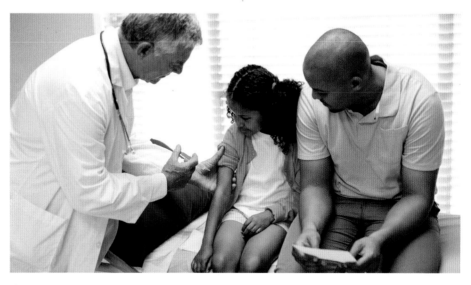

△ A child is given the tetanus vaccine (combined with diphtheria and pertussis vaccines). When dealing with anyone with a wound, no matter how clean it looks, always try to check if their immunization against tetanus is up to date. Older people in particular may never have had any routine tetanus boosters.

Dealing with major wounds

SEE ALSO

➤ Controlling severe bleeding, p138

➤ Recognizing internal bleeding, p140

➤ Managing rib fractures, p160

The two main priorities when treating major wounds are to stop the bleeding and get help as fast as possible. You must call the emergency services as fast as possible because large blood loss is very serious, and because the wound may conceal further internal injury. Try to dress the wound effectively if you can, although large wounds will usually need professional cleaning and stitching in a hospital's accident and emergency department. While you wait for paramedics to arrive, keep the casualty warm and reassure them that help is on the way.

Large wounds may bleed profusely and signify greater problems internally. When wounds are over the abdomen or chest, particular care must be taken to avoid exacerbating the situation. You should not attempt to remove an object embedded in a wound (see page 130), nor should you try to stop the bleeding by applying a tourniquet (see page 136).

If possible, wear protective gloves before treating the bleeding; otherwise wash your hands well both before and afterwards. Once you have stopped the bleeding, cleaned any debris from the wound (do not wash it) and dressed it, call for an ambulance if this has not already been done by a helper.

The casualty may lose consciousness and may also develop symptoms of shock. Do not leave them alone except to call for help. Keep the person warm while you wait for the emergency services to arrive.

BASIC FIRST AID FOR MAJOR WOUNDS

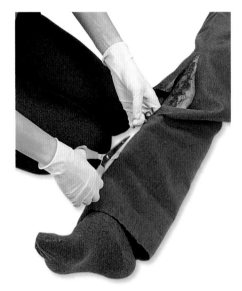

1 Wear protective gloves. Expose the wound. Do not drag clothing over the wound, but cut or lift aside the clothing.

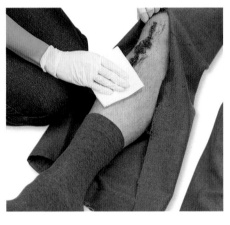

2 Using a wet gauze pad, gently clear the wound surface of any obvious debris such as large shards of glass, lumps of grit or mud. If necessary rinse the wound under clean running tap water, but if particles remain embedded, leave them for the hospital to deal with.

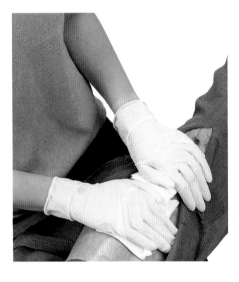

3 Control bleeding with direct pressure and then by elevating the limb.

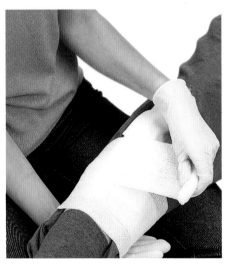

4 Apply a bandage to the wound. If blood seeps through, add a second dressing on top.

5 Keep the casualty warm and rested until help arrives. (If the casualty is suffering from shock, keep both legs raised above heart level, comfortably supported.)

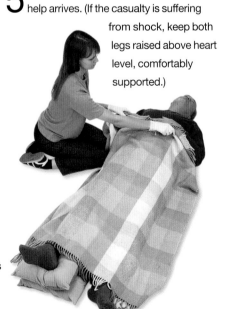

ABDOMINAL WOUNDS

There are many organs within the abdominal cavity, all of which may become injured and bleed profusely with little sign of external damage. Any penetrating injury to the abdomen could damage the internal organs, and might also introduce infection into the abdominal cavity, leading to peritonitis. If a penetrating object – such as a knife or a piece of metal – remains in the wound, it should be left where it is, or even more damage may be inflicted pulling it out.

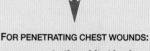

△ When dealing with abdominal wounds, try to keep the casualty's legs elevated at about this height or slightly higher, with knees bent.

CHEST WOUNDS

Take great care when dealing with any injury in the chest area. Look out for breathing difficulty, a penetrating wound, or a "flail chest" (multiple rib fractures causing unusual movement). These conditions can indicate life-threatening damage that needs emergency attention.

In many cases, especially after a high-speed car accident or a fall, the casualty may have fluid or bruising in the lungs, which will make them very short of breath. Keep them warm, sitting up and supported, and reassure them, until the emergency services arrive.

First-aid efforts are potentially life-saving where a casualty has an injury that penetrates the chest wall. This may occur as a result of a rib fracture (even a person with a simple rib fracture may perforate a lung if they bend at an awkward angle), a stabbing or a gunshot injury, for example. The casualty may end up with air entering the lung cavity as they breathe in, and this will eventually lead to lung collapse. If the lung is perforated, air escapes out of the lung into the space between the lung and the chest wall, and will again cause the lung to collapse. These cases need urgent help.

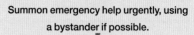
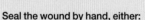

Coping with severed body parts

SEE ALSO

➤ What is first aid?, p12

➤ Full resuscitation sequence, p33

➤ Dealing with shock, p68

➤ Controlling severe bleeding, p138

When a person loses a finger, hand, toe, ear or limb as the result of an accident, there may be considerable bleeding and the person is likely to suffer shock. Your priorities are to stop the bleeding and to get the person to hospital or summon the emergency services immediately.

It is vital that you take the body part with you, if you can, as it may be possible for it to be reattached. Keeping it cool improves the chances of this, but you should not freeze or place ice directly next to the body part. It is also important that you do your best to keep the casualty calm.

A severing of a body part by whatever means, whether accidental or surgical, is known as an amputation. Accidental amputations are most commonly the result of occupational injuries inflicted by power tools or industrial machinery; they also can often occur during a road accident. The body part may be torn, crushed or sliced off. The smaller parts of the body such as fingers and toes are most likely to be involved.

The main priority in the case of an amputation is to stop the bleeding, but also to remember to take the amputated body part to the hospital with the casualty. If a

body part is kept at 4°C (39.2°F), there is still a chance that it can be sewn back or "re-implanted" within 12–24 hours.

If you have to take a severed body part to hospital, keep it dry and cool – wrapped in plastic, then protected with padding and placed in ice (see flowchart). **Do not**:

• Let ice or water come into direct contact with the part – this causes tissue damage.

• Use dry ice or chemical additives.

• Freeze the part.

• Use cotton wool or fluffy dressings, as the fibres may stick to the part.

• Wash the part, especially not with soap or disinfectant.

WARNING

Tourniquets are emergency devices for stemming bleeding – the simplest form is a very tight bandage. Tourniquets risk making the tissue damage even worse by cutting off its blood supply, and thus necessitating even more of the limb being amputated. They also lessen the chances of successful re-implantation. This is why they should never be used in first aid, except by highly trained professionals under specific circumstances.

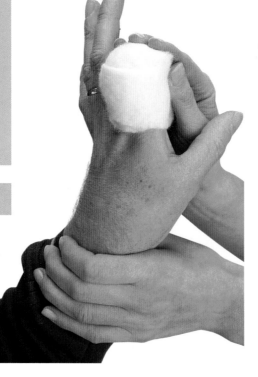

FIRST AID AFTER AN AMPUTATION

Follow DRABC and if necessary, administer basic life support.

⬇

Control bleeding by applying pressure directly to the wound using gauze cloths, and elevation. If you have a sterile dressing, place it on the wound.

⬇

Call the emergency services and tell them that the case involves amputation. Treat the casualty for shock.

⬇

If pressure does not stop the bleeding, press harder and elevate higher. Do not consider using a tourniquet unless you are a trained professional (see Warning box).

⬇

Keep the amputated part dry, protected and cool: double-wrap it in plastic, then add padding and place in a container or bag of ice. Do not allow the part to come into direct contact with water or ice.

◁ Pressure and elevation are the key things for a first-aider to remember when trying to stop bleeding after an amputation.

Managing crush injuries

SEE ALSO
➤ Full resuscitation sequence, p33
➤ Dealing with shock, p68
➤ BONE AND MUSCLE INJURIES, p147

A casualty who has suffered a crush injury requires the urgent attention of paramedics, and immediate ambulance transfer to hospital. Crush injuries can occur in road accidents, from falling heavy furniture in buildings that suffer structural damage, and in industrial and agricultural accidents when someone is crushed by heavy machinery. The crush injury may result in serious complications, so it is essential to call the emergency services as quickly as possible, and to control any external bleeding until help arrives.

In all cases involving trapped casualties or crush injuries, call the emergency services immediately. As well as paramedics, the fire service may be needed to release the casualty. Only attempt to do so yourself if you can do so safely.

CRUSHED HANDS, FINGERS, FEET AND TOES

If these are caught in machinery or tricky to release, leave this to the professionals. If the crushed part has already been released:
- Deal with any bleeding, and apply a sterile dressing.
- Treat as for fractures, with padding, immobilization and elevation.

CRUSHED LIMBS

The offending object may be just bulky enough to cut off the blood supply, or a hard impact or very heavy object may have caused fractures and severe tissue damage.

If left for too long, toxins, waste products and blood clots can develop in crushed limbs. When released, these may lead to fatal kidney and heart failure. However, this usually takes well over 30 minutes to occur, by which time emergency helpers will hopefully be in control. Where a crushed limb has been released, treat it as a fracture.

CRUSHED ABDOMEN AND PELVIS

Any crushing or blunt impact to the abdomen can cause severe internal bleeding and damage. The casualty may show no outward signs at first, so the accident history could be your only clue to a potentially severe condition.

The ideal first-aid position here is the "shock" position, with legs raised – unless this might worsen damage, in which case keep them still. If they need to vomit, you may need to turn them on their side. Do not sit them up. Treat a crushed pelvis as a fracture, and get help very quickly.

CRUSHED CHEST

A heavy weight on the chest can cause a casualty's breathing to stop. Check that nothing under the object is penetrating the chest and then carefully lift the object off, if you can. If breathing has stopped, start chest compressions. Conscious casualties may find it easier to breathe sitting up, but keeping them in their current position until help arrives will often prevent further damage.

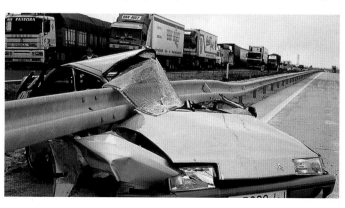

◁ Road accidents are a major cause of crush injuries. Such accidents also have great potential for further disaster. Never step into a dangerous environment or try to release anyone if you are risking your own safety or could cause them further harm.

FIRST AID FOR CRUSH INJURIES

Make any threatening structures/objects safe/stable, but only if this will not endanger yourself or the casualty.

Check the casualty's ABC and contact the emergency services.

Release the victim if possible, but **do not endanger yourself or further endanger the casualty.** If the crushing force has been in place for some time, be prepared for the casualty's condition to deteriorate rapidly: keep monitoring ABC and start resuscitation if necessary.

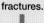

Treat any injuries in order of their importance and severity. If injuries involve the head or neck, make sure that these are kept still (to avoid worsening any possible spinal injury). Treat any bleeding or fractures.

Treat for shock, but only raise the legs if pretty certain there are no leg fractures.

Keep the casualty warm, still and as comfortable as possible. Continue to monitor them until help arrives.

Controlling severe bleeding

SEE ALSO

➤ Dealing with head injury, p80

➤ Dealing with major wounds, p134

Stemming blood flow from a large wound is a life-saving procedure. The main method used combines pressure and elevation. Apply direct pressure to the site of the blood loss with your hand or the casualty's hand, unless the wound contains foreign matter such as glass. In this case, squeeze the edges of the wound together. Elevating the wounded area also helps to stem blood loss – even if a limb is fractured, your priority is to stop the bleeding, especially if it is heavy, and then worry about the fracture. However, try to handle fractured limbs gently.

Injury to an artery can lead to a life-threatening loss of blood in a very short time. Stemming the blood flow may save the casualty's life and is your main priority as a first-aider (once you have dealt with the casualty's ABC, that is).

With more superficial wounds, bleeding may sometimes seem profuse without, in fact, being too dangerous. Head wounds are a good case in point here. The scalp has a very rich blood supply, so head wounds often bleed profusely, even if they are quite superficial. Do not, however, automatically go to the other extreme and assume that it is not serious. Also, always try to assess any underlying damage – especially important with head wounds.

CONTROLLING BLEEDING ON A HEAD WOUND

Dealing with heavy bleeding from a head wound varies slightly in some details from tackling heavy bleeding from other sites (see text elsewhere on other types of wound).

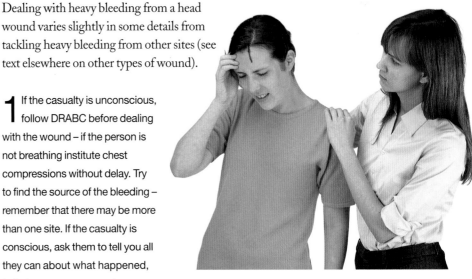

1 If the casualty is unconscious, follow DRABC before dealing with the wound – if the person is not breathing institute chest compressions without delay. Try to find the source of the bleeding – remember that there may be more than one site. If the casualty is conscious, ask them to tell you all they can about what happened, to help your assessment.

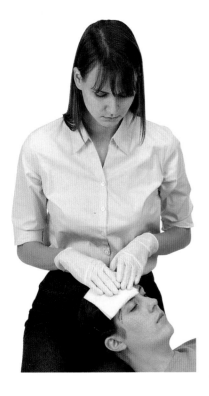

2 To control bleeding, place firm pressure directly over the wound using a clean pad (a sterile first-aid dressing or a towel, sanitary towel, tea towel or T-shirt). Use gentle pressure if you suspect a fracture. Getting the casualty to lie down with head and shoulders raised (and supported) helps to reduce pressure within the head. Send for emergency help, if you have not already done so.

3 Secure the dressing with a roller bandage or equivalent. If the casualty's general condition seems good, sitting them up may reduce bleeding, but don't get them sitting up and lying down like a yo-yo. Make sure that the dressing covers the whole wound. If blood starts oozing through the dressing, don't take the original dressing off but place another one on top.

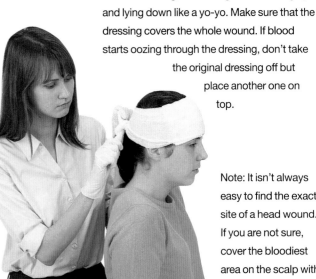

Note: It isn't always easy to find the exact site of a head wound. If you are not sure, cover the bloodiest area on the scalp with a dressing.

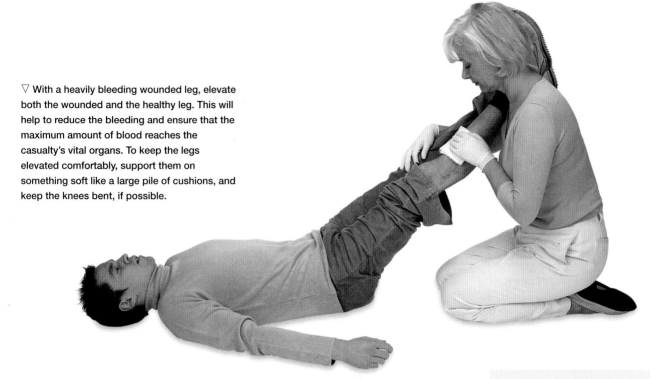

▽ With a heavily bleeding wounded leg, elevate both the wounded and the healthy leg. This will help to reduce the bleeding and ensure that the maximum amount of blood reaches the casualty's vital organs. To keep the legs elevated comfortably, support them on something soft like a large pile of cushions, and keep the knees bent, if possible.

FIRST AID FOR CONTROLLING SEVERE BLEEDING

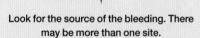

↓

Look for the source of the bleeding. There may be more than one site.

↓

Lay the person down. Elevate their legs, and the bleeding part if possible. Place firm pressure over the wound using a clean pad large enough to cover the whole wound area. For the pad, use a sterile first-aid dressing or improvise with a towel, sanitary towel, tea towel or T-shirt. Call the emergency services.

Secure your pad with a bandage or equivalent; make sure that the dressing covers the whole wound.

If blood starts oozing through the dressing, don't take the original dressing off but place another dressing on top.

STEMMING BLOOD FLOW

The most effective method is applying direct pressure to the wound and, where possible, keeping the body part elevated – gravity naturally lessens the flow. If an object is embedded in the wound, compress the edges on either side of the object. Stemming blood flow by applying pressure to the main arteries supplying the bleeding site is not advised for the average first-aider – this can be tricky.

Bleeding may be copious in a head injury, and you may be hampered by the person's hair. Apply a dressing larger than the wound, bandage it in place and get medical help rapidly. If a limb is bleeding

THIGH INJURIES

A cut on the thigh can easily sever an artery with life-threatening results. The use of very sharp knives by butchers can lead to an injury known as "butcher's thigh". The artery running down the front of the thigh is close to the skin's surface. If the butcher's knife slips and cuts through this artery, rapid and sometimes fatal blood loss follows. Many butchers have bled to death in this way over the centuries. These days, however, the injury is more likely to be caused by knives used in crafts or DIY.

TYPES OF BLEEDING

From arteries

➤ Blood spurts rhythmically with the beat of the heart.

➤ Blood is bright red.

➤ Blood loss is rapid and quickly leads to shock.

From veins

➤ Blood is darker red with a bluish hue.

➤ Blood oozes steadily.

➤ Blood loss is slower but can eventually cause shock.

heavily, elevate it to reduce the blood flow to the area. If the wound is on a leg, lift both legs to maximize blood flow to the casualty's vital organs, especially their brain. Even a fractured limb should be elevated if it is bleeding very profusely.

AVOID TOURNIQUETS

These should never be used to control serious bleeding except by fully trained medical professionals, and only by them as an absolute last resort. The scenario in which use of a tourniquet is most likely to occur is when a limb has been partially or wholly severed, when it has very little chance of survival anyway.

Recognizing internal bleeding

SEE ALSO
➤ Dealing with shock, p68
➤ Bleeding from orifices, p142

It is vital that the first-aider is able to recognize the signs of internal bleeding and take appropriate action. Internal bleeding can be caused by stabbing or shooting, which also cause external bleeding, or by a fall, a crush injury, a punch or kick, a fractured bone or an ulcer, which may not. The signs include cold and clammy, pale skin, weakness, thirst, and blood coming from an orifice. Internal bleeding is a medical emergency and if you suspect it you should call the emergency services at once.

Unlike external bleeding, internal bleeding is a difficult condition to assess. It may be unclear what is happening until the problem is at a late stage, when the casualty has already bled a great deal and is going into shock. Detecting internal bleeding early on, and calling an ambulance, is by far the most helpful action you can perform under these circumstances.

CAUSES OF INTERNAL BLEEDING

Stabbing and shooting are obvious causes of internal bleeding, and the size of an external wound is often no indicator of the extent of the internal damage. Internal blood vessels and organs can tear and rupture without any obvious external damage.

An injury caused by an object that is not sharp enough to penetrate the skin is called "blunt trauma". This may be due to any number of causes – from a fall, a car accident or crush injury to direct punches or kicks. A warning sign of possible internal damage would be bruising on the skin, especially if it is over the abdomen or chest.

Another common cause of internal bleeding is fractured bones, especially the femur and pelvis, which quickly lead to serious blood loss. Conditions such as duodenal and gastric ulcers may lead to profuse internal bleeding. People with blood-clotting abnormalities such as haemophilia, or who are on anti-clotting treatment such as warfarin, may bleed heavily after relatively minor injuries. Many diseases affecting the liver may adversely affect the blood's ability to clot, and may also cause varices, which are like internal varicose veins – these can bleed catastrophically.

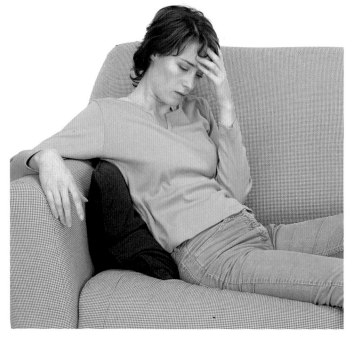

◁ Internal bleeding could be indicated if a casualty has just had a fall or a period of abdominal pain and exhibits the following symptoms: cold, clammy, pale skin, weakness and inability to stand up.

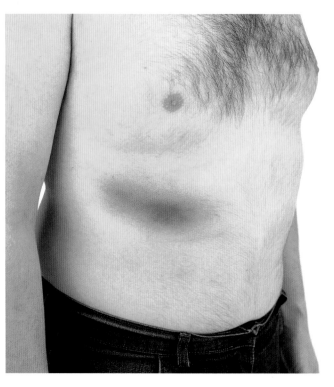

◁ Bruising on the skin, especially if it is over the abdomen or chest, may indicate internal bleeding.

SIGNS AND SYMPTOMS OF INTERNAL BLEEDING

➤ If someone shows signs of shock. This is indicated by: cold, clammy, pale skin; loss of consciousness on sitting or standing up; thirst and general weakness; a fast, weak pulse.

➤ If the victim coughs up blood or vomits blood or anything that looks like blood (bits of gritty brown vomit that look like coffee grounds are a classic sign of a bleeding duodenal ulcer).

➤ If they have passed blood from their rectum (back passage), especially black tar-like stools that smell strongly. This is likely to be due to a bleeding ulcer in the stomach or duodenum.

➤ If they have been in an accident where they fell from a height, or stopped suddenly, as in a car accident, or fell off a bicycle on to the handle bars.

➤ If there is profuse bleeding from the vagina with no obvious cause.

➤ If the casualty has bruising, tenderness and/or swelling, especially if it is over the abdominal area. The kidney, spleen and liver may bleed after an accident. There may be blood in the urine, abdominal pain, and the abdomen may be visibly swollen.

➤ If a woman is in the early stages of pregnancy, particularly between 6 and 8 weeks. A pregnancy in the Fallopian tube (known as an ectopic pregnancy) may cause profuse internal bleeding that is life-threatening. The woman may have warning pains low in her abdomen, but not invariably.

➤ If there is blood coming from the nose, ear or mouth after a head injury. This may be due to a fracture of the skull.

▷ Call for the emergency services the minute you suspect internal bleeding. The casualty needs urgent medical attention.

WARNING
Signs of internal bleeding may not appear for some time after the incident that caused it, and it may be after considerable blood is lost from the circulation. This is why, if there is any risk that an accident or condition could cause internal bleeding, the casualty should be checked over promptly by a medical professional.

FIRST AID FOR SUSPECTED INTERNAL BLEEDING

If the injury is caused by an object that is still penetrating the skin, do not try to take the object out. You could do as much or more damage as occurred when it went in, and it may be "plugging" the wound.

Call the emergency services immediately.

Initiate the DRABC procedures and monitor the casualty's breathing – they may vomit, so make sure this cannot choke them. If they stop breathing, start chest compressions.

If the casualty is conscious, lie them flat and raise up their legs, to alleviate shock – ideally raised significantly and supported comfortably (on a pile of cushions, say), with knees bent. If they become unconscious, place them into the recovery position, but still keep their legs elevated.

Do not let them eat or drink anything.

Keep the casualty warm and loosen any tight clothing.

Bleeding from orifices

SEE ALSO

➤ Dealing with shock, p68

➤ Recognizing internal bleeding, p140

➤ Tackling skull and facial fractures, p152

Bleeding can occur from the mouth, nose, ear, urethra, rectum or vagina (though menstrual bleeding is normal, obviously). These may require first aid to staunch the flow if possible, and you should also check for signs of shock. Bear in mind that dealing with another person's body fluids puts you and them at risk of infection, so use gloves, if they are available. If you do not have gloves, wash your hands well both before and afterwards. Bleeding from orifices with no obvious cause may indicate internal bleeding, which requires urgent medical attention.

VAGINAL BLEEDING

There can be many reasons for non-menstrual vaginal bleeding, including pregnancy problems and sexual assault.

Bleeding in early pregnancy is a warning that miscarriage may be imminent or might already have occurred, and the bleeding can be very heavy, including clots that look like lumps of liver. When the bleeding is this heavy, you must get medical aid urgently.

In cases of sexual assault, the casualty is likely to be very distressed, so use great tact and care. Ideally, the casualty should not get undressed or wash until seen by the police, to aid collection of forensic evidence. Your priorities are to staunch the flow, reassure the victim and contact the emergency services.

BLEEDING FROM ORIFICES – POSSIBLE SITES

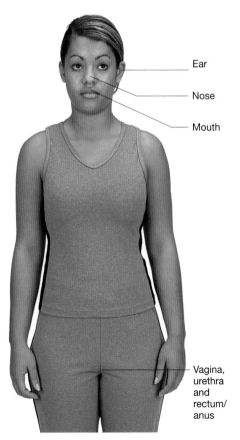

- Ear
- Nose
- Mouth
- Vagina, urethra and rectum/anus

RECTAL BLEEDING

Bleeding from the rectum can be divided into two types. Bright red blood is usually due to problems lower down in the gut, most commonly piles or a small tear after passing a difficult motion, although there may be more sinister causes. Dark, sticky, black motions indicate old blood from higher up in the gut. It is the dark blood that requires the most urgent action, as it signifies heavy bleeding that could be life-threatening.

VOMITING BLOOD

Bleeding from the stomach and upper digestive system may be bright red or resemble coffee grounds (it may also come from a swallowed nosebleed). The casualty may appear in shock, or seem almost normal. All vomiting of blood should be treated as serious. Sit the casualty down, or if pale or shocked lie them on their side, and seek urgent medical help.

COUGHING UP BLOOD

This usually appears as small spots mixed in sputum, and causes include lung disease and lung damage. Sit the casualty up, supported and quiet. If their breathing is distressed, or their history suggests lung damage, get help fast. Anyone who coughs up blood must be seen by a medical professional.

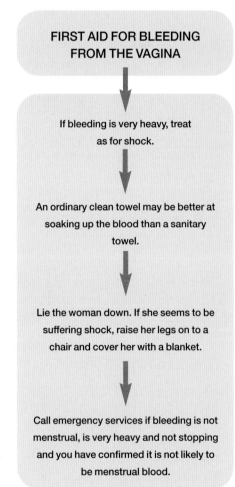

FIRST AID FOR BLEEDING FROM THE VAGINA

If bleeding is very heavy, treat as for shock.

An ordinary clean towel may be better at soaking up the blood than a sanitary towel.

Lie the woman down. If she seems to be suffering shock, raise her legs on to a chair and cover her with a blanket.

Call emergency services if bleeding is not menstrual, is very heavy and not stopping and you have confirmed it is not likely to be menstrual blood.

FIRST AID FOR RECTAL BLEEDING

Check the casualty for signs of shock and act accordingly, then seek urgent medical attention.

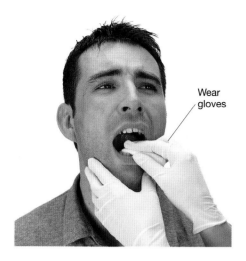

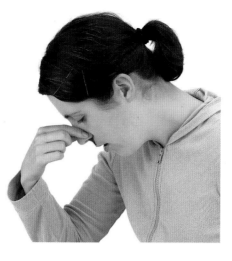

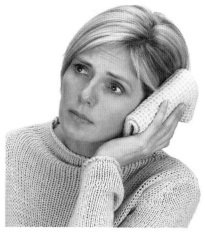

Wear gloves

△ Bleeding from the mouth: place a wad of sterile gauze in the mouth and ask the casualty to bite down on it to soak up the blood.

△ Nosebleed: the casualty should breathe though the mouth and pinch the soft end of the nose. If it still bleeds, they should pinch harder.

△ Bleeding from the ear: place a sterile pad or clean towel over the ear and tilt the head to drain out the blood. Call a doctor immediately.

BLEEDING FROM THE MOUTH

This may arise from biting the inside of the mouth, or after a tooth has fallen out or been extracted. It can occur after violent impact, along with possible concussion or jaw fracture. The main concern should be keeping the airway clear of blood, especially if the person is unconscious.

FIRST AID FOR BLEEDING FROM THE MOUTH

Wear gloves. If the person has lost a tooth or had one extracted, place a wad of sterile gauze against the tooth socket and get them to bite down on it. Change it if it becomes soaked. With a mouth wound, ask the person to apply pressure with their finger and thumb until bleeding stops. Make sure they replace the pad every 10 minutes.

Tell the person to spit out the blood – they may vomit if they swallow it. If the bleeding ceases, they should avoid hot drinks for at least 12 hours.

If bleeding persists, seek medical or dental advice.

BLEEDING FROM THE NOSE

Nosebleeds usually start at the lower end of the nose, although in older people or those with very high blood pressure, they may come from the back of the nose and be harder to stop. Nosebleeds often occur during or after a cold when the lining is inflamed. Other causes are a direct impact (which may also have caused concussion or head or facial fractures), violent nose-blowing and nose-picking. Watery blood or clear fluid from the nose may arise from a fracture at the base of the skull.

FIRST AID FOR A NOSEBLEED

Casualty must lean forwards, breathe through the mouth and pinch the soft end of their nose. If bleeding persists, they must pinch harder. Pinch for at least 10 minutes, then check to see if the bleeding has stopped. Place a bag of frozen peas (wrapped in a towel or similar to prevent damage to the skin) over the nose.

Get the person to rest for several hours, and avoid sniffing, blowing or picking their nose. If bleeding continues for 30 minutes, take them to hospital (lots of swallowing may indicate blood still going down the back of the throat). If it is very heavy and shock symptoms set in, call for an ambulance.

BLEEDING FROM THE EAR

Like a nosebleed, watery blood or clear fluid from the ear may be a sign of a fractured base of the skull if it happens after a head injury. However, it is usually due to local causes – often a hairgrip or other foreign body has been inserted into the ear and has perforated the eardrum. Other causes of a perforated eardrum are loud explosions, blows to the head and, most commonly, an infection in the middle ear. The person will always have experienced severe ear pain when this happens, which will often be relieved once the drum perforates. Ear infections may need antibiotics.

FIRST AID FOR BLEEDING FROM THE EAR

Put a pad over the ear, and get the sufferer to tilt their heads to allow the blood to drain out.

If there is no head injury they may take pain relief if needed and then seek medical attention. If bleeding follows a head injury, take the casualty to the emergency department or call an ambulance.

Miscellaneous foreign bodies

SEE ALSO

➤ Coping with choking 1, p38, p50

➤ Treating infected wounds, p132

➤ Bleeding from orifices, p142

As well as becoming embedded in wounds, foreign bodies of all kinds – from an insect flying into the ear to a piece of grit caught under an eyelid – can become lodged in the body's orifices. Such objects may cause injury, bleeding, infection and other problems. Children are notorious for putting things in their mouths and ears and up their noses, as they explore the world around them, when they are too young to realize the potential danger. Foreign bodies must be removed safely and cleanly, to avoid the risk of damage or infection.

It is usually young children and people with psychiatric problems who place foreign bodies inside their orifices deliberately. But foreign bodies can become lodged in parts of the body accidentally as well.

SWALLOWING OBJECTS

Children often put things in their mouths without thinking and then swallow them – plastic toys, pen lids, money and paper clips, to name a few. If this occurs, the child may have a choking episode and then fully recover – but with a noticeable absence of the object that was in their hand. Adults may also accidentally swallow small, whole items of food, such as peanuts, whole grapes or sweets, if they are eating while talking or laughing.

If, instead of being swallowed, the object sticks in the windpipe, it may cause partial or complete obstruction and choking. Because this will impede breathing, it is a life-threatening emergency (see pp 38-41 for adults and p50-51 for children). If the object sticks in the oesophagus, the upper gullet leading down to the stomach, the person may drool, gag or be unable to eat or drink anything – also a medical emergency.

Once in the stomach, inedible objects usually pass through the gut and out in the faeces with no problems. Unless a child develops acute stomach pain or vomiting, or stops opening their bowels, nothing needs to be done. However, if they have swallowed a battery or a sharp object such as a pin, these can damage the digestive tract and must be removed; they will show up on an X-ray.

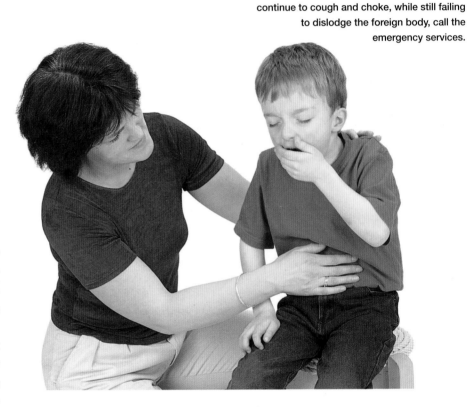

▽ If a swallowed object makes a child or adult continue to cough and choke, while still failing to dislodge the foreign body, call the emergency services.

GENITALS AND RECTUM

People may end up with objects lodged in the penis, the female urethra, the vagina or the rectum. In any of these cases, never try to retrieve the object, as this can cause damage to these delicate areas. Take the person to an accident and emergency department for treatment by a doctor or nurse.

NOSES

Children often put small objects up their noses. The child may develop a foul-smelling discharge from one nostril after a few days. Blocking the other nostril and getting the child to blow their nose often brings out the foreign body. There is a danger that the child will inhale the foreign body into their airway, so if you do not succeed in removing it, take them to hospital immediately.

EYES

People often get things in their eyes – dust on a windy day, a bit of ash from a bonfire or even a fragment of metal hammered off a metal object. They can often feel the object in the eye, or the eye may feel irritated and painful, and it will usually water profusely and look red. An X-ray may be needed if any metal hits the eye at speed, as it may end up at the back of the eye.

HOW TO EXAMINE THE EYES FOR SMALL PARTICLES

1 If there is any chance of a fragment that has penetrated the eye, do not touch it – seek immediate medical advice. Otherwise, examine the person's eye either in natural daylight or under a direct ray from a lamp. Stand behind the person, so that you are looking down on them. Keeping their head very still, ask them to look from side to side and then up and down. In each direction, have a good look at the white of the eye, called the conjunctiva, then look at the coloured part of the eye, the iris.

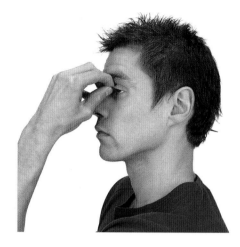

2 Ask them to look down and then get them to gently pull out their upper lid by the lashes. Look on the underside of the upper lid – specks of grit often stick here.

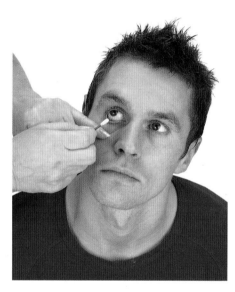

3 If you see a speck, try to remove it with a cotton bud moistened in water. Only touch the white area of the eyeball very gently, and only once. Or flush the eye with cooled, boiled water or a sterile eye-wash solution. If all this fails, cover the eye with an eye pad and take them to a doctor or ophthamologist.

EARS

Insects flying into ears is a fairly common occurrence, and this can be alarming for people of any age. Deafness is the main symptom of a foreign body in the ear, or there may be a loud buzzing from a trapped fly. Whatever the culprit, do not attempt to prise it out.

Try filling the ear with lukewarm water or olive oil. This will kill any insects, and small foreign bodies may float out. If not, ask the person to turn their head so that the ear containing the foreign body points downwards – this may lead to the foreign body dropping out. If all fails, take them to a doctor.

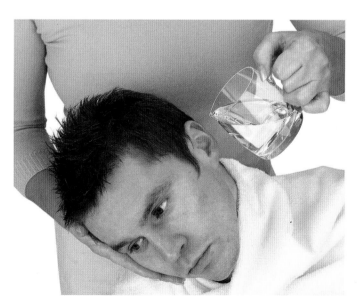

◁ **Flush out a foreign body in the ear with lukewarm water or with olive oil. Never try to dig or poke it out as you may cause damage to the eardrum.**

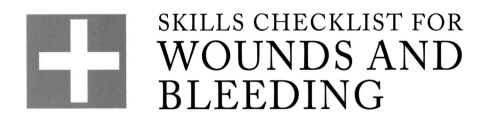

SKILLS CHECKLIST FOR
WOUNDS AND BLEEDING

KEY POINTS

- The basic issues of wound-care are stemming blood loss and preventing infection. For major wounds, the priorities (after assessing ABC) are stopping bleeding and getting help ☐

- Heavy blood loss can lead rapidly to serious consequences ☐

- Foreign objects can cause severe damage and infection and must be dealt with promptly ☐

- Any infected wound must be closely monitored ☐

- Wounds may mask underlying damage – which is why getting help fast is so vital ☐

- If you release a crushed/trapped casualty, you need to monitor them closely and be prepared for sudden deterioration ☐

- Stem heavy blood loss by using pressure and elevation ☐

- Internal bleeding often shows few clear outward signs. Urgent medical help is vital ☐

SKILLS LEARNED

- How to recognize different types of wound and follow appropriate treatment ☐

- How to control bleeding and deal with infection ☐

- What to do with severe wounds and injuries ☐

- When to suspect internal bleeding ☐

- How to tackle embedded and lodged foreign bodies ☐

BONE AND MUSCLE INJURIES

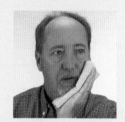

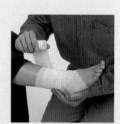

It is not always easy to distinguish a fracture from a dislocation or a sprain. This chapter explains how to help a casualty in the event of various types of fracture, sprains, dislocations and back pain. It is essential if there is any possibility of a neck or spinal injury that the casualty is not moved, unless not moving them would put them in further danger. The main priorities in dealing with bone and muscle injuries are to immobilize the affected limb, cover any open wounds and alert the emergency services.

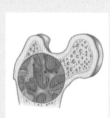

CONTENTS

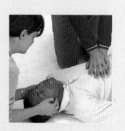

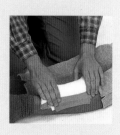

Understanding the skeleton

SEE ALSO
➤ Removing clothing and helmets, p18
➤ Moving and handling safely 1 and 2, pp20, 22
➤ Dealing with broken bones, p150

The body's bones come in all shapes and sizes, and it is the muscles that are attached at multiple points all over the skeleton that enable us to move about. If any of the 206 bones in the body are injured through fracture (a clean break, a messy break, a chip, a splinter, or a crack), our ability to move properly can be substantially diminished, and pain and swelling may occur around the site of the injured bone. Initial first aid, followed by professional treatment in hospital, is vital for optimum healing of all such bone injuries or fractures.

Bone is a living tissue that continuously builds, degrades, and rebuilds itself throughout life. The skeleton's bony framework has many functions: bones protect the organs from damage; muscles attach to bones so that we can move; many types of blood cell are produced in the bone's marrow; and bone acts as a store of the minerals calcium and phosphate.

As we grow older, the strength of our bones – bone density – declines as bones lose calcium, so they become easy to break. Many older people break bones after minor bumps or falls.

WHAT IS BONE MADE OF?

Bone is made of a meshwork of a protein (collagen) into which calcium is deposited to give hardness and strength. Although bone is extremely strong it is not completely solid. The outer layer is hard and compact, but beneath it lies a centre of spongy bone. The spaces within the spongy bone allow room for the skeleton's immense blood supply and nerves.

INSIDE A TYPICAL BONE

▽ The circle section shows a close-up view of the internal meshwork of the spongy bone.

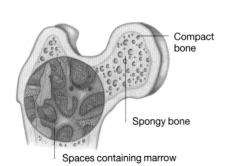

Compact bone

Spongy bone

Spaces containing marrow

THE SKELETON

▷ The many bones of the skeleton give the body shape and structure. Bones that are commonly fractured are named on this illustration.

Scapula (shoulder blade)

Humerus

Radius

Ulna

Skull

Mandible (jaw)

Sternum (breastbone)

Clavicle (collarbone)

Rib

Vertebral column

Ilium
Ischium
(all three together known as the pelvis)

Femur (thighbone)

Tibia

Fibula

Calcaneus (heel bone)

WHAT HEALTHY BONES NEED

➤ Calcium – Your diet should include plenty of calcium-rich foods such as milk, cheese and yogurt. Good sources of calcium for vegans are green, leafy vegetables and calcium-fortified soy milk. During childhood, pregnancy and breastfeeding, a higher calcium intake may be needed to avoid your body raiding the skeleton's stores calcium.

➤ Vitamin D – The body makes vitamin D in the skin when it is exposed to sunlight. This vitamin allows the body to absorb calcium and phosphorus from food. Vitamin D occurs in fatty fish, such as tuna, mackerel and salmon. There are also foods fortified with vitamin D such as soy milk and cereals.

➤ Exercise – Weight-bearing exercise promotes bone growth and bone density.

HOW BONES CAN FRACTURE

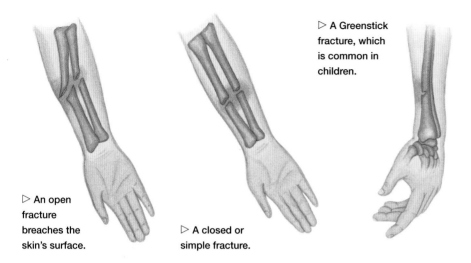

▷ An open fracture breaches the skin's surface.

▷ A closed or simple fracture.

▷ A Greenstick fracture, which is common in children.

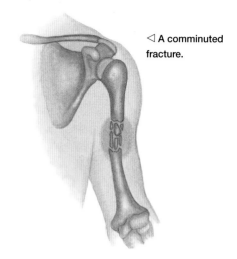

◁ A comminuted fracture.

WHAT CAUSES A FRACTURE?

A bone may break because of a direct blow, such as a punch or kick, or from indirect forces. Bones fracture indirectly when, for example, a person falls on to a hand that they have stretched out to break their fall. The forces from the fall may travel up the arm (which remains unharmed) and cause the collarbone to break. Bones may also fracture from rotating movements – when someone twists an ankle, for example.

OPEN OR CLOSED FRACTURES?

There are two basic types of fracture known as open and closed. Open fractures (also called compound fractures) occur when the broken ends of bone stick out through the skin. In open fractures, the risk of developing an infection is much higher, as are the chances of nerve or blood vessel damage. Closed fractures (also called simple fractures) are fractures in which the skin is not broken over the fracture site.

HOW BONES HEAL

Different bones heal at different rates, so while a fractured collarbone may heal fully in six weeks, a broken thighbone (femur) may take up to six months before it is mended completely. The rate of bone regeneration in children is much faster than in most adults, and so broken bones in children tend to heal much more quickly.

COMMON FRACTURE TYPES

Bones fracture in different ways in different people and depending on how an incident came about. Common types of fracture are:

➤ Greenstick fracture – Children sometimes fracture only one side of a bone. The other side bends like a new tree branch.

➤ Comminuted fracture – The bone is splintered at the fracture site, and smaller fragments of bone are found between the two main fragments.

➤ Fracture-dislocation – This type of fracture occurs when a bone breaks or cracks at the same time as a nearby joint dislocates.

➤ Avulsion fracture – When a ligament or muscle attached to a bone is ripped off, it often takes a piece of bone with it.

➤ Pathological fractures – Certain medical conditions, such as osteoporosis and osteogenesis imperfecta, make bones more likely to break.

Bone-healing has several stages:

• Six to eight hours after injury – In this inflammatory period, blood seeps out of the broken bone ends and forms a clot.

• After two days – Bone-making cells migrate to the blood clot and start to form new bone, called callus, to bridge the gap between the bones.

• A few weeks to several months – The original shape of the bone is restored.

WHAT DELAYS HEALING?

Although infection increases the blood supply to a fracture site, it brings the wrong kind of cells, so healing is delayed. Also, if the bones are not in alignment with one another, they are not going to heal well. This is one reason why splinting, or at least immobilization, of a fracture is vitally important for proper and speedy bone healing.

HOW BONE HEALS

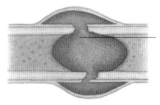

Blood clot fills the gap between the broken bones

△ Six to eight hours after the injury.

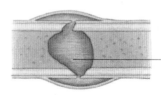

New spongy bone (callus) starts to form

△ Two days after the injury.

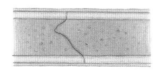

△ A few weeks or months afterwards.

Dealing with broken bones

SEE ALSO

➤ What is first aid?, p12
➤ Dealing with shock, p68
➤ Fixing slings, p206

Bones tend to break as the result of a huge impact or force. A fracture casualty may be able to tell you that they heard or felt a crack when the accident occurred or that they can feel bones grating over one another when they try to move. Such clues are important information for the first-aider. Bear in mind that the casualty could be in great pain, and also watch for signs of shock – this may develop, for example, if the fracture causes heavy internal bleeding. Never move a casualty unless you have to in order to remove them from other serious dangers.

When managing any accident victim, always monitor ABC procedures in case resuscitation is needed before dealing with possible fractures and always assess the person as a whole – there could well be other injuries.

In the short term, the various methods used to deal with fractures focus on preventing the fracture from becoming worse, and they all achieve this by immobilization – keeping the fracture still. The general idea is to immobilize the fracture and the joints above and below the fracture. Movement of a fracture can cause increased pain, damage to surrounding tissue and structures and possibly even severe complications such as shock from increased bleeding or from bone penetrating through skin, nerves or blood vessels. In the long term, a broken bone needs to be left clean and undisturbed for proper healing.

SHOULD SPLINTS BE USED?

Using splints (rigid supports) for a fracture is little used by most first-aiders today, unless in very remote locations, or where the first-aider is forced to transport the casualty to help. Improvised examples of splints include umbrellas and broom handles. Except for simple, undisplaced arm fractures, transporting a splinted fracture casualty is not recommended unless you have proper training and practice, and a suitable vehicle.

IMMOBILIZATION STRATEGIES

There are two major types of immediate first aid for fractures:
• Basic hand immobilization. Try to imagine the break that has occurred in the normally rigid bone. Use your hands

BASIC CARE FOR A CLOSED OR SIMPLE FRACTURE

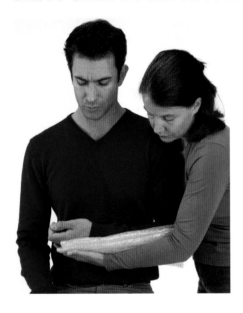

1 Having assessed the casualty, ask them to keep the fracture area still. Support the fracture and apply light padding, such as some folded bubble wrap or a small towel or tea towel (nothing too bulky).

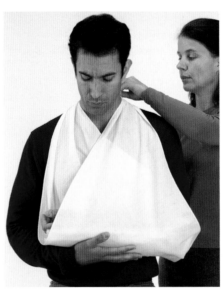

2 Depending on the part of the body involved, you should usually attempt to immobilize the area. Do this here by applying a broad arm sling, as shown, keeping the light padding in place within the sling.

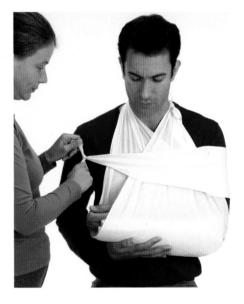

3 Immobilize the arm further by tying a triangular bandage (folded into a long strip), or equivalent, across the chest. This will prevent movement when the casualty is in transit to hospital. Phone for medical help.

and arms to cradle the limb in order to stop all movement. This method is most appropriate when help will arrive fairly quickly, or where no other equipment or materials of any kind are available.

• Using padding and boxes. These first-aid props are used mostly for leg fractures or for arm fractures where bending the elbow to put the arm in a sling would cause further damage. For this method, hold the limb still. Roll large, loose sausages from objects such as blankets, coats or towels and place these carefully against the fractured limb. Any gaps beneath the limb, such as from a bent knee, should be carefully filled with just enough padding material to provide support under the area without moving the limb at all. Boxes or other weighted items are now placed carefully but firmly either side of the limb to hold the padding in place.

The padding and boxes method is ideal in most populated areas with good ambulance response times. It frees the first-aider to concentrate on taking care of the casualty and on simply minimizing any movement.

It also means that paramedics arriving on the scene do not need to waste time removing a first-aider's bandages in order to replace them with their own, superior, equipment.

COMMON SIGNS AND SYMPTOMS OF A FRACTURE

➤ There may be a history of impact or trauma at the site.

➤ Swelling, bruising or deformity at fracture site.

➤ Pain on moving.

➤ Numbness or tingling in injured area.

➤ Wound site at or near fracture site.

➤ The casualty may have heard the bones grating on one another as the accident happened.

FIRST AID FOR FRACTURES

First, assess the situation and reassure the casualty. Prevent movement at the injury site and stem bleeding if an open fracture.

Support the joint above and below the fracture.

Phone the emergency services and arrange transport to hospital.

Monitor the casualty's condition, paying particular attention to the circulation beyond any tied bandages.

FIRST AID FOR AN OPEN FRACTURE

When you are dealing with an open fracture, it is important to prevent blood loss and infection at the injury site as well as immobilizing the area.

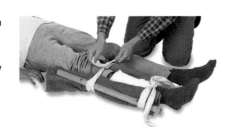

▷ Call the emergency services urgently. Carefully place a dressing or sterile pad over the wound site, and apply hand pressure either side of the protruding bone to control the bleeding. Never press on the protruding bone itself. Build up padding alongside the bone if it is sticking out of the skin. You may want to secure the dressing and padding firmly with a bandage, but do not do so if it causes any movement of the limb, and never bandage too tightly. Monitor the casualty's condition, specifically their ABC, and be alert for signs of shock.

▷ In more extreme circumstances – if you are in a very remote location, emergency help is seriously delayed, or you are forced to take the casualty to a doctor/hospital yourself – you may need to splint the fracture. Add extra padding around the limb and fix with tied bandages or equivalent. Keep any movement to a minimum.

WARNING

In most cases, a first aider must never straighten or move the fractured limb. If a foot looks blue or bloodless, always tell the paramedics; they may manipulate the fracture in order to restore circulation.

Tackling skull and facial fractures

SEE ALSO

➤ Responsiveness and the airway, p28

➤ Dealing with head injury, p80

➤ Dealing with broken bones, p150

Suspected head injury is always a serious situation. The spinal cord, brain or organs within the head, such as the eye or ear, may also be damaged – not only by the impact of the injury but also by the potential bleeding into the brain or swelling that such an injury can cause. It is vital to monitor someone with a suspected skull fracture as they may lose consciousness and/or may have a neck or spinal injury. The main point to bear in mind with any facial fracture is that swollen tissues, blood and saliva may impair breathing by obstructing the airway.

Skull fractures are worrying because an impact large enough to fracture skull bones might also injure the delicate brain beneath. The fracture itself may cause no damage, but if a slab of skull bone is crushed inwards (a "depressed fracture") it may put pressure on the brain. Skull fractures may also cause internal bleeding into the brain area.

Call the emergency services as promptly as possible. Assume there may be a neck or spinal injury as well and treat the casualty with extreme care. Keep them totally still if possible.

SKULL AND FACIAL FRACTURES

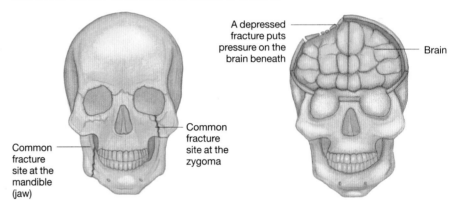

Common fracture site at the mandible (jaw)

Common fracture site at the zygoma

A depressed fracture puts pressure on the brain beneath

Brain

△ The tough skull and facial bones can be fractured; common injury sites are shown above.

△ A serious skull fracture could mean that the vulnerable tissues of the brain directly beneath are also damaged. If there is also a wound over the fracture site, then the brain may become exposed to the possibility of infection.

SIGNS OF A SKULL FRACTURE

➤ A "boggy" soft swelling or egg-shaped bruise on the head.

➤ Bruising around eye and/or ear area.

➤ A noticeably lopsided appearance to the head – very serious sign.

➤ A deteriorating level of consciousness (remember AVPU) – very serious sign.

➤ Any blood visible in the whites of the eyes – very serious sign.

➤ Clear or blood-stained fluid leaking from the nose or ears – very serious sign.

Signs of possible internal bleeding:

➤ One-sided, worsening headache; headache that worsens with lying flat/making any effort.

➤ Any visual problems.

➤ Change in/loss of consciousness.

➤ Vomiting.

FIRST AID FOR SUSPECTED SKULL FRACTURE

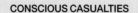

CONSCIOUS CASUALTIES

Call for an ambulance and make sure the casualty is comfortably seated.
Dress any open scalp wounds.
Watch out for drowsiness/loss of consciousness or profuse vomiting and try to keep them awake.
If they have a headache, do not give any medication, or anything else by mouth, until a doctor has assessed them.

UNCONSCIOUS CASUALTIES

Call an ambulance.
Check DRABC and begin CPR if needed.
If breathing, with signs of circulation, place in recovery position, and dress any open head wounds.

FRACTURES TO THE FACE

Facial injuries are not often fatal, but they are worrying because of their potential to obstruct the airway and result in breathing problems. Compulsory seat-belt wearing has dramatically cut down facial injuries due to road traffic accidents, and the main causes of injuries now are sport, falls and assaults. Heavy force is needed to fracture a bone in the face, and there will often be other injuries of the neck, chest and skull to look out for.

Suspect a facial fracture if:

• The face looks asymmetrical or deformed in any way.

• There is bruising and/or a black eye.

• There is bleeding from the mouth or nose.

• The person cannot clench their teeth.

• There is difficulty breathing, or the casualty is snoring if unconscious.

Ensure that the casualty's airway is clear.
If necessary, remove any debris from
the mouth.

If there is a lot of bleeding or you think
they may lose consciousness, place
them in the recovery position.
(Be aware of the risk of neck injury.)

Call the emergency services promptly.
Place ice, wrapped in a clean towel, on
any swelling of the face.

FRACTURES TO THE JAW

The jaw is a common bone to break. Any
blow to the chin may break one or both
sides of the jaw. If both sides fracture, then
the tongue can become unstable and may
block the airway. Suspect a fractured jaw if:
• There is pain, nausea and/or swelling of
the jaw area.
• The person cannot bite and is dribbling.
• The casualty has difficulty swallowing,
breathing or speaking.

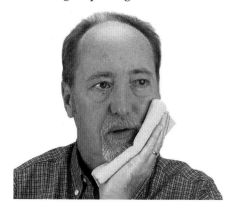

△ In a suspected jaw fracture, ask the casualty
to hold a soft cloth against the injured site to
protect it, and then transport them to hospital
without delay.

FIRST AID FOR A
FRACTURED JAW

If there is bleeding in the mouth and
they have potentially broken both sides
of the jaw, lie them down, place them
in the recovery position and keep a
careful eye on their airway.

Call the emergency services promptly.

If only one side of the jaw is painful and
swollen, get them to hold a soft cloth
against the area to keep it still.

NOSE AND CHEEKBONE
FRACTURES

Fractures of the nose and cheekbone are
generally not serious unless the cheekbone
injury involves the eye socket. A direct
blow to the eye, especially common in
squash games, may cause what is called a
"blow-out fracture", making it impossible
for the person to look upwards.

If you suspect either a nose or
cheekbone (or eye socket) fracture, do not
let the person blow their nose. This is
because it may cause air to track through
broken bones into the skin or into the brain.

Action to take if you suspect a fracture
of a cheekbone or nose is to:
• check carefully to see whether the
casualty's airway is clear and that it is not
obstructed by swollen tissues
• apply a cold compress to the injured site to
reduce pain and swelling
• get the casualty to hospital.
If the casualty has a nosebleed, you should
try to stop the bleeding; if the liquid is
either clear or yellow, then treat as you
would for a skull fracture.

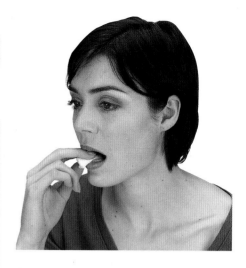

△ The casualty should hold the dislodged tooth
in its socket either by keeping the mouth shut
or by pressing on it with a pad.

KNOCKED-OUT TEETH

Tooth injuries are especially common in
children, and any loose first teeth should
be taken out by a dentist, to avoid possible
inhalation. Adult teeth can be damaged
permanently by fracture or by being
dislodged from a socket. If the tooth can
be put back into its socket within 30
minutes to an hour's time, a dentist may be
able to save it.

FIRST AID FOR A
KNOCKED-OUT TOOTH

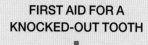

Pop the tooth back into its socket
and ask the casualty to hold the
tooth in place.

If they cannot hold it firmly in place, get
them to keep it in their cheek or
put the tooth in a beaker or a small plastic
bag of milk to prevent it drying out.

Take them to a hospital or dentist
as soon as possible.

Managing spinal injuries

SEE ALSO

➤ LIFE-SAVING
  PRIORITIES, p25
➤ Coping with neck
  injuries, p156

The golden rule with spinal injuries (and neck injuries) is that the casualty must not be moved unless it is vital to do so. People with head injuries of any kind often have spinal injuries as well. The spinal cord, housed within the vertebrae, is commonly damaged at the most mobile parts of the backbone such as the neck and lower back. Road accidents, rugby and diving are notorious causes of spinal injuries; other causes include falling from a height, being thrown from a horse, and impact to the head and/or face.

The term spinal injury can refer to damage to the bones of the spine (vertebrae), the spinal cord, the discs between the backbones or any muscles and ligaments attached to the spine. The most serious type of injury is to the spinal cord, as a partial or complete break can result in permanent paralysis. If a splinter of bone or swollen tissue compresses a nerve, a person may suffer a temporary paralysis but sensation and movement return once the injury is treated.

THE BACKBONE

There are 24 moving vertebrae in the spine, and these form a column between the skull and the pelvis. The spinal cord travels down through a channel formed by the vertebral arches. Nerves supplying the arms pass out at the highest level, then those to the trunk, and then those to the legs. Between each vertebra and the next is a disc, which cushions any force or pressure on the vertebrae. Ligaments and muscles also protect and strengthen the spine.

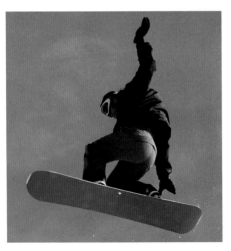

◁ Sport and recreational pursuits are common causes of spinal injury.

THE SPINE OR VERTEBRAL COLUMN

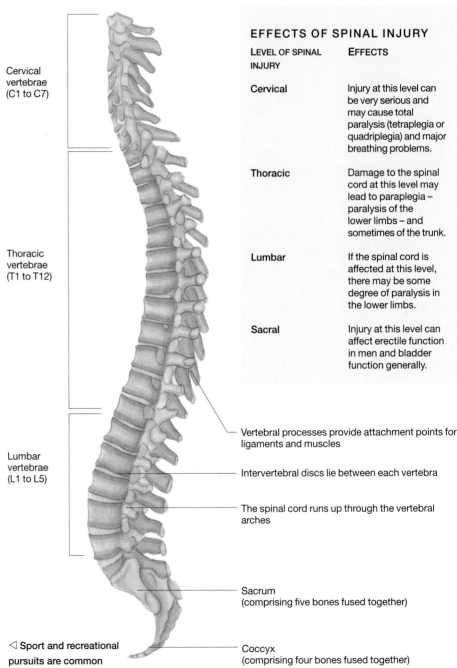

Cervical vertebrae (C1 to C7)

Thoracic vertebrae (T1 to T12)

Lumbar vertebrae (L1 to L5)

Vertebral processes provide attachment points for ligaments and muscles

Intervertebral discs lie between each vertebra

The spinal cord runs up through the vertebral arches

Sacrum (comprising five bones fused together)

Coccyx (comprising four bones fused together)

EFFECTS OF SPINAL INJURY

LEVEL OF SPINAL INJURY	EFFECTS
Cervical	Injury at this level can be very serious and may cause total paralysis (tetraplegia or quadriplegia) and major breathing problems.
Thoracic	Damage to the spinal cord at this level may lead to paraplegia – paralysis of the lower limbs – and sometimes of the trunk.
Lumbar	If the spinal cord is affected at this level, there may be some degree of paralysis in the lower limbs.
Sacral	Injury at this level can affect erectile function in men and bladder function generally.

FIRST AID FOR SPINAL INJURY IN AN UNCONSCIOUS PERSON

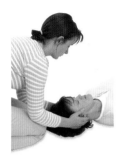

1 Keep the casualty still, in the position in which they are found. Hold the head still, as shown here, in its current position. Ask others to support the rest of the body using hands and blankets, coats or towels. Continue to keep the casualty as still as possible. If the casualty is already on their back, and the airway is clear, with nothing in the mouth and no signs of possible bleeding or vomiting, keep them in that position. If the tongue is falling back and blocking the airway, bring it forward by pushing up at the angles of the jaws, as already explained on page 29. Do not use a head tilt unless absolutely necessary to clear the airway.

2 With both unconscious and conscious casualties, blood, vomit or other substances in the mouth or throat can block the airway (listen for gurgling). Only if this is a risk, make sure that they are in a position that allows these to drain out of the mouth. If you need to move them for this, be gentle, keep movement minimal, and keep the head still as you do so. Use a "log roll" if turning them from their back to their side.

▽ **Using the "log roll" – for draining the mouth or resuscitation.**

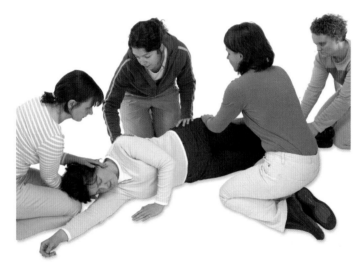

3 If the breathing or heartbeat stops, and the person is not already on their back, you must turn them on to their back to perform CPR. Use the "log roll" technique (see page 157), so that there is no change in the spine or head position.

4 To resuscitate, one person holds the head still while another performs resuscitation.

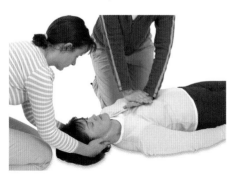

WARNING

Only move a casualty with a suspected or certain spinal injury if you need to: remove them from further serious danger; carry out resuscitation techniques (for which they must be on their back); drain the mouth (for which they need to be on their side). Any moving ideally needs at least three people – to make sure that the spine and the head do not change position.

SIGNS AND SYMPTOMS OF A SPINAL INJURY

Suspect a spinal injury if a person:

➤ Has suffered a significant impact/fall.

➤ Is unconscious after a head injury.

➤ Has fallen from a height and injured their face or head.

➤ Says that their neck hurts.

➤ Holds their neck in an odd position.

➤ Has any paralysis (loss of movement and sensation), loss of sensation or tingling or numbness in their arms and/or legs.

➤ Is confused or uncooperative.

➤ Has lost bowel or bladder control.

➤ Has difficulty breathing, with only small amounts of movement in the abdomen.

➤ Is lying flat on their back with arms stretched above the head, or with arms and hands curled to the chest.

FIRST AID FOR A CONSCIOUS SPINAL INJURY CASUALTY

Reassure the casualty. Unless there is an urgent reason to move them, such as breathing difficulties, do not do so. Call the emergency services promptly.

Ask the casualty to keep absolutely still. Kneel behind their head and hold their head still, in the position in which you found it.

Support the head at all times and ask someone to help monitor their condition until medical help arrives. Be prepared to resuscitate if necessary.

Coping with neck injuries

SEE ALSO

➤ Removing clothing and helmets, p18

➤ Full resuscitation sequence, p33

➤ Managing spinal injuries, p154

The most important rule for dealing with a casualty with a suspected neck injury is that they are not to be moved, unless they would be in great danger, for example lying in the middle of a road or in the path of a spreading fire. A first-aider's priorities in such accidents are to prevent any further injury and phone the emergency services immediately. If a casualty absolutely has to be moved for safety then the "log roll" technique, which requires at least four people and preferably more, must be used to keep the spine straight and supported at all times.

Fractures of the bones in the neck may be life-threatening because the nerves that supply your main breathing muscle (the diaphragm) pass out of the spinal cord here; if these nerves are damaged by a fractured vertebra, your breathing may stop. Unlike other vertebrae in your backbone, the bones in the neck are vulnerable and are easily damaged.

IF RESUSCITATION IS NECESSARY

Keeping the neck still is extremely important in a neck injury, but a pumping heart is even more important. If a person is not breathing, then you must start chest compressions at once. It is perfectly possible to perform CPR and mouth-to-mouth on a person with a possible neck injury. Ideally, you should get someone else to keep the casualty's head steady and supported, while you start resuscitation.

FIRST AID FOR A NECK INJURY

In any injury affecting the spine, but especially the neck, it is vital to keep the head still. Another helper should phone for help while you deal with the casualty. You may well find the casualty on their back, as shown here. If not, do not move them on to their back unless you need to in order to start resuscitation.

IF YOU ARE ALONE...
If you are a lone first-aider, and have to leave the casualty to get help, immobilize their neck before you go with something like rolled-up towels, held in place by heavier objects. Tell the casualty to stay still and reassure them that you will return as soon as possible.

▽ Place your hands either side of the casualty's head to steady and support it.

HOW A NECK INJURY CAN DAMAGE BREATHING

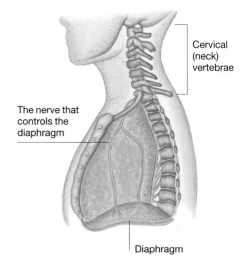

Cervical (neck) vertebrae

The nerve that controls the diaphragm

Diaphragm

▷ The nerve that controls the diaphragm exits the spine in the neck area. If this is damaged by a neck injury, breathing could cease.

THE "LOG ROLL" TECHNIQUE

If you absolutely must move a casualty with a spinal injury you should only use the "log roll" technique. By moving them "as one piece", with everyone in synchronicity, you avoid their head twisting on their shoulders or their body rotating on their pelvis. This minimizes the chances of any of the spinal vertebrae moving and causing more damage. There should be a minimum of four people, ideally six, present to carry out this technique. One person should be in charge of the head and should dictate everyone else's movements. There should always be one helper at the casualty's feet. The other helpers are positioned along the body at close intervals and act as a team. To be absolutely safe, the log roll needs training and team practise.

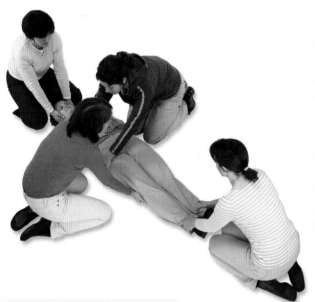

1 To move someone from their back on to their side (if they want to vomit or if blood, vomit or other substances are blocking their mouth/throat): cross their arms over in front. Then, while one person supports the head, the other people stagger themselves along the body, gently straighten out the limbs and prepare to make the "log roll".

FIRST AID FOR A SUSPECTED NECK INJURY

Don't try to straighten or pull on the neck. Keep it in the position found, and as still as possible.

Ask a helper to get some towels or clothing and place these rolled-up items either side of the neck, all the time keeping it still.

Monitor their breathing and pulse and if either start to stop, be prepared to start resuscitation procedures. If they vomit, "log roll" them on to their side.

PREVENTING NECK/SPINAL INJURIES

Most spinal injuries occur in men aged 18 to 30 – the "risk-takers". Certain simple measures can prevent many such injuries:

➤ Always wear proper protective clothing when participating in a sport.

➤ Never dive into water until you know the depth, especially in tidal waters.

➤ Never dive into a swimming pool unless the water is at least 2.7 m (9 ft) deep.

➤ Always wear a seat-belt in any moving vehicle.

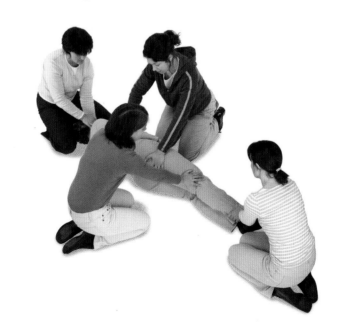

2 The head is supported all the time, and the helpers must hold the body and legs steady. The casualty's head, body and toes must align and all face in the same direction. Once turned on to their side, keep them there, perfectly still, until professional help arrives. Only move them (on to their back again) if they stop breathing or their heart stops and resuscitation becomes necessary.

Tackling upper limb fractures

SEE ALSO

➤ Fixing slings, p206

The bones of the shoulder, upper arm, forearm, wrist and hand can all be fractured, and such fractures are relatively common. An outstretched hand or wrist often takes the brunt of forces from a fall but such forces can also travel up the arm and fracture one of the collarbones. With any upper limb fracture, the first-aider's main aims are to immobilize the injured limb (as it may well be unstable) and arrange transport to hospital. Skill in applying various types of slings and bandages is crucial for dealing with such injuries.

When you arrive at an accident scene, watch out for these common signs of a potential fracture:

- Pain and tenderness at the site of injury, which is worse on moving.
- Swelling and deformity.
- Attempts by the casualty to support the injured arm by holding it in a certain way.

A FRACTURED COLLARBONE

The collarbones, also known as the clavicles, are one of the commonest bones to break, especially among young people doing sports. Sometimes the broken ends of the collarbone can pierce surrounding tissues and result in bleeding and swelling.

Most collarbone fractures knit together well simply by fixing the arm in a sling, which uses the weight of the arm to slowly pull the fractured bones back into line.

▽ By immobilizing the arm in a high (or "elevation") sling, pain and discomfort from collarbone fractures can be minimized until arrival at hospital.

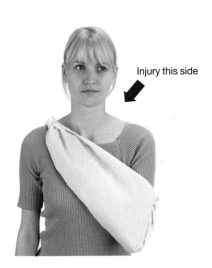

Injury this side

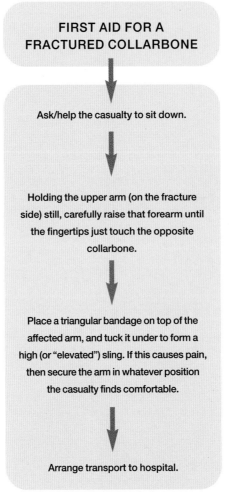

FIRST AID FOR A FRACTURED COLLARBONE

Ask/help the casualty to sit down.

↓

Holding the upper arm (on the fracture side) still, carefully raise that forearm until the fingertips just touch the opposite collarbone.

↓

Place a triangular bandage on top of the affected arm, and tuck it under to form a high (or "elevated") sling. If this causes pain, then secure the arm in whatever position the casualty finds comfortable.

↓

Arrange transport to hospital.

FRACTURES OF THE UPPER ARM

The long bone that joins the shoulder to the elbow – known as the humerus – fractures most frequently at the top end nearest the shoulder, which is its weakest part. This is a serious form of fracture because it may actually go unnoticed by an observer as it is usually a stable fracture. The casualty may well be feeling some pain but may not seek medical assistance for some time.

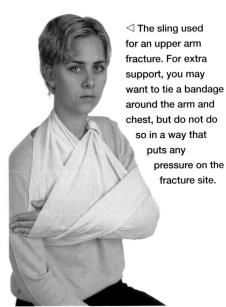

◁ The sling used for an upper arm fracture. For extra support, you may want to tie a bandage around the arm and chest, but do not do so in a way that puts any pressure on the fracture site.

FIRST AID FOR AN UPPER ARM FRACTURE

↓

Ask the casualty to hold the injured arm across their body with their good hand.

↓

Place a triangular bandage in between the arm and the chest and tie a sling.

↓

Tie a broad-band bandage around the chest to secure the sling before transporting the casualty to hospital. Do this very low down the bent arm, so no pressure is put on the fracture site.

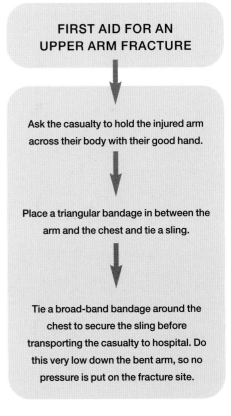

HUMERUS FRACTURE

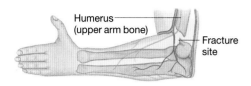

Humerus
(upper arm bone)

Fracture site

△ Fractures of the humerus above the elbow are common in children. Adults tend to fracture the shoulder end of this bone.

AN INJURED ELBOW

Elbows are highly sensitive when injured, even without fractures, and may be painful and stiff for weeks after an injury.

Dealing with elbow injuries depends on whether or not the elbow can be bent. For elbows that can bend, follow the advice for an upper arm injury. Non-bending elbows need completely different first aid.

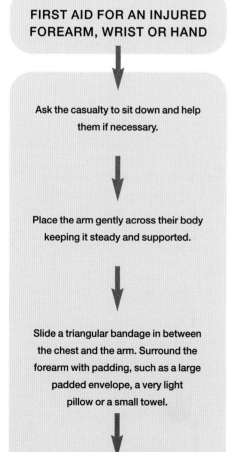

FIRST AID FOR AN INJURED FOREARM, WRIST OR HAND

↓

Ask the casualty to sit down and help them if necessary.

↓

Place the arm gently across their body keeping it steady and supported.

↓

Slide a triangular bandage in between the chest and the arm. Surround the forearm with padding, such as a large padded envelope, a very light pillow or a small towel.

↓

Finish tying the arm sling and arrange transport to hospital.

DEALING WITH AN ELBOW THAT CANNOT BEND

1 Help the casualty to lie down. Position soft padding to support and cushion the arm, as shown below. Now add weighted boxes or objects at the side to hold the padding in place. Phone the emergency services. (Note: If you are in a remote location and are forced to transport the casualty to hospital yourself, then use broad bandages tied around the body to secure and immobilize the limb. However, never do this under normal circumstances, as it causes pain and potentially harmful further movement.)

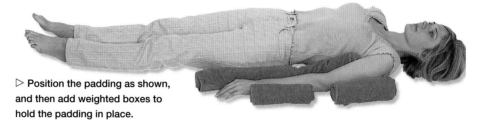

▷ Position the padding as shown, and then add weighted boxes to hold the padding in place.

FRACTURES TO THE FOREARM, WRIST OR HAND

It may be obvious when there is a fracture of the radius or ulna bones of the forearm, as there can be swelling and extreme tenderness. In children, whose soft, new bones often bend rather than break, there may only be a small crack called a greenstick fracture, and minimal swelling in the forearm.

A Colles fracture – a break of the radius bone near the wrist – is a common wrist fracture, often affecting older women.

The most common type of hand fracture affects the knuckle, often from a punch, but the hand can also be crushed, resulting in open fractures with profuse bleeding and swelling. As with any fracture, always compare the suspected injured side with the healthy side.

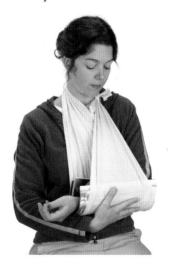

SIGNS AND SYMPTOMS OF A HAND INJURY

➤ An uninjured hand has a natural look called the "cascade" when it rests palm upwards on a flat surface. Each finger curls naturally just under the larger finger next to it. If one finger lies straight or is very bent, serious tendon, bone or nerve injury is likely.

➤ Ask the casualty to make a fist. Do all the fingers work together or do any seem to be out of line? If so, a bone may be broken.

➤ Numbness of any part of the hand beyond a wound is an ominous sign of nerve damage, as is lack of sweating.

FRACTURES TO THE FINGERS

For fractured fingers, apply padding around the hand, elevate in a high sling and take to hospital. Avoid taping fingers together to splint them, as the tape will only have to be removed by hospital staff, causing pain and possible movement. Only splint if help will be delayed for more than 12 hours.

◁ Fractures to the forearm or wrist require supportive padding and a secure sling. Make sure that the support is lightweight – you must not use anything that will strain the neck.

Managing rib fractures

SEE ALSO
➤ Dealing with shock, p68
➤ Dealing with major wounds, p134
➤ Fixing slings, p206

While a cracked rib usually constitutes a relatively minor accident, multiple rib fractures can lead to a collapsed lung (a pneumothorax) or later to pneumonia. If part of the chest wall caves in completely an injury known as a "flail chest" may occur, which may cause severe breathing difficulties and is potentially life-threatening. If ribs lower down the ribcage are fractured they may damage internal organs nearby, such as the liver and spleen, causing internal bleeding, which could cause the casualty to go into shock.

A human ribcage has 12 pairs of ribs. All ribs connect with the spine at the back and all but the lowest pair attach to the breastbone at the front. The ribs are joined together by muscles, which expand and contract in order to move the ribcage. This movement, along with the movement of the diaphragm muscle, allows us to breathe.

The upper ribs protect the heart, lungs and vital blood vessels in this area. The lower ribs help to protect internal organs such as the liver, stomach and spleen.

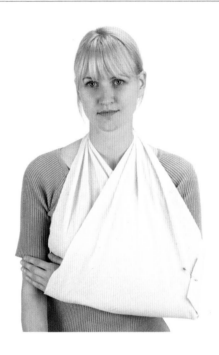

▷ For a fractured rib, use this type of sling to support the arm on the injured side. This prevents certain muscles (ones that are attached to the chest and help to move the arm) from pulling on the ribs.

TYPES OF RIB FRACTURE

There is a difference between a cracked rib caused by a badly aimed kick during a football match, and the sort of fractures that might occur from a steering wheel on the driver's chest after a road traffic accident. Although a single rib fracture can be excruciatingly painful and may remain so for up to ten days after the injury, there is little chance that it could cause serious internal damage. Sometimes, although it is

FIRST AID FOR A FRACTURED RIB

YOUR AIMS:
For a minor rib fracture you need to prevent further damage, such as from bending forward. For rib injury with possible complications (e.g. lung damage), call the emergency services and sit the casualty up, supported and encourage them to relax, so that they can breathe more easily and oxygen demand is reduced.

For all cases: keep the casualty comfortable and supported and apply a broad arm sling to support the arm on the injured side.

For more serious cases, call an ambulance or transport the casualty straight to hospital, keeping the chest supported.

SIGNS AND SYMPTOMS OF A FRACTURED RIB OR RIBS

As fractured ribs can cause a collapsed lung, possible internal bleeding and/or breathing difficulties, it is vital to know which symptoms indicate the severity of the injury so that the right help can be given.

Signs of fractured ribs:

➤ Sharp pain at the site of fracture.

➤ Painful breathing, especially when taking a deep breath in.

➤ Shallow breathing or breathlessness.

➤ Swelling or bruising over the fracture site.

➤ A crackling sensation affecting the chest wall.

➤ "Sucked in" air sounds through an open wound over the fracture site.

Signs of internal bleeding:

➤ Bright red, frothy coughed-up blood in the mouth.

Signs of shock (due to internal bleeding):

➤ Pale skin, and/or a blueness just inside the lips.

➤ Dizziness.

➤ Nausea, possibly vomiting.

➤ Rapid shallow breathing or gasping for air.

➤ Any degree of deteriorating level of consciousness.

unusual, the jagged edge of a fractured rib may penetrate a lung and cause it to collapse (a pneumothorax).

Multiple rib fractures are a different story, however. These not only indicate the greater forces involved (and thus an increased chance that internal organs may be damaged) but also pose a potential danger in that the damaged section of the chest wall may lead to a pneumothorax and later to pneumonia. If damaged ribs become detached from the chest wall, part of the chest wall can cave in completely and form what is known as a "flail chest". Such a condition can cause serious breathing problems and is a potentially life-threatening situation.

In cases of rib fracture, especially if the casualty has been crushed, there is increased chance of internal bleeding and, in turn, of developing shock. Be aware of such events, monitor the casualty's ABC and be prepared to give first aid accordingly until medical help arrives.

PARADOXICAL BREATHING

This is a condition that occurs with some flail chest casualties. Usually, as you breathe in, your ribcage moves up and out and as you breathe out it returns to a lower position. If part of the chest wall is damaged, then it will move in on inspiration and out on breathing out – paradoxical breathing.

OPEN CHEST WOUNDS

If there is a deep chest wound at the fracture site, call the emergency services promptly. Apply a totally airtight dressing consisting of plastic first, then a pad and then a bandage.

If there is an object such as a knife embedded in the wound DO NOT remove it – tape it in place. Get the casualty to sit up – they should be supported and preferably leaning towards the injured side. Apply a sling as in a simple rib fracture, keep the casualty supported and relaxed and await medical help.

FIRST AID FOR FLAIL CHEST

When two or more consecutive ribs on the same side of the chest are fractured in two places, the injured part of the chest wall is known as a "flail segment". The casualty will display all the symptoms of a rib fracture, and may also have paradoxical breathing.

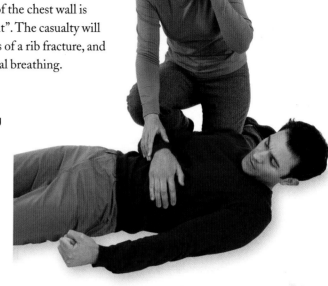

1 First assess the casualty, including their ABC, and be prepared to resuscitate if necessary. Whatever their condition, phone the emergency services promptly.

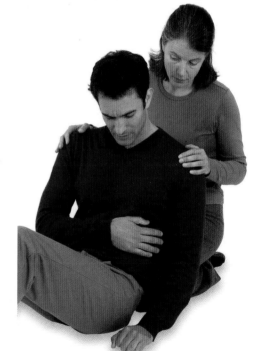

2 ▷ IF THE CASUALTY IS CONSCIOUS: Keep them sitting up as much as possible, relaxed and supported from behind. This means they can breathe more easily and reduces the body's oxygen demand.

▽ IF THE CASUALTY IS UNCONSCIOUS: Place in the recovery position, injured side down. This lets the uninjured side of the ribcage expand. Place padding, in the form of folded blankets, towels or clothes, either side of the flail area, in order to take pressure off the flail site itself. Always try to avoid moving the casualty and then tucking padding underneath. You should place the padding on the floor first and then roll the casualty very carefully on to it.

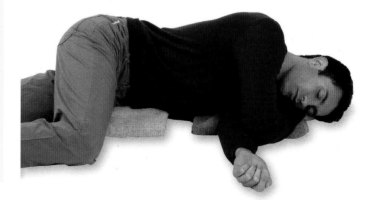

Coping with pelvic and upper-leg injuries

SEE ALSO
➤ Full resuscitation sequence, p33
➤ Dealing with shock, p68
➤ Recognizing internal bleeding, p140

The pelvis, hips and thighbones all have a huge nerve and blood supply; what's more the pelvis contains many vital organs. Damage to any of these regions is an emergency. If fractured, the pelvis and/or thighbone can bleed profusely; multiple pelvic fractures are often fatal. Pelvic fracture may be caused by a crush injury, such as from a steering wheel in a road accident, or by indirect forces of the type occurring during traffic collisions. A horse rider may suffer pelvic injury if they are thrown off, and/or are then kicked by, their horse.

PELVIC FRACTURES

Injuries to the pelvis must be taken seriously. Major blood vessels might be damaged, leading to profuse and even life-threatening internal blood loss. The bladder and urethra may be damaged by the fractured bones, as may the reproductive organs.

Pelvic fractures tend to result from high-speed accidents, and so there will often be other injuries too, including internal damage and spinal injuries. All of these factors may quickly lead to signs of shock developing.

SIGNS AND SYMPTOMS OF A FRACTURED PELVIS

➤ Pain and tenderness in the pelvis, groin or hip especially on moving.

➤ Inability to walk or stand or to lift their legs while lying flat on the floor.

➤ An obviously deformed pelvis.

➤ Blood seeping from the penis or urethra (urinary outlet).

➤ Signs of shock or internal bleeding.

THE PELVIC REGION

▽ The pelvis comprises the ilium, pubis and ischium bones. The head of the femur (thighbone) fits into the pelvis at the hip.

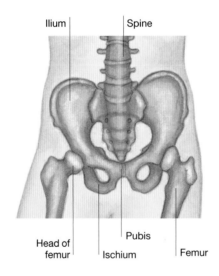

Ilium | Spine

Head of femur | Ischium | Pubis | Femur

WARNING

You should never attempt to move a casualty if you suspect a fractured pelvis unless they are in immediate danger – you could risk further serious damage.

STABILIZING A FRACTURED PELVIS

▷ Place padding as shown. Padding either side of the body should extend above the pelvis and should be held in place by weighted objects. Make sure that the feet cannot rotate in either direction – this rotates the head of the femur in the pelvis.

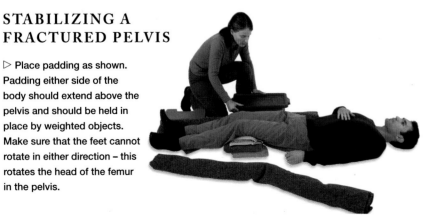

FIRST AID FOR A FRACTURED PELVIS

Call the emergency services urgently.

Move the casualty as little as possible; try to keep their feet in the position found.

Stabilize the pelvis by immobilizing the legs: place rolled blankets or similar under the knees and either side of the legs, held in place by weighted boxes, or similar.

Monitor the casualty's condition, and keep a close eye out for signs of shock.

Only if you are in a very remote location and need to take the casualty to a hospital yourself, tie bandages around the padding and legs at the lower thigh, knees and ankles. However, do not do this if it causes more pain.

FRACTURES TO THE THIGHBONE

The thighbone (femur) forms a large ball and socket joint – the hip – where it meets the pelvis. Any fracture to the thighbone is a serious emergency as it can lead to profuse bleeding if the broken bones pierce the large blood vessels nearby. Shock, then, is a distinct possibility and the casualty should be monitored closely for any such signs that appear.

The thighbone can fracture anywhere but common sites include the long shaft and the neck (top) of the bone, near the hip joint. Fractures to the long shaft would occur after the considerable force involved in traumas such as a traffic accident; fractures of the neck of the bone (that is, at the hip) are common in older people whose bones tend to become weaker and more fragile with age, or the brittle bone disease osteoporosis. If such a fracture is stable, an older person may hobble about on the injured leg. When combined with confusion or dementia, such a fracture may go unnoticed for some time as they may forget that they have fallen or are in pain.

FEMUR FRACTURES

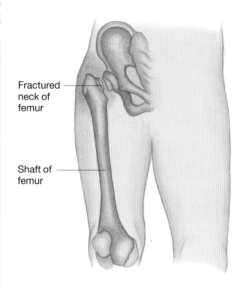

Fractured neck of femur

Shaft of femur

△ The thighbone (femur) commonly fractures at the top and along its shaft.

SIGNS AND SYMPTOMS OF A FRACTURED THIGHBONE

➤ Pain and tenderness at the site of injury or at the knee.

➤ An inability to walk or put weight on the affected leg.

➤ Deformity in the affected leg, making it look shorter than the unaffected one.

➤ An awkward-looking leg that is noticeably bent at the knee and also turned outwards at the ankle.

➤ Signs of shock.

FIRST AID FOR A FRACTURED THIGHBONE

Call the emergency services promptly.

Keep the area still by using your hands or by placing padding (such as blankets or towels) around the hip, leg and body, held in place with weighted objects. Ideally, padding should extend above the pelvis and below the knee.

Monitor the casualty and keep a close eye out for signs of shock.

Only if you are in a very remote location, and need to transport the casualty to hospital yourself, splint the body (ideally from armpit to below the feet) on the injured side and secure the body and limb to the splint with bandages, tied at regular intervals.

FIRST AID FOR A FRACTURED THIGHBONE

▷ If a fractured thighbone casualty is found on their side, keep them in that position (always try to treat in the position found), but support their back in some way. Essentially, a fractured thighbone is treated in the same way as a fractured pelvis, using support and padding. This picture shows an alternative manual method of support, where the first-aider's arm is being used as a splint – suitable for fracture cases where help will arrive quickly or there are few materials to hand.

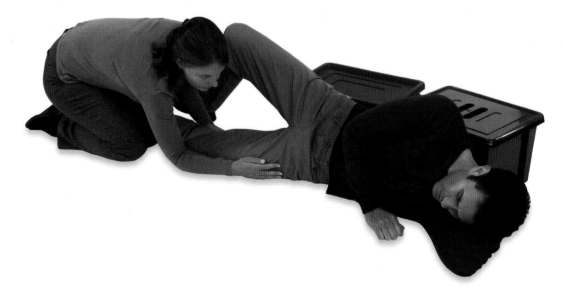

Handling knee and lower-leg injuries

SEE ALSO

➤ Managing sprains and strains, p168

The knee is the body's largest joint. It can perform complex movements and is structured so that it remains stable while bearing the body's weight. The knee has sets of ligaments to hold the bones in place, including the patella (kneecap) at the front. Broken bones, tears or impacts to the knee joint can produce incredible pain and swelling. Any fracture or tear requires immobilization and open wounds should also be dealt with. Your first-aid aims are to immobilize limbs, minimize swelling and arrange for urgent transport to hospital.

INJURIES TO THE KNEE

There are two cruciate ligaments in the knee joint, so called because they cross over each other as they pass diagonally down from the thighbone to the shinbone. These ligaments are most commonly damaged in accidents when the knee is twisted. Other tissues in the knee that can suffer injury include the cartilage and the bony patella (kneecap).

SIGNS AND SYMPTOMS OF A LOWER-LEG INJURY

➤ Pain deep within the knee or localized pain to the injury site, often made worse by trying to move the limb or put weight on it.

➤ Swelling and/or bruising around the knee or injury.

➤ Great pain when trying to straighten the leg (gently) if the knee has "locked".

➤ Broken bones protruding through the skin at the fracture site.

➤ Inability to bear weight on the affected side.

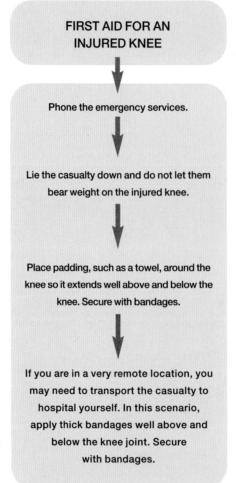

FIRST AID FOR AN INJURED KNEE

Phone the emergency services.

Lie the casualty down and do not let them bear weight on the injured knee.

Place padding, such as a towel, around the knee so it extends well above and below the knee. Secure with bandages.

If you are in a very remote location, you may need to transport the casualty to hospital yourself. In this scenario, apply thick bandages well above and below the knee joint. Secure with bandages.

INJURIES TO THE LOWER LEG

The fibula is a spindly bone that fractures easily without necessarily stopping a person from weight bearing. Fractures of the fibula, therefore, may not be initially obvious. However, if the larger, load-bearing tibia (shinbone) is broken, a person cannot usually stand up or bear weight. A fracture of the tibia may cause bleeding and circulation problems in the area beyond the fracture site. Other injuries include tears to muscles, tendons and ligaments of the lower leg.

LOWER-LEG FRACTURES

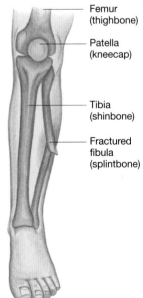

▷ Any of the lower leg bones – patella, tibia or fibula – may be fractured in an accident. This illustration shows a fracture site in the thinner fibula.

Femur (thighbone)

Patella (kneecap)

Tibia (shinbone)

Fractured fibula (splintbone)

FIRST AID FOR AN INJURED KNEE

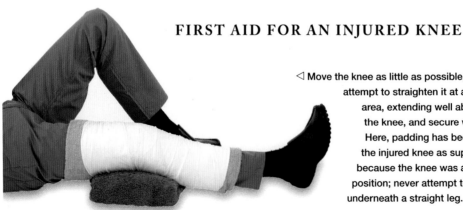

◁ Move the knee as little as possible, and never attempt to straighten it at all. Pad a wide area, extending well above and below the knee, and secure with bandages. Here, padding has been slid under the injured knee as support only because the knee was already in a bent position; never attempt to force padding underneath a straight leg.

FIRST AID FOR A LOWER-LEG FRACTURE

1 Lay the casualty down while supporting the injured leg. Remove shoes in case of swelling and feel the foot and lower leg for warmth and to check that the casualty can sense your touch.

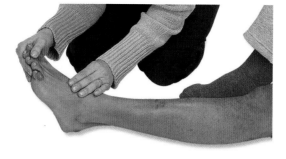

2 Phone for the emergency services. Place some soft padding on both sides of the legs, extending well above the knees and held in place by objects such as heavy boxes. Ensure that the foot is supported in the position found.

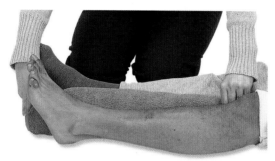

▷ If you are in a remote location and have to take the casualty to a hospital or doctor yourself, then secure the padding with bandages. Place them well above and below the fracture site.

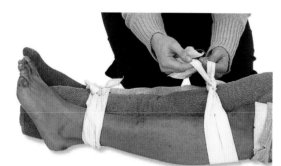

ANKLE INJURIES

By far the most common ankle injury is a sprain, which is dealt with elsewhere using the RICE guidelines (RICE stands for rest, ice, compression and elevation). Any fracture to the ankle bone should be treated as for a lower-leg fracture.

A BROKEN FOOT

There are many small bones in the foot, any of which could be broken during an accident, most often one of a crushing nature. A fracture of the calcaneum (heelbone) is particularly common after a fall from a height on to the feet.

Individual toes may also suffer injury, but unless a toe is twisted right out of its usual alignment, even broken toes generally heal extremely well after professional medical treatment.

FIRST AID FOR A FRACTURE OF THE FOOT

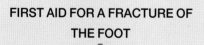

Sit or lay the casualty down. Elevate and support the injured foot immediately to minimize swelling.

↓

Applying a cold compress may further reduce swelling, but do not do if painful.

↓

Get the casualty to hospital by either car or ambulance.

▽ Elevate and comfortably support a fractured foot. Only apply a cold compress (such as ice wrapped in a towel) to reduce swelling if this does not cause pain – extreme temperatures can be very uncomfortable for fracture casualties. Elevate the leg above horizontal if possible and comfortable.

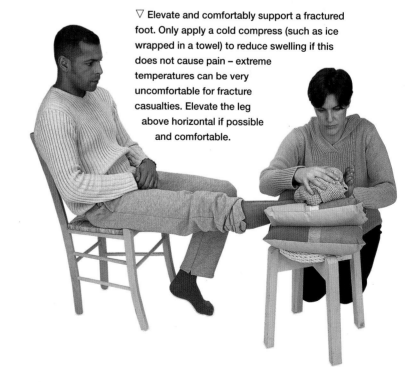

Coping with dislocations

SEE ALSO
➤ Moving and handling safely 1 and 2, pp20, 22
➤ Understanding the skeleton, p148

Any joint may become dislocated due to a violent wrenching action. In dislocated joints, surrounding muscles, ligaments, tendons and blood vessels may be disturbed or damaged as a result. The force of dislocation can sometimes also produce a fracture nearby. Any dislocated joint looks misshapen, and the casualty experiences extreme pain and the joint soon becomes swollen, discoloured and immobile. First-aiders should try to immobilize the injured joint, to prevent further injury and reduce pain, and seek emergency medical help.

Dislocations may occur within any joint, when the end of a bone is pulled or pushed out of place and thus out of the joint. It can be a very distressing experience as the muscles around a dislocated joint often go into spasm, causing intense pain. Nerves and blood vessels around the joint may also be damaged.

It is not always possible to distinguish between a fracture and a dislocation, and both may occur within a joint at the same time. If in doubt, treat a dislocation as if it were a fracture.

The most common joints for dislocation are the shoulder, hip, elbow, jaw and joints of the thumbs and fingers.

WARNING

Never try to relocate the bone of a dislocated joint or attempt any strategies to get the bone to "pop" back in again. It is easy to inflict further serious damage.

SIGNS AND SYMPTOMS OF A DISLOCATED SHOULDER

➤ It may be possible to feel the "popped out" rounded head of the humerus (upper arm bone) in front of the shoulder joint.

➤ Distortion in the shoulder joint; the upper arm may look flat.

➤ Severe pain in the shoulder, which is also difficult to move.

➤ Swelling and/or bruising in the joint.

FIRST AID FOR A DISLOCATED SHOULDER

Get the casualty to sit down and make them as comfortable as possible. Let them hold their arm in whatever position is least painful. Calm and reassure the casualty – dislocations can be sudden and acutely painful and so may be highly distressing.

Slide a triangular bandage between the arm of the affected shoulder and the casualty's chest – as for an arm sling. Very gently place some padding underneath the affected arm.

Tie the padded arm sling so that the affected arm is well supported.

Arrange transport to hospital. In transit, the casualty should stay seated.

SHOULDER DISLOCATION

Some people are unlucky enough to suffer from this common injury recurrently. For these unfortunate few, the condition is often just as painful as for one-off or occasional cases, but the shoulder does "pop" back in much more easily.

IMMEDIATE HELP FOR A DISLOCATED SHOULDER

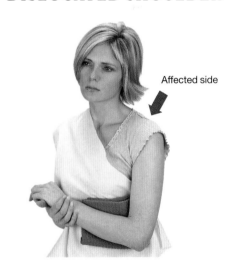

Affected side

1 Carefully place a sling and some soft padding between the arm of the affected shoulder and the body.

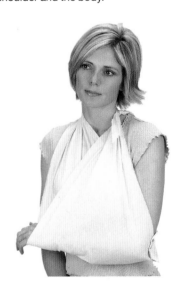

2 Once the padding is in place, tie the sling so that the joint is supported. Get the casualty to hospital straight away.

HOW TO DEAL WITH A DISLOCATED HIP

The hip joint may dislocate, for example, when the knee hits the dashboard in a car accident. This sort of accident often results in a fractured pelvis and damage to nearby nerves as well, resulting in paralysis. The head of the thighbone usually moves backwards, and the leg rotates outwards and is bent at the knee. The bony end of the thighbone may be easily felt or seen sticking out under the skin at or near the hip.

▽ Treatment for a dislocated hip is essentially the same as for a fractured pelvis or thighbone. Treat the casualty in the position found and do not move them if at all possible. Immobilize the immediate and surrounding area by padding and supporting it – using rolled blankets, towels and so on located under the knees and either side of the body and held in place by heavy objects such as boxes or briefcases.

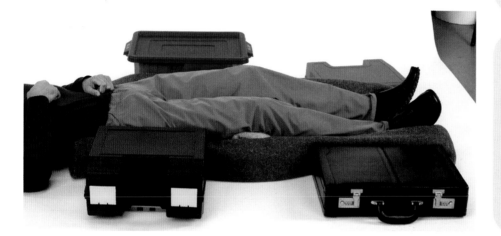

A DISLOCATED ELBOW

Children very easily stretch ligaments. In the elbow, the top of one of the forearm bones (the radius) sometimes "pops out" of the elbow joint, especially if a child's arm is yanked suddenly as might happen in a fall. Suspect a pulled elbow if:
- The child suddenly stops using the affected arm.
- The child cries when the arm is moved or touched at all, especially in the elbow area.

HOW TO DEAL WITH A CHILD'S PULLED ELBOW

Reassure the child and allow them to hold their arm in whatever position they find comfortable.

Do not try to "pop" the lower arm back into place. Phone the emergency services or take the child to hospital.

A DISLOCATED JAW

This is a fairly common occurrence and may be caused by an everyday action of the jaw, such as yawning. In cases of a dislocated jaw, a person will not be able to close their jaw at all so they will be unable to speak properly and may drool. The jaw will have to be relocated in hospital, after which it will be bandaged to keep it immobile for two to three days.

HAND DISLOCATIONS

Contact sports, such as martial arts, and skiing accidents can often lead to the dislocation of one of the many joints in the hand, especially the thumb. The best action to take is to pad up the hand and elevate it in a high sling before taking the casualty to hospital for medical treatment. Never attempt to change the position of any damaged fingers.

HOW TO DEAL WITH A DISLOCATED HAND

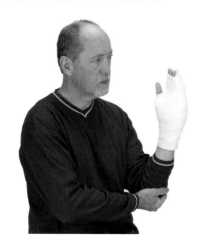

1 Remove any rings, watches or bracelets before the hand starts to swell, but only if you can avoid bending affected fingers. Ask the casualty to support their arm while you wrap the hand in padding.

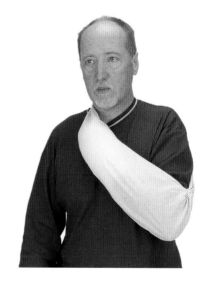

2 Once the casualty is comfortable and the arm supported, immobilize the joint using a high sling (and more padding if necessary). Firmer support could be given by tying another bandage around the sling to attach it to the body. Get the casualty to a doctor.

Managing sprains and strains

SEE ALSO
➤ Moving and handling safely 1 and 2, pp20, 22
➤ Applying dressings & bandages, p200
➤ Applying bandages 1, p202

The soft tissues – muscles, tendons and ligaments – that attach to or support the bones of the skeleton can also be injured or damaged in an accident. Such injuries are generally called sprains and strains and happen most often during sporting activities. The first-aid aims of treating such soft-tissue injuries are to reduce pain and swelling and to seek medical help if necessary. It can sometimes be tricky to distinguish between a sprain and a fracture, and so medical advice should be sought if there is any shadow of a doubt.

For the skeleton to be able to move the body about, it needs the help of essential soft tissues – muscles, tendons and ligaments. Muscles attach to bones via tendons, while ligaments are the tough fibrous cords that hold bones together at joints and allow joints to function properly. Together the bones, muscles and joints are known as the musculoskeletal system.

When there are no broken bones, the injury is called a soft-tissue injury. These are perceived to be less serious than fractures but can still cause a great deal of pain and disability. If they are not dealt with properly in the initial stages, they may lead to long-term weakness and malfunction in a muscle or joint.

"GOING OVER"

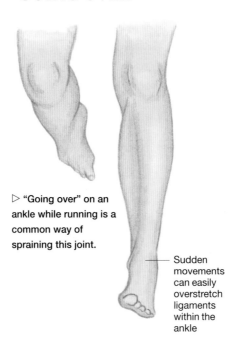

▷ "Going over" on an ankle while running is a common way of spraining this joint.

Sudden movements can easily overstretch ligaments within the ankle

TORN LIGAMENTS

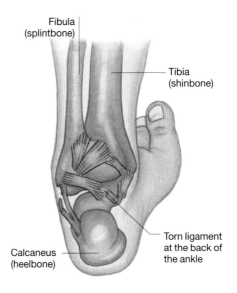

Fibula (splintbone)

Tibia (shinbone)

Torn ligament at the back of the ankle

Calcaneus (heelbone)

△ In a sprained ankle, one or more of the ligaments are partially or completely torn.

DIFFERENT TYPES OF SOFT-TISSUE INJURY

➤ Sprain – A common form of ligament injury resulting in tearing or overstretching of the ligament.

➤ Strain – The tearing or overstretching of a muscle. Strains often happen near the junction of the muscle and its tendon, which tethers the muscle to the nearby bone.

➤ Rupture – The complete tearing of a ligament or a muscle.

➤ Bruise – The swelling, pain and bleeding below the skin that result from a direct blow to the body. A large amount of blood that collects as a result of damage is known as a haematoma.

SIGNS AND SYMPTOMS OF A SPRAIN OR STRAIN

Bear in mind that it can be difficult to distinguish between a sprain or strain and a fracture. There are a few clues, though, to watch out for.

Symptoms of a sprain or strain include:

➤ Pain and tenderness. (If the casualty heard or felt a crack at the time of the incident, the injury is more likely to be a fracture.)

➤ Inability to use the injured part. (However, an immediate inability to bear weight on the injured part points to a fracture.)

➤ Swelling and bruising. (If the swelling takes several hours to appear it's more likely to be a soft-tissue injury; swelling after a fracture is immediate.)

HOW TO TREAT SPRAINS AND STRAINS

After following the RICE guidelines (opposite), you may decide to seek medical attention. After following RICE, minor soft-tissue injuries should be followed by gentle, controlled exercise as soon as symptoms allow. Many sprains remain stiff, swollen and painful even after 48 hours of RICE treatment. This is normal, and it is important to start using the joint or muscle, as it can easily stiffen up and recover slowly. If not properly treated in the first few weeks after injury, a sprain can cause recurrent problems in the long term – even more so than a simple fracture in the same area.

FIRST AID FOR SPRAINS AND STRAINS

Follow the RICE guidelines – Rest, Ice, Compress and Elevate.

Rest – Most soft-tissue injuries need to be rested for 24–48 hours while being kept as comfortable as possible.

Ice – Reduce the pain and swelling associated with soft-tissue injuries using ice or a packet of frozen peas wrapped in a cloth. Apply initially and then for short periods of 10–15 minutes at a time for the first 24–48 hours. Do not apply ice or anything frozen directly to the skin; it will be painful and may damage the skin.

Compress – Applying pressure to the injured part may make the casualty more comfortable. Elasticated tubular bandages give the best compression, although crepe bandages over layers of cotton wool also work well.

Elevate – Rest the injured part above horizontal and ideally above the level of the heart, which will reduce swelling.

WARNING

If you are in any doubt as to the severity of injury, it is always best to get a medical opinion about any sprain or strain. An X-ray may be needed to find out whether it is indeed a sprain, or a fracture has occurred. The casualty may need physiotherapy, or referral to a clinic for regular checks.

HOW TO DEAL WITH A SPRAINED ANKLE

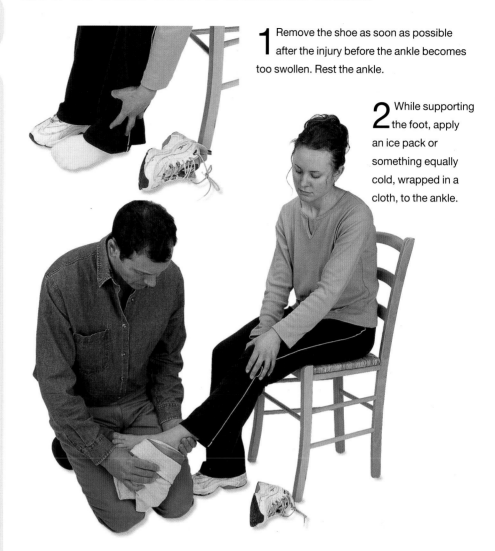

1 Remove the shoe as soon as possible after the injury before the ankle becomes too swollen. Rest the ankle.

2 While supporting the foot, apply an ice pack or something equally cold, wrapped in a cloth, to the ankle.

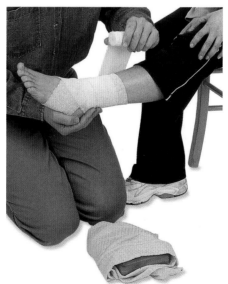

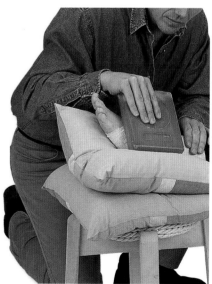

3 Use a crepe or elasticated bandage to apply compression to the injured ankle. Keep supporting the ankle all the time.

4 Carefully place the injured ankle in a position that keeps it rested, comfortable and elevated. Apply a cold compress regularly.

Alleviating back pain

SEE ALSO

➤ Moving and handling safely 1 and 2, pp20, 22

➤ Managing spinal injuries, p154

Back pain varies enormously from person to person. Even an excruciating bout of back pain can resolve itself in a matter of a few weeks. However, anyone who is worried about what is causing the pain in their back should consult their doctor. When approaching an incident where someone complains of back pain, be alert to the danger signs that could indicate some form of spinal injury. Much back pain resolves with painkillers and, contrary to popular opinion, staying active – resting can make the back stiff and immobile.

Most people suffer from back pain at some point in their lives. In the vast majority of cases, the pain is in the lower back, or lumbar region. The lumbar spine has to be strong as it bears the weight of the body as well as any other loads it has to carry.

It is reassuring to know that back pain is not usually due to any serious disease. Most cases of low back pain resolve quickly, although they may take up to 6–8 weeks to settle down completely. Upper back pain is more unusual.

▷ Pain in the mobile regions of the spine – the neck and lower back – is the most common form of back pain.

COMMON PAIN SITES

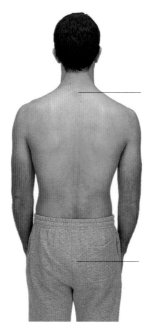

Pain at the top of the spine – the neck – will often cause headaches, and the sufferer may not realize their root cause

Lower back pain that spreads into one or both buttocks and one or both legs is due to impingement of the sciatic nerve

CAUSES OF BACK PAIN

Frustratingly for the sufferer, the exact cause of most back pain is rarely discovered. Back pain tends to originate in the muscles, ligaments and joints of the back, but pinpointing exactly which ones is often impossible. Rarely, there is an underlying cause, such as a tumour, kidney problems, a collapsed vertebra due to the bone-thinning condition osteoporosis, scoliosis (where the spine develops an abnormal curvature to the side) or a slipped intervertebral disc.

SPINAL COMPRESSION

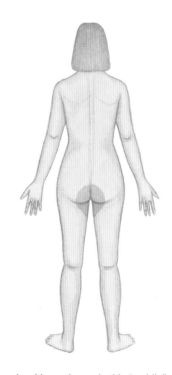

△ People with numbness in this "saddle" area may have spinal compression and should see a doctor immediately. (Sphincter disturbance and lower limb weakness are other signs.)

SIGNS AND SYMPTOMS OF BACK PAIN

Signs of back pain:

➤ Pain, which may vary from dull to severe, across the lower back is particularly common. Sometimes this pain spreads into the buttock and shoots down the leg (sciatica); such pain is due to pressure on the sciatic nerve.

➤ Inability to move the back, especially bending and leaning back.

➤ Muscle spasm in the back muscles, causing a rigid or stiff neck.

➤ Tenderness in the back muscles themselves.

Seek medical help if there is also:

➤ Pain in the buttocks, legs or arms.

➤ Any numbness or tingling in the limbs.

➤ Weight loss.

➤ Fever.

➤ Any loss of sensation or movement.

➤ General feeling of being unwell.

➤ Incontinence or inability to open bowels. Urinary problems such as low output, pain on urinating, unusual colour, smell or cloudiness.

➤ Unremitting/increasing back pain.

➤ If the person is under 20 or over 50.

WHAT YOU CAN DO AT HOME

Most people find it useful to use pain-controlling medication of some kind but your doctor may prescribe a muscle relaxant if your pain is not relieved by painkillers alone. You can also modify your physical activities to avoid potential problems in the first place:

• Lifting – Never twist the back, but turn with your feet instead. Always bend at the knees to grasp the object and use your legs to help you lift rather than relying solely on the strength of your back. Keep the heaviest side of the object close to your body and get help if needed.

HOW TO DEAL WITH BACK PAIN

You may choose to take your regular painkillers to ease backache. Non-steroidal anti-inflammatory drugs such as ibuprofen, paracetamol-based painkillers and prescription muscle relaxants can all help.

In the first 24 hours, apply a bag of frozen peas wrapped in a towel on the back for regular periods of 10 minutes. Or try a soak in a warm bath or a hot-water bottle, or alternate hot and cold applications.

Back manipulation – Physical therapies such as osteopathy and chiropractic can help relieve back pain and solve many back-related problems.

Complementary treatments – Acupuncture and massage therapy have both been shown to help alleviate some types of back pain.

PAIN IN THE OVER-50S

The sudden onset of severe and unremitting back pain in anyone over 50 should be taken seriously, especially if it is not in the lower back, but higher up. The bones of the back are a common place for various cancers to spread, and there are also cancers that develop in the bones of the back.

• Sitting – Sit in an upright chair for no longer than 20 or 30 minutes at a time. Also, a lumbar support helps to keep you sitting "tall" rather than slumping.
• Driving – Travelling of any kind can make back pain a lot worse, especially when undertaking long-distance journeys.
• Sleeping – Get a good night's sleep and lie on a fairly firm, flat surface. Too soft and too hard are both bad for the back.
• Working – Make sure all working surfaces are at a good height for you, so that you are not straining.

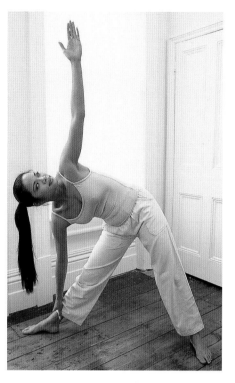

△ When trying out a new activity, such as yoga, take it easy on your back and stretch slowly and gradually.

STAY ACTIVE

People who are physically fit suffer from less back pain and generally recover faster than those who are unfit and overweight. Regular gentle activity helps to strengthen a painful back, and the sooner this exercise is started the better. Swimming, walking and cycling are all good low-impact exercises that will not damage the back.

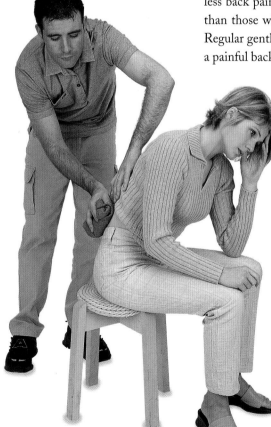

◁ One tip that helps to ease back pain, is to ask a friend or partner to apply an ice pack or bag of frozen peas – wrapped in a towel – to the site of the pain.

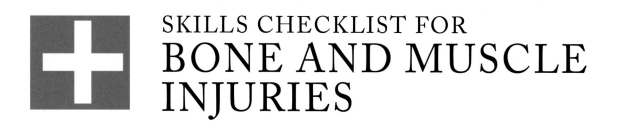

SKILLS CHECKLIST FOR
BONE AND MUSCLE INJURIES

KEY POINTS

- Take great care over the how and when of moving a casualty with a bone or muscle injury, especially if they have a definite/suspected head or spinal injury; keeping affected parts still and supported is key ☐

- Splinting is best reserved for extreme situations where you are forced to take the casualty to the nearest doctor/hospital yourself ☐

- Be alert to the possibility of a spinal injury after any accident ☐

- Do not try to relocate a dislocated joint ☐

- Back pain usually resolves itself within six to eight weeks ☐

SKILLS LEARNED

- How to tackle both "open" and "closed" fractures ☐

- How to deal with the many different types of fractures, all over the body ☐

- How to recognize and manage potential spinal problems ☐

- How to "log roll" a casualty ☐

- How to deal with dislocations, strains and sprains ☐

- How to relieve back pain ☐

BURNS AND SCALDS

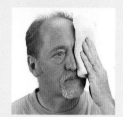

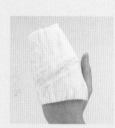

First aid is of paramount importance for the burn casualty. The first-aider can significantly limit the pain, damage and trauma of a burn by cooling the area as quickly as possible. Reducing the skin's temperature helps to limit the depth and severity of damage to underlying tissues. Burns range from a straightforward, relatively superficial injury to a very deep injury that penetrates muscles, nerves and bone. Home safety has a major part to play in preventing burn accidents. Domestic fires are responsible for over three-quarters of civilian deaths from burns, and many of these might be avoided through installing and maintaining smoke detectors.

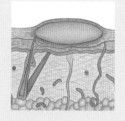

CONTENTS

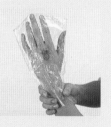

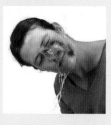

Understanding and assessing burns 1

SEE ALSO

➤ Assessing burns 2, p176

➤ Safety in the home, p224

➤ Safety in the kitchen, p226

Initial action with any burn, however severe, is the same – remove the source of the burn and cool the burnt area under cold running water for at least 10 minutes. Burns weaken and damage the skin so do not turn on the tap to full power. Cooling the skin as quickly as possible reduces any pain and swelling and also helps to prevent damage to underlying tissues. Remove any constricting articles, such as jewellery. If a burn is larger than the size of the casualty's palm, is deep, or is on the face, hands or feet the casualty should be seen at a hospital.

The skin is the body's largest organ, covering the entire surface of the body. It forms a barrier against infection and also helps protect against injury and maintain body temperature. Burns to the skin cause instant damage but quick thinking and rapid first-aid action can make all the difference to the outcome. If deep layers of the skin are damaged, they will not heal easily and may even require skin grafts.

COMPLICATIONS OF BURNS

When giving first aid for a serious burn, bear in mind the following life-threatening burn-related complications:

- If the casualty's airway becomes burnt, it may swell, resulting in potentially fatal breathing problems.
- The casualty may have other injuries (if they have jumped to escape a fire or have been in an explosion, for example).
- If the entire circumference of their chest is burnt, they will not be able to move their chest in order to breathe.
- Severe burns lead to large amounts of fluid loss and therefore can lead to shock.

GIVING ALL THE DETAILS

When speaking to the emergency services, it is essential to give them any known information about the cause of the burn. If there was an explosion, for example, the casualty may have other injuries. And, if there was burning material, or the fire was in an enclosed space, there is a risk of inhalation poisoning and airway swelling. Knowing how long the casualty was exposed to the material helps paramedics to assess the extent of any damage.

THE SKIN'S STRUCTURE

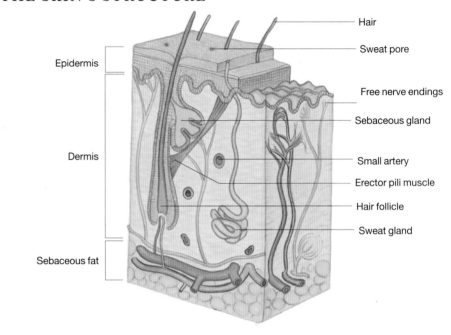

Epidermis

Dermis

Sebaceous fat

Hair

Sweat pore

Free nerve endings

Sebaceous gland

Small artery

Erector pili muscle

Hair follicle

Sweat gland

DIFFERENT TYPES OF BURNS

➤ Dry burns – Such injuries are caused by any form of flame or hot surface, such as lighted cigarettes, hot irons and hobs, bonfires and hot barbecue coals.

➤ Wet burns – Also called scalds, these are caused by boiling liquids, steam and cooking fat or oil.

➤ Cold burns – The skin can also be burnt by extreme cold, such as contact with ice-cold metal.

➤ Friction burns – These are the result of a surface (especially of a synthetic material) rubbing against the skin at speed. A moving rope or wire, revolving brushes and machine belts are common culprits.

➤ Radiation burns – Most commonly from over-exposure to ultraviolet light, such as in sunburn.

➤ Chemical burns – Many common household products and work chemicals (such as bleach, ammonia, oven cleaners, drain fluids, caustic soda, wood preserver and treatments for wet and dry rot) contain chemicals that can burn skin. Appropriate safety gloves and goggles should be worn when using such products, and protective clothing should be worn by anyone dealing with industrial chemicals.

➤ Electrical burns – These burns are caused by contact with electricity in any form, including lightning.

ESSENTIALS OF BURN MANAGEMENT

Cooling the burnt area is the major principle to remember when dealing with burns and scalds. Cooling will not only reduce pain but it will also limit the extent of the burn and any damage. Do not wrap the burn in a damp dressing as it may stick and promote infection.

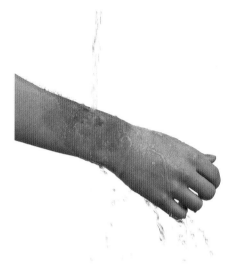

1 Cooling the burnt or scalded area is a top priority. Hold the affected area under a stream of cold water for at least 10 minutes. You should only cool the burnt area; do not over-cool the casualty.

2 Once the burn or scald is cooled, cover with a clear food wrap, or a loose, clean plastic bag.

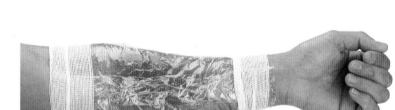

△ To use clear food wrap, discard an initial length of wrap (it will be dirty). Place a layer of wrap on top of the area with the ends running lengthways and secure them loosely, rather than winding the wrap around the limb, in case the burn swells.

ASSESSING BURNS

One important aspect of dealing with burns is deciding how severe the problem is. You need to assess whether a burn is minor or major. Factors affecting this include the depth, extent and site of the burns. For example, burns in the neck and head area can compromise the airway, while burns in the genital area may lead to large amounts of swelling and serious problems with passing water.

MINOR AND MAJOR BURNS

Use the following summary when assessing whether a burn is minor or major and deciding what to do. (However, if you are at all unsure, always seek expert help.)

Minor/superficial burns

If the burn seems relatively small and superficial and there is no risk of infection or scarring, then you should simply get the casualty to make an appointment with a practice doctor or nurse.

Superficial/mild partial-thickness burns

(Note: thickness of burns is dealt with in more detail on the following pages.) If the burn is of this type, and there are other symptoms present – such as dizziness, headache or fainting – the casualty should be seen by a doctor or emergency department without delay.

Serious burns

These include:
- Non-superficial burns with an area greater than the size of the victim's palm.
- Burns in young children, older people and pregnant women.
- Electrical and chemical burns.
- Deep/full-thickness burns of any size.
- Burns that go all around a limb or the

chest ("circumferential" burns).
- Burns to the face, hands, feet or the genitals.

Potentially life-threatening burns

These include:
- Burns to the airway, face or neck.
- Anyone who has inhaled either smoke, fumes or flames.
- A burn over a large area (more than the size of the casualty's palm) or any deeper than superficial.

You must get these burns seen by emergency medical help immediately.

Understanding and assessing burns 2

SEE ALSO

➤ Understanding and assessing burns 1, p174

➤ Safety in the kitchen, p226

It can be hard to judge exactly how severe burns are, but understanding a little more about burn depth and area will help. If you are in any doubt about the severity of any kind of burn, seek medical help as fast as possible. If the casualty is clearly in distress and some pain, call the emergency services immediately, or get the casualty to a local hospital's accident and emergency department. If the burns are severe or over a large surface area, then the casualty may go into shock, so watch for shock signs and be prepared to resuscitate if necessary.

ASSESSING A BURN'S DEPTH

The depth of a burn depends upon the intensity of, and length of exposure to, the burn agent (such as heat, cold or chemicals). The skin has two layers: a surface layer called the epidermis and a deeper layer called the dermis. How deeply a burn has damaged the skin is an indicator of potential complications – fewer such events occur with superficial burns compared with partial- or full-thickness burns.

SUPERFICIAL BURNS

Formerly known as first-degree burns, this type of burn involves only the very uppermost layer of the skin – the epidermis. Typical features of a superficial burn include:

- Red-looking skin that may be a little puffy but with no blistering; it will feel very sensitive and painful.
- Blanching of the skin when pressed.
- Fairly fast healing – usually within 10 days and without leaving a scar.

PARTIAL-THICKNESS BURNS

Burns of this kind used to be called second-degree burns. They destroy areas of the epidermis and result in blistering. Large amounts of fluid may be lost from partial-thickness burns if they cover a large area of the body.

- The skin is red or white, blistered and extremely painful.
- The burn may heal within 21 days and cause little scarring, but very deep burns may take up to 60 days and leave more extensive scars.

DEPTHS OF BURN

▷ **Superficial burns involve only the outermost layer of skin – the epidermis. Underlying layers and the structures they contain, such as nerve endings, are unaffected.**

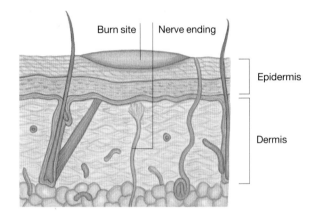

Burn site | Nerve ending

Epidermis

Dermis

▷ **A partial-thickness burn is again limited to the epidermis layer. The skin will look red and raw and will be blistered because tissue fluid from damaged tissues accumulates.**

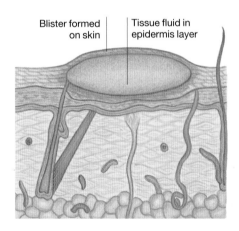

Blister formed on skin | Tissue fluid in epidermis layer

▷ **A full-thickness burn affects both layers of the skin. Because of the burn's severity, fat, nerves, muscle and blood vessels may also be damaged.**

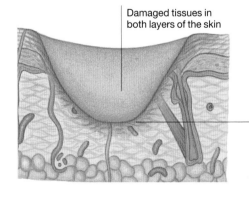

Damaged tissues in both layers of the skin

Pain sensation may be lost as nerve endings are damaged

FULL-THICKNESS BURNS

This type of burn was previously known as a third-degree burn. Such serious burns extend into the skin's dermis and beyond. Hair follicles, nerves and sweat glands, which lie within the dermis, may never recover if they are badly burned. Fluid is unable to ooze through the damaged dermis but is lost internally. In a full-thickness burn:

• The skin is white, black or brown.
• The skin appears leathery or waxy (do not touch it to see how it feels).

• The burnt area is numb and therefore, paradoxically, less painful than a less serious burn.
• The affected skin will never heal on its own and requires a skin graft.

THE EXTENT OF THE BURN

When assessing burns, it is vital to judge how much of the body's surface area is affected, as this will indicate likely fluid losses. When tissue is damaged by burns, tissue fluid leaks from tiny capillaries in the skin as a response and forms blisters or seeps out of the skin blood vessels. The bigger the burn, the bigger the fluid loss and thus the higher the risk of shock.

When trying to assess just how serious a casualty's burns are, it can be helpful to think of the palm of the casualty's hand (including their fingers) as representing 1 per cent of their total body surface. As a good general guide, any partial-thickness burn of 1 per cent or more should be seen urgently by a doctor. Any suspected full-thickness burn, no matter what size, is an emergency and must be seen immediately.

ASSESSING THE BURN AREA

▽ Professional medical personnel have traditionally used the "rule of nines" as a way of accurately assessing the area, and therefore the potential severity, of a burn. Under this rule, parts of the body can be assigned 9 per cent or multiples of 9 per cent. However, the average first-aider should never waste valuable time trying to make such a detailed assessment. Instead, they can quickly compare it to the size of the inner surface of the hand (see right).

▽ Using the burn casualty's hand as a guide is now a common way for first-aiders to assess a burn area. The area of the inner surface of a casualty's hand, including the fingers, represents about 1% of their body area. If a burn is deeper than superficial and has an area of 1% or more, the casualty must be seen urgently at a hospital.

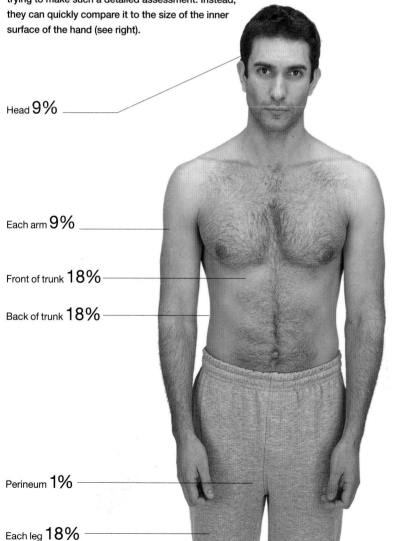

Head 9%

Each arm 9%

Front of trunk 18%

Back of trunk 18%

Perineum 1%

Each leg 18%

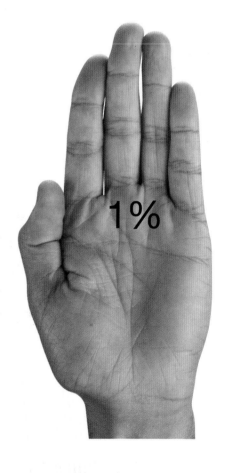

1%

Managing burns

SEE ALSO

➤ Dealing with shock, p68

➤ Understanding and assessing burns 1, p174

➤ Assessing burns 2, p176

Time is of the essence when giving first aid to a casualty with burns. You must ensure that the person is no longer in danger of further burns and then cool the affected area of skin. Do not turn the tap on full force as a powerful jet of water may further damage the delicate skin of the burnt area. Reassure the casualty and phone the emergency services if necessary. If you think the burns are deep or cover a large proportion of the body, watch the casualty carefully and be ready to deal with signs of further problems, such as shock.

As already mentioned, a major priority in all burn cases is to cool the skin. This not only eases much of the pain, but also ultimately reduces the amount of damage done to the skin, so that it heals faster and scars less. However, be careful about making the person too cold and causing hypothermia. If in doubt, cover the casualty with a coat or light blanket.

COVERING BURNS

Skin damage allows potential infection to enter, so burns must be covered. Dry dressings, even non-fluffy ones, tend to stick to burns, so your best options are: gel burn dressings, if available, clean plastic bags, or clear food wrap film.

DEALING WITH CLOTHING ON FIRE

Dousing a victim in water may be impossible if there is no water nearby or if the flames are too strong. If so, get the casualty down to the floor (to stop them running around and fanning the flames) and wrap them in a heavy, non-synthetic material (for example, a cotton or wool rug, coat or curtain) to exclude the air and smother the flames. This is known as the Stop-Drop-Roll technique (see page 232).

BURNS: BASIC PRIORITIES

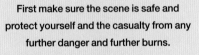

First make sure the scene is safe and protect yourself and the casualty from any further danger and further burns.

Check the casualty's responsiveness and breathing and be prepared to resuscitate if necessary. Continue to monitor the casualty for noisy or difficult breathing.

Cool down the burnt skin. For serious burns, call the emergency services.

Cover the burn, to prevent infection.

Minimize shock and check for any other injuries.

WHAT TO DO WITH SMALL BURNS AND SCALDS

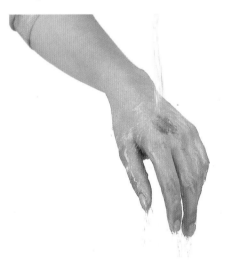

1 Run cold water over the burn site for at least 10 minutes. If the burn is on a hand or arm, remove any watches, rings or bracelets while you are cooling the skin, as the burn may cause some swelling of tissues.

2 After cooling, help prevent infection by wrapping the area with a gel burn dressing or with clear food wrap or a clean plastic bag (ideal for hands and feet). When using a plastic bag, fill the bag with air (do not blow into it, as that will introduce germs), gently place the hand or foot in the open bag, then hold loosely in place at the wrist or ankle with a length of dressing, a bandage or similar – never use rubber bands.

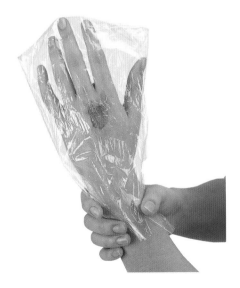

FIRST AID FOR ALL MAJOR BURNS AND SCALDS

1 Having controlled or eliminated any dangers, put the casualty into a safe position. This is usually lying flat, unless there is breathing difficulty, in which case they should sit upright and supported. Prevent the burn from touching the ground. Send for the emergency services and cool the burnt area with cold water for at least 10 minutes. While cooling, remove any constricting items such as watches and bracelets in case swelling cuts off the circulation. See box for advice on clothes removal.

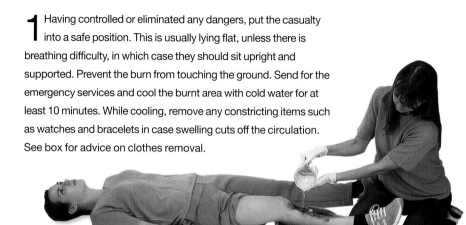

2 If the emergency services have not arrived after 20 minutes of cooling, cover the burnt area to prevent infection. Observe the casualty for breathing problems or worsening shock. Carefully check for other injuries.

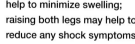

▷ Raising a burnt limb may help to minimize swelling; raising both legs may help to reduce any shock symptoms.

REMOVAL OF CLOTHING

Dry burns (from flames, for example):
Douse any smouldering clothes with water to extinguish and cool. Try to cool burns directly onto the skin, but do not remove the clothing unless it is impeding the cooling (in this case, cut around any adhered clothing, leaving the adhered material in place).

Wet burns (scalds from boiling water, for example):
Flood water under the clothing to start cooling and separate it from the skin. Scalded skin is often fragile, so remove clothing carefully by

cutting it first some distance away from the scalded area. Continue to cool the affected area gently.

Chemical burns (caustics, acids or alkalis, for example):
Use a shower or hose to drench the area. Remove affected clothing in the shower. In the absence of water, use scissors to remove affected clothing quickly. At any stage, avoid contact with the chemical, the contaminated area, or with "run-off" water used for dousing. Wear suitable protective gloves – do not risk a chemical burn yourself.

Chemical, electrical and inhalation burns

SEE ALSO
➤ Understanding and assessing burns 1, p174
➤ Assessing burns 2, p176
➤ Keeping yourself safe, p220

Chemical and electrical burns are especially hazardous, as further injury is possible both for casualty and helper. With a chemical incident, make the area safe or remove the casualty to safety and then get someone to inform the fire service about the chemical in question.

Electrical burns can look deceptively mild at skin level while underlying muscles, nerves and organs may be badly burned. With both chemical and electrical burns, the casualty could go into shock, so monitor their vital signs until medical help arrives.

BURNS FROM CHEMICALS

Corrosive chemicals will continue to damage the skin while in contact with it so dispersing the harmful chemical as soon as possible is a priority. Chemical burns tend to develop more slowly than those from other causes. They may also be particularly hazardous to the first-aider (because you may easily become burnt yourself) and they may give off fumes that could be inhaled. If there is any doubt about the chemical, move everyone away from the casualty and summon expert help.

You may recognize a burn as a chemical burn because:
- The casualty informs you what happened.
- There are containers of chemicals nearby.
- The casualty is suffering intense, stinging pain around the burnt area.
- After some time, blistering and discolouration may develop, along with swollen tissues in the affected area.

▽ While wearing protective gloves and goggles, in case of splashes to the eye, flood the burnt area with cold water to cool the skin and disperse the chemical.

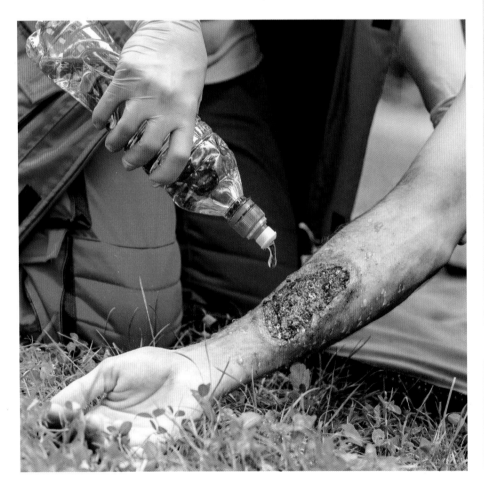

FIRST AID FOR CHEMICAL BURNS

Phone the emergency services or arrange urgent transport to hospital.

⬇

Get the casualty out of the contaminated area as soon as possible, without exposing yourself to danger.

⬇

Protect yourself. Wear appropriate gloves and an apron if readily available; open windows and doors for ventilation.

⬇

Flood the injured part with water, for at least 20 minutes or until help arrives. Pour the water so that contaminated water neither runs on to other parts of the casualty's body nor on to you.

⬇

Remove any contaminated clothing, unless it is stuck fast to the skin.

WARNING

Do not try to "neutralize" the chemical (by putting alkali on acid or vice versa) as the resulting reaction may produce heat or exacerbate the existing burn.

COMMON CAUSES OF CHEMICAL BURNS

Certain chemicals can irritate, burn or even penetrate the skin's protective layer. Many chemical-related accidents are in industry but the following are all common household chemicals that are corrosive.

➤ Dishwasher products.

➤ Oven cleaners.

➤ Bleach.

➤ Ammonia.

➤ Caustic soda.

BURNS FROM ELECTRICITY

Electrical burns can occur from all kinds of electric current – from lightning strikes and overhead power cables to domestic current. There are three distinct types of electrical burn:

• A flash burn, caused by electricity arcing over a distance, and which leaves a distinctive residue on the skin that is sometimes coppery in appearance.

• Burns from flames caused by electricity.

• Direct burning of the tissues by an electric current.

ELECTRICITY-RELATED DAMAGE

Electrical burns can look deceptively mild. Like chemical burns, the extent of the burn may not be immediately obvious and often looks quite innocuous. There may be entry and exit wounds, which give an idea of the path of the electric current, but these are often hard to find.

Underneath the fairly normal-looking skin, the muscle, blood vessels and nerves may have literally "fried". What's more, the jolt of electricity could have affected the casualty's heartbeat.

If you arrive at the scene of an electrical accident do not touch the casualty until you are sure that they are not still in contact with a live power source. Disconnect the supply or remove the casualty from the source by safe means (see page 233). In the case of a high voltage supply such as from power lines

FIRST AID FOR ELECTRICAL BURNS

Do not touch the casualty unless and until you know they are no longer connected to a live electrical source.

If the casualty is unconscious, check their ABC and start resuscitation if necessary. Call the emergency services.

Treat as for a dry burn.

Watch for any signs of shock, or for any effects on the heartbeat.
Note: Anyone who has suffered more than a mild tingling sensation should be seen at hospital – electricity can affect the heart some time after the initial exposure.

▽ Difficulty with breathing is one of the main problems suffered by someone who has inhaled toxic and burning fumes. Urgent medical attention is vital for such an injury.

or pylons, stay at least 20 metres away and do not approach the casualty – call for help.

Once it is safe to do so, check the casualty's ABC and be prepared to start resuscitation techniques immediately and to continue until emergency medical assistance arrives.

INHALATION BURNS

Breathing in dangerous fumes may affect the respiratory system – the trachea (windpipe), bronchi and lung tissue – and can cause serious damage. Such fumes include car exhaust emissions (including carbon monoxide), smoke from a fire, fumes from faulty domestic appliances (such as a gas heater) and fumes from smouldering foam-filled upholstered furniture. Certain chemicals, including dry-cleaning solvents, may also give off toxic or irritant fumes.

Signs of inhalation burns:

• Soot and singed hairs around the mouth and nose area.

• Breathing difficulties.

• Headache.

• Dizziness.

• Shock.

The best first-aid approach is as follows: Send for the emergency services; get the casualty to a safe place in clean air if you can do so without exposing yourself to fire, smoke or fumes; position the casualty sitting up and supported; monitor the casualty for changes in consciousness or breathing; be prepared to resuscitate if necessary and if you can do so safely. Do not use mouth-to-mouth if there is any possibility that chemicals may have been inhaled – use chest compressions only.

Coping with facial burns

SEE ALSO

➤ Dealing with shock, p68

➤ Assessing burns 2, p176

➤ Managing burns, p178

Any type of facial burn is an emergency because it can result in possible blindness, breathing difficulties and obvious scarring. The priorities are to cool the burnt area with cold water and to convey the casualty to hospital. Do remember to reassure the casualty throughout and keep an eye out for any signs of shock. It's a good idea to gather details on what has caused the burn in the first place so that you can relay this information to medical personnel so that they can take prompt and appropriate action.

Burns to the face can have further, highly serious, implications. They strongly suggest that there may be other burns – to the casualty's airway, nose and mouth –

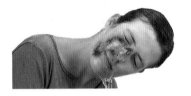

◁ Flood a facial burn with cold water and continue to do so for at least 10 minutes.

and there is a danger they may compromise the casualty's breathing. Also, it is vital to take rapid action in order to minimize any scars from a facial burn, as significant scarring can cause psychological difficulties.

BURNS TO THE EYE

Facial burns to the eye area are especially painful and are prone to significant amounts of swelling, which can make it difficult for the casualty to see and for you to examine the eyeball.

It is vital to get the person to a doctor or hospital very quickly as any burns to the eyelid or cornea can lead to scarring that may cause blindness. Reassure the casualty throughout as they may think that they are going blind and panic. Keep them calm and remind them that it is just the swelling that is obstructing their vision.

CHEMICAL BURNS TO THE EYE

Chemicals can burn the delicate tissues of the eye and cause scarring, which may lead to blindness. The main first-aid priority is to irrigate the eye to remove as much of the chemical as possible. The casualty's eye may be very painful, red and watery, making it difficult to prise open and flush out.

FIRST AID FOR FACIAL BURNS

↓

Sit the casualty up in case breathing problems develop.

↓

Keep a careful watch on their breathing throughout.

↓

Phone the emergency services.

↓

Apply cold compresses or pour cold water over the burn if this is possible.

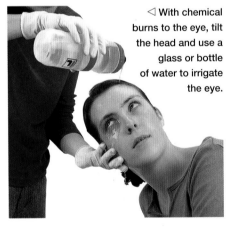

◁ With chemical burns to the eye, tilt the head and use a glass or bottle of water to irrigate the eye.

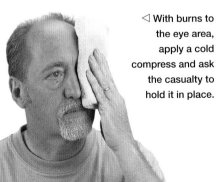

◁ With burns to the eye area, apply a cold compress and ask the casualty to hold it in place.

FIRST AID FOR CHEMICAL BURNS TO THE EYE

↓

Turn the person's head to one side with the affected eye below the good eye so that no chemical runs into the good eye.

↓

Hold the eyelid open under a gently running tap or pour water from a glass or bottle. Flush both sides of the eye; don't splash contaminated water into the good eye.

↓

Cover the eye with a sterile eye pad and secure loosely. Try to find out what chemical has caused the burn and always take the casualty to hospital.

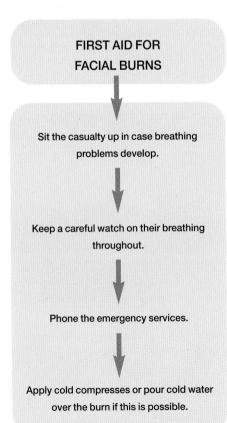
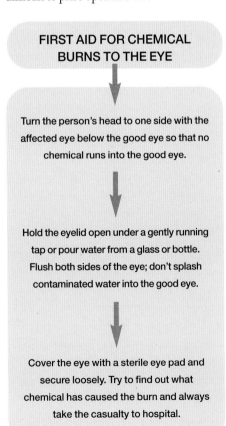

Tackling sunburn

SEE ALSO
➤ Understanding burns, p174
➤ Assessing the severity of burns, p176

Burns caused by the ultraviolet rays of the sun can be painful and potentially dangerous. First, the skin reddens and may start to itch; then it becomes tender and painful. Severe sunburn may eventually lead to blistering and flaking of the skin, and in the long term can lead to skin cancer. Sunbeds and tanning lamps can inflict the same or more damage as natural sunlight, and so are best avoided. Taking sensible precautions when out in the sun at any time of year can ensure that a holiday is a happy and healthy one.

Sunburn can not only cause severe skin damage but may also be accompanied by the serious conditions of heat exhaustion or even heat stroke. The sun's ultraviolet radiation can also be harmful to the eyes, so sunglasses should be worn when outside, especially in areas where there is a lot of reflected light such as on the sea or in snow. The effects of too much sun are not immediately obvious and can take 12–24 hours to develop.

Many people don't realize that you can get sunburn even on a cloudy day. There are also other factors that make sunburn more likely, including:

- High altitudes – The thinner the atmosphere, the greater the risk of even small amounts of sunlight causing burning.
- Reflective surfaces – Water, sand, wind, snow and pavements increase the sun's strength by reflecting its rays.
- Sweat and water on the skin – Such moisture increases the chances of burning and stops sunscreens from working well.

PREVENTING SUNBURN

A few sensible precautions can prevent sunburn in the first place. Take on board the following advice.

➤ Use a sunscreen on all exposed skin, especially when in open areas with little shade. Reapply regularly.

➤ Wear a wide-brimmed hat ideally with a neck flap.

➤ Always wear sunglasses, especially near snow or expanses of water.

➤ Stay out of the midday sun altogether, especially when in hot countries close to the equator. Make a siesta part of any holiday; resurface at around 3pm when the sun's rays are less damaging.

➤ Remember that no sun tan has to be better than risking skin cancer. If you must sunbathe, build up exposure to the sun very slowly, staying in the sun for no longer than 20 minutes on the first day. Never use low-factor sunscreens.

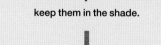

FIRST AID FOR SUNBURN

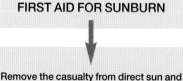

Remove the casualty from direct sun and keep them in the shade.

Apply cold compresses to the burnt area to cool the skin or immerse the affected area in a cold bath for at least 10 minutes.

As the casualty may be dehydrated, encourage them to take frequent small sips of water.

If the sunburn is mild, apply some soothing calamine lotion; for severe sunburn take the casualty to see a doctor straightaway.

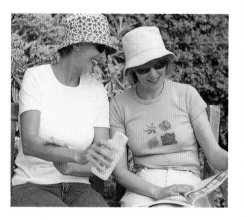

△ To prevent sunburn, wear a T-shirt and a hat and apply some sunscreen.

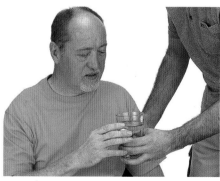

△ Encourage the sunburnt casualty to sip water frequently as they may be dehydrated.

USING A SUNSCREEN

All sunscreens have an SPF (Sun Protection Factor), which is measured by timing how long skin covered with the sunscreen takes to burn compared with unprotected skin. If your skin normally burns after 10 minutes, then an SPF 15 sunscreen should allow protection for 150 minutes; an SPF8 offers 80 minutes' protection. Even "waterproof" or "water resistant" sunscreens lose their effectiveness once you have been in the water for 40 minutes. The minimum recommended sunscreen is SPF15.

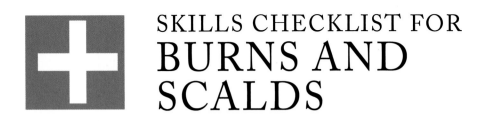

SKILLS CHECKLIST FOR
BURNS AND
SCALDS

KEY POINTS

- Burns must be cooled as fast as possible – run cold water over a burn site for a minimum of 10 minutes in order to limit the internal damage ☐

- Do not touch burnt skin, to avoid inflicting further injury ☐

- Use non-adhesive dressings – either dedicated gel burn dressings or clear food wrap or clean plastic bags – never adhesive or fluffy materials ☐

- Approximately three-quarters of deaths from burns occur in domestic house fires that could often have been prevented. ☐

SKILLS LEARNED

- How to treat minor burns and scalds ☐

- How to treat more extensive burns or scalding ☐

- Assessing the depth, extent and seriousness of a burn ☐

- Recognizing the possibilities of breathing difficulties, shock and internal injury as a consequence of burns ☐

- Avoiding sunburn ☐

ACTION ON POISONING

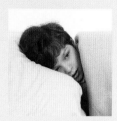

There are some substances that the human body cannot tolerate. These poisons – which include toxins (harmful substances produced by living things) – include a wide variety of plants and fungi, chemicals (including household products), contaminated food, medicines in overdose and illicit drugs. The body's defence system often recognizes such poisons as threats to survival and tries to get rid of the offending substance – by vomiting and/or diarrhoea, for example. When encountering a poisoning incident, the first-aider is limited to calling for medical emergency services and to gathering any evidence on what the poison could have been. Do not under any circumstances try to make the casualty vomit up the poison.

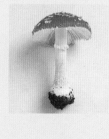

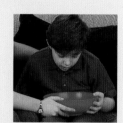

CONTENTS

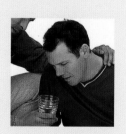

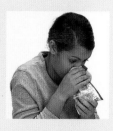

Understanding poisoning

SEE ALSO
➤ Managing drug poisoning, p188
➤ Managing poisoning in children, p194

The golden rule in giving first aid for a suspected poisoning is never to attempt to treat them yourself. In particular do not try to induce vomiting, as this could damage the oesophagus (gullet) if the poison is a corrosive chemical, or cause lung damage by breathing in certain fumes. Poisons can get into the body in many ways – via the skin, digestive system, lungs or bloodstream. The mode of entry influences the speed of reaction; for instance if a poison is injected into the bloodstream, it can reach all parts of the body within a minute or so.

A poison is any substance that can cause temporary or permanent damage to the body if taken in sufficient quantities. Poisoning may occur accidentally or intentionally. Suicide attempts often involve more than one poisonous agent, and the casualty may resist any help that is offered. Some drugs have no obvious immediate effects when taken in overdose but ultimately are fatal.

Accidental poisoning is most often seen in children and older people. There are fewer deaths from such incidents in children, but some agents may wreak havoc in a child. Older people may get confused and take the wrong medicine or the wrong amount.

There is a wide variety of poisons:
• Noxious gases or fumes.
• Cleaning products.
• Toxins in plants and fungi.
• Bacterial and viral toxins (in food).
• Drugs and alcohol.
• Toxins from bites and stings.

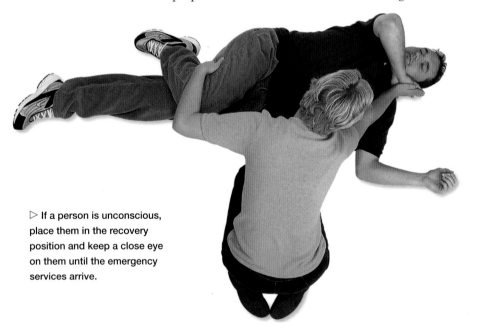

▷ If a person is unconscious, place them in the recovery position and keep a close eye on them until the emergency services arrive.

BASIC GUIDELINES FOR DEALING WITH POISONING

Assess the casualty's ABC (airway, breathing and circulation). If they are breathing but unconscious, put them in the recovery position.

If they are not breathing, start resuscitation with compression-only CPR. Do not give mouth-to-mouth, in case there is poison on the casualty's face, in the mouth, or in their breath.

Phone or get someone to phone the emergency services.

If they start to have a fit, do not restrain them. Keep them out of danger and ensure a clear airway.

Look around to see if you can find any clues to the identity of the poison that has been taken. If the casualty has vomited, take a sample of the vomit to hospital as there is a good chance it will help doctors identify the appropriate treatment.

IDENTIFYING THE CAUSE OF THE POISONING

Once you have dealt with the casualty's immediate needs, gather information to try to identify the poison.

➤ Look for empty pill bottles or loose pills or capsules on the floor. Bag them and give to the emergency services.

➤ Search for codes on containers that will identify any chemical.

➤ Scan the area for a dead insect or snake to bag up and take to hospital.

➤ Cast your eye around for any potentially poisonous foods.

HOW POISONS AFFECT THE BODY

▷ Poisons can have wide-ranging effects on different parts of the body. Effects depend on how the poison gets into the system and how much poison has been taken.

Brain
Once in the bloodstream, drugs can easily reach the brain causing confusion, drowsiness, fits and, at worst, coma. If the part of the brain that controls breathing is affected, a person's breathing can stop altogether.

Blood
Poisonous gases such as cyanide and carbon monoxide react with the blood, so that there is not enough oxygen in the circulation, leading to potentially lethal effects on the body.

Lungs
Inhaled fumes or drugs quickly reach the lungs and then travel in the bloodstream. Such poisons cause breathing difficulties (which are especially dangerous in people with asthma) and lead to blue skin (cyanosis) – a sign that there's too little oxygen in the body.

Digestive tract
Most cases of poisoning result from ingestion (swallowing), including chemicals, drugs and food poisoning. Toxins from bacteria or viruses in contaminated food commonly cause nausea, vomiting and diarrhoea.

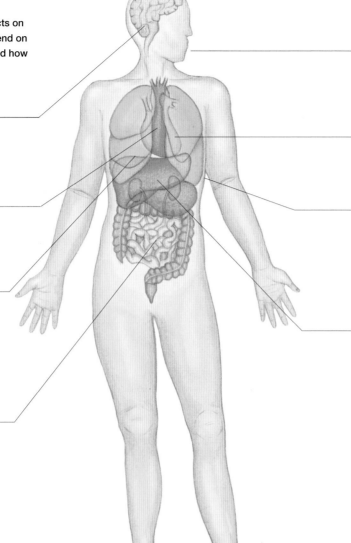

Mouth
Corrosive substances such as bleach and dishwashing powder may burn the tissues lining the throat and oesophagus (gullet) and cause nausea and vomiting.

Heart
Injected and swallowed poisons can result in an irregular heartbeat or in the heart beating too fast or too slowly.

Chest wall
Certain snake venom, certain garden fertilizers and botulinum toxin can lead to paralysis of the muscles in the chest wall and therefore cause suffocation.

Liver
This is the body's vital detoxifying centre. Toxins from some wild mushrooms may cause severe liver damage and the everyday painkiller paracetamol can destroy liver cells if taken in excess (even relatively small amounts over the recommended dosage).

COMMON POISONS

Food:
➤ Contaminated food, especially with poor hygiene or inadequate cooking.

➤ Certain types of toadstools and mushrooms can be lethal – even if only tiny quantities have been eaten.

Household:
➤ Bleach, caustic soda, household cleaning products, perfume, aftershave, hair spray, nail varnish remover, lighter fuel, turpentine, white spirit and all kinds of solvents, including dry cleaning solvents, mercury-filled thermometer, child's play "putty", shoe creams and polishes, slug pellets, tobacco, weedkiller, glues, wood preservative, lead paint (in old houses), antifreeze, bug and rodent killers.

Drugs and chemicals:
➤ Medicines in excess of stated dose (or if taken by someone who suffers from an allergic reaction to them), large amounts of vitamins A and D, large amounts of Epsom salts, iodine.

Bites and stings:
➤ From insects, jellyfish and snakes, among others.

Plants:
➤ For example, laburnum, foxglove, holly berries, monkshood and yew.

Gases:
➤ Carbon monoxide may leak from faulty gas heaters, boilers and the vents of air conditioning systems.

Managing drug poisoning

SEE ALSO

➤ What is first aid?, p12

➤ Understanding poisoning, p186

➤ Tackling alcohol and illicit drug poisoning, p190

Most drugs produce specific signs and symptoms fairly quickly when taken in overdose; the exception here is excess paracetamol, which can take a few days to produce recognizable symptoms. The effects of the drugs depend on the type of drug and how it is taken (swallowed, inhaled or injected). The basic first-aid aims when dealing with drug poisoning are to maintain breathing, call the emergency services and look for any information at the scene that could provide vital clues for the medics treating the casualty.

Drug poisoning can result from overdosage of prescription or over-the-counter medicines or from abuse of illicit drugs. It may also be caused by two or more drugs interacting.

If it is possible for the first aider to identify what substances have been taken, such information may be incredibly helpful, especially if the casualty is drowsy or unconscious by the time they reach the hospital.

PARACETAMOL-BASED PAINKILLERS

Such painkilling medicine can be commonly bought over the counter and is a basic part of most home medicine cupboards. If paracetamol is taken in overdosage, even just a relatively small amount, destruction of the liver can occur.

The casualty may feel fine for the first few days, until liver (or, less commonly, kidney) damage starts to take effect. Then,

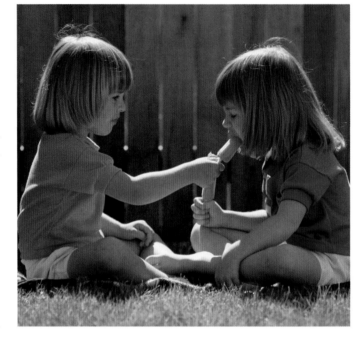

◁ Children love to experiment with tasting things, but if unsupervised, their natural curiosity may result in a poisoning incident. Keep all medicines and household chemicals well out of the reach of small children.

the following symptoms may appear:
• Nausea and profuse vomiting.
• Pain in the upper right-hand abdomen after 24 hours (a sign of liver damage).

Irreversible liver damage can occur within three to four days so prompt recognition and transfer to hospital is vital.

ASPIRIN-BASED PAINKILLERS

If these common painkillers are taken in excessive amounts they can cause the following symptoms:
• Upper abdominal pain.
• Nausea and vomiting.
• Fever, with sweating and dizziness.
• Deep "sighing" breaths.
• Deafness and/or loud noises heard in the ears (tinnitus).
• Restlessness and confusion.
• Deterioration in consciousness or fitting.

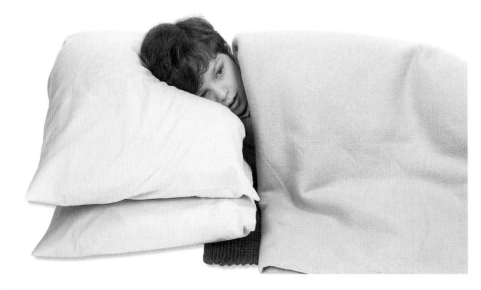

◁ Drowsiness followed by loss of consciousness can be a sign of poisoning. Seek immediate medical help.

FIRST AID FOR POISONING

↓

If the casualty is conscious, then let them rest in a comfortable position. Reassure them and ask if they can tell you what they have taken.

↓

Phone the emergency services and tell them you suspect drug poisoning.

↓

Monitor their breathing and talk to them until help arrives.

↓

Keep samples of any vomit. Look for any clues as to the identity of poisons.

ANTIDEPRESSANT DRUGS

There are many different types of antidepressant medicine available on prescription. If taken in excess, the older type of tricyclic antidepressants, such as amitriptyline, initially cause:

• Blurred vision.
• Dilated pupils.
• Dry mouth.
• An inability to pass urine.

They can then result in:

• Drowsiness.
• Drops in blood pressure and temperature.
• Fits, followed by cardiac arrest.

The newer-style antidepressants, such as fluoxetine and sertraline, may cause agitation, drowsiness or an erratic heart rate.

TRANQUILLISERS

Tranquillizing and sedative drugs may be prescribed for anxiety and sleeping problems. Older barbiturate drugs have largely been replaced with benzo-diazepines, though barbiturates may still be encountered as drugs of abuse. If tranquillisers are taken in overdose, they can result in the following:

• Slurred speech.
• Drowsiness and lethargy, leading to a loss of consciousness.
• Weak, irregular or slow or fast heartbeat.
• Slow breathing rate (breathing may actually stop altogether).

If tranquillisers are taken in combination with excessive alcohol the situation is much more dangerous. Older people often take sleeping tablets; when taken in excess, these may produce hypothermia (dangerously cold body temperature).

IRON SUPPLEMENTS

Women often take an iron supplement (commonly as iron tablets) during pregnancy and while breastfeeding. Children can mistake such tablets for candies and eat them. The signs of iron overdosage include:

• Stomach pain.
• Vomiting and diarrhoea.
• Blood in the vomit or the stool.

Excessive iron can cause severe damage to a child's liver and this is one of the types of tablet that children accidentally take that can turn out to be lethal.

POISON HELP

In any case of suspected poisoning, you can get advice from your national poison helpline or be put through to your local poison control centre.

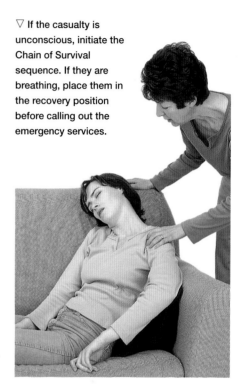

▽ If the casualty is unconscious, initiate the Chain of Survival sequence. If they are breathing, place them in the recovery position before calling out the emergency services.

▽ Iron poisoning causes vomiting and severe stomach pain in children. They should be taken straight to hospital.

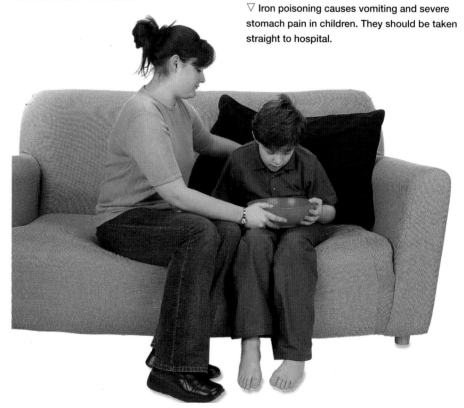

Tackling alcohol and illicit drug poisoning

SEE ALSO

➤ Understanding poisoning, p186

➤ Managing drug poisoning, p188

➤ Managing poisoning in children, p194

Alcohol in moderate amounts is easily detoxified by the liver; but in very large quantities alcohol becomes a poison that the body's organs can no longer deal with – and it can prove fatal.

Even relatively small amounts of an illicit drug such as cocaine or fumes from a substance like glue can result in severe effects on the body. Emergency medical treatment is vital, especially the casualty is a child, because their smaller bodies mean the effects are greater than in adults.

Taking illicit substances and drinking large quantities of alcohol is socially acceptable in some parts of society, but such practices are potentially dangerous and can lead to medical crises and even fatalities.

ALCOHOL POISONING

Alcohol is a poison when drunk in sufficient quantities. Consumption of half a litre (1 pint) of a spirit, such as vodka, is enough to cause severe alcohol poisoning. Alcohol-related risks include:

• Depression of the central nervous system, most seriously the brain.

• Widening of blood vessels, making the body lose heat and risking hypothermia.

• The inebriated person may choke on their vomit while unconscious.

SIGNS AND SYMPTOMS OF ALCOHOL INTOXICATION

It is usually fairly obvious when someone is intoxicated with alcohol, but similar symptoms may be caused by a head injury or a diabetic hypoglycaemic (low blood sugar) condition.

➤ A smell of alcohol on the breath.

➤ Empty bottles or cans nearby.

➤ Flushed and warm skin.

➤ Actions are aggressive or passive.

➤ Speech and actions are slow and become less coordinated.

➤ Deep, noisy breathing.

➤ Low level of consciousness; they may often slip into unconsciousness.

HOW TO DEAL WITH ALCOHOL INTOXICATION

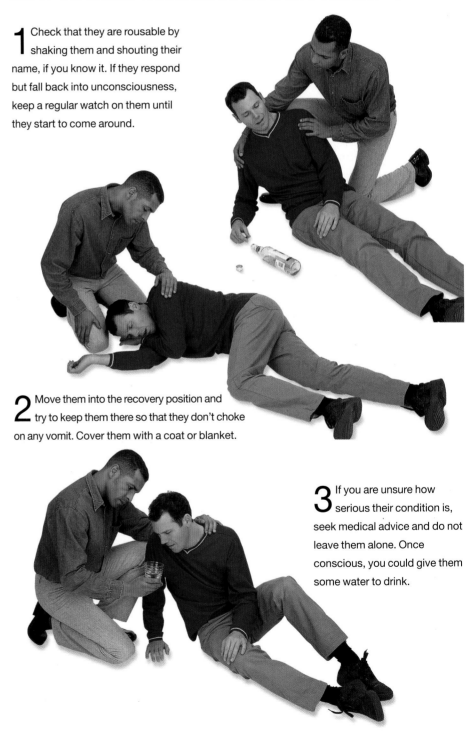

1 Check that they are rousable by shaking them and shouting their name, if you know it. If they respond but fall back into unconsciousness, keep a regular watch on them until they start to come around.

2 Move them into the recovery position and try to keep them there so that they don't choke on any vomit. Cover them with a coat or blanket.

3 If you are unsure how serious their condition is, seek medical advice and do not leave them alone. Once conscious, you could give them some water to drink.

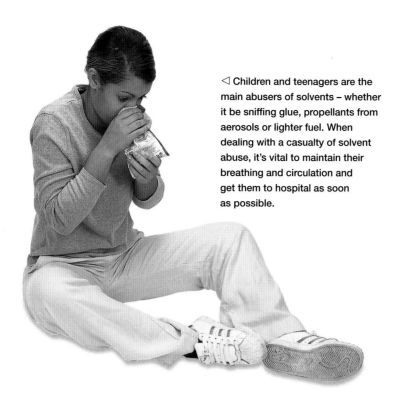

◁ Children and teenagers are the main abusers of solvents – whether it be sniffing glue, propellants from aerosols or lighter fuel. When dealing with a casualty of solvent abuse, it's vital to maintain their breathing and circulation and get them to hospital as soon as possible.

ILLICIT DRUGS

Illicit stimulant drugs include Ecstasy, cocaine, amphetamines and LSD. If you suspect someone has taken any of these drugs, watch out for the following signs:

• Excitable and hyperactive behaviour.
• Sweating.
• Shaking hands.
• Hallucinations.

These drugs can occasionally be fatal. Ecstasy interferes with the brain's ability to control body temperature, which can rise to over 42°C (107.6°F) and cause heat exhaustion. Ecstasy-takers often drink lots of water, which can cause kidney malfunction and abnormal heart rhythms. Cocaine's main effects are on the heart rate – with the potential to lead to abnormal rhythms and even cardiac arrest.

Opiate drugs such as heroin and codeine may depress the respiratory system, causing breathing to stop. Rapid recovery occurs if a particular antidote is given intravenously, but this must be done urgently, by trained medical personnel.

POISONING VIA SOLVENT ABUSE

Children and adolescents are the main solvent abusers – they may inhale fumes from glue, paint, lighter fuel, cleaning fluids, aerosols and nail polish to "get high". All such solvents depress breathing and heart activity, and may cause respiratory and cardiac arrest.

FIRST AID FOR SOLVENT ABUSE POISONING

↓

If the casualty has stopped breathing or their heart has stopped beating, start resuscitation immediately.

↓

If unconscious but their breathing is normal, place them in the fresh air in the recovery position.

↓

Phone the emergency services and monitor the casualty at regular intervals.

↓

It may prove useful to collect a sample of the casualty's vomit to help identify the type of drug taken.

↓

Often, the casualty starts to "come round" quickly and may seem normal after 20 minutes. Stay with them until help arrives.

SIGNS AND SYMPTOMS OF SOLVENT POISONING

➤ The casualty has a dry throat and cough.

➤ Their chest feels tight and they may be breathless.

➤ They have a headache.

➤ They feel nauseous and may vomit.

➤ They have hallucinations – they "hear voices" or "see things".

➤ Their breathing becomes faster and more laboured as fluid builds up in their lungs.

➤ They become drowsy and confused and eventually may lose consciousness.

➤ They have episodes of fits (convulsions), which may lead to coma and eventually to death.

FIRST AID FOR ILLICIT DRUG POISONING

↓

Do not try to make the casualty vomit.

↓

Place them in the recovery position.

↓

Phone the emergency services.

↓

Monitor their condition continually until help arrives.

Dealing with food and plant poisoning

SEE ALSO
➤ Dealing with shock, p68
➤ Understanding poisoning, p186
➤ Managing poisoning in children, p194

Potentially poisonous things to eat are all around us: in the garden, the kitchen, the bathroom or a nearby wood. Make your garden safe if you have young children by ensuring that all plants are harmless or that any toxic plants are inaccessible. Never be tempted to try a wild mushroom; it may look harmless but it could give you severe, or even fatal, poisoning. Always practise good food hygiene to avoid food poisoning at home. If you have any worries or doubts at all about a potential poisoning incident, you should always call the emergency services.

Young children are the most likely group to eat poisonous plants as they find brightly coloured seeds and berries attractive. Adults may eat poisonous mushrooms by mistaking them for an edible species. The effects of plant poisoning can be almost anything depending on the plant. While many fungi are relatively harmless, the common death cap mushroom, for example, contains a toxin that causes nausea and vomiting around 24 hours after ingestion and destroys the liver after a delay of several days.

First-aid priorities for poisoning, whether it is from a plant or a fungus, are to:
• Identify the poisonous agent, if possible.
• Manage any fitting episodes.
• Call the emergency services.

MUSHROOM POISONING

Serious poisoning through eating poisonous mushrooms is rare. Some species of fungus may cause some less serious digestive symptoms, but eating a species such as the death cap can be fatal.

Suspect mushroom poisoning if you notice these signs and symptoms:
• Nausea and vomiting.
• Crampy abdominal pain and diarrhoea.
• Episodes of fitting.
• Deterioration in level of consciousness.

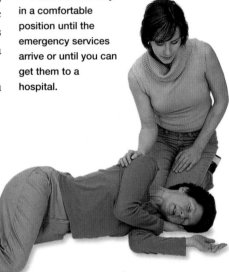

▽ Place the casualty in a comfortable position until the emergency services arrive or until you can get them to a hospital.

SOME COMMON POISONOUS PLANTS

➤ Autumn crocus (*Colchicum*) – all parts are very toxic and can prove to be fatal.

➤ Californian glory (*Fremontodendron*) – little hairs on the stem and leaves can cause skin irritation and itching.

➤ Castor oil plant (*Ricinus communis*) – all parts of this plant – especially the seeds – are very toxic if eaten and could be fatal.

➤ Daffodil (*Narcissus*) – if a bulb is eaten (a child can mistake it for an onion), it causes vomiting, stomach ache and diarrhoea.

➤ Deadly nightshade (*Atropa belladonna*) – toxic if eaten and can irritate skin.

➤ Dumb cane or Leopard lily (*Dieffenbachia*) – eating any part of the plant, even a small quantity, can make the tongue, mouth and throat swell and interfere with breathing. Skin contact with the sap causes irritation.

➤ Foxglove (*Digitalis purpurea*) – all parts can be very toxic. As this bitter plant often causes vomiting first, poisoning is rare.

➤ Holly (*Ilex aquifolium*) – red berries are poisonous.

➤ Hyacinth (*Hyacinthus*) – if the bulbs are mistaken for onions and eaten, they will make a person sick and can sometimes cause a skin rash.

➤ Laburnum (*Laburnum anagyroides*) – all parts are toxic, especially the seeds.

➤ Lantana (*Lantana camara*) – all parts of this plant are toxic. The unripe berries, in particular, are attractive to young children.

➤ Lupin (*Lupinus*) – the seeds and pods are poisonous but would have to be eaten in large quantities to do real harm.

➤ Monkshood (*Aconitum*) – all parts are highly toxic if eaten and contact with the sap can cause skin irritation.

➤ Spurge laurel (*Daphne laureola*) – all parts are highly poisonous if eaten.

➤ Umbrella tree (*Schefflera*) – any contact with cut stems or leaves causes skin irritation.

➤ Winter cherry (*Solanum capsicastrum*) – the fruit is poisonous but not fatal.

➤ Woody nightshade (*Solanum dulcamara*) – the berries of this plant are poisonous and when eaten can cause stomachache, vomiting and diarrhoea.

➤ Yew tree (*Taxus*) – all parts of this tree are toxic if eaten.

FIRST AID FOR PLANT OR MUSHROOM POISONING

If the casualty is conscious, ask them what they have eaten.

If they are breathing but unconscious, place them in the recovery position. If not breathing, start CPR.

Try to identify what poisonous plant or mushroom they could have eaten.

Phone the emergency services or take the casualty to hospital. Take a sample of the plant with you to the hospital, if possible.

FIRST AID FOR FOOD POISONING

Encourage the casualty to rest and drink plenty of water.

Do not give them solid food for 24 hours or until their symptoms settle.

If symptoms persist or worsen for more than a few days, or if the victim is an older person, a child or a pregnant woman, call your doctor for medical advice.

FOOD POISONING

Symptoms of food poisoning may develop within an hour after consuming the tainted food, although it can sometimes take days or even weeks. Contaminated food often tastes and smells entirely normal. The commonest culprits of food poisoning are bacteria and viruses, including *E. coli*, *Campylobacter*, *Salmonella* and *Listeria*. Common sources of food poisoning include shellfish and other protein-containing foods, such as poultry, meat or fish, that have been handled with improper hygiene, badly stored, left too long or inadequately cooked.

Food poisoning may cause such severe fluid losses, through vomiting and diarrhoea, that dehydration develops. If the lost fluids are not replaced quickly enough, then a further danger is the development of shock.

Typical signs of food poisoning are:
• Nausea and vomiting.
• Crampy abdominal pain.
• Diarrhoea, which may be blood-stained.
• Fever and shivering and/or headache.
• Signs of shock.

SOME EXAMPLES OF POISONOUS MUSHROOM

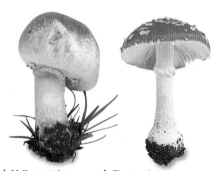

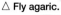
△ Yellow stainer.   △ Fly agaric.

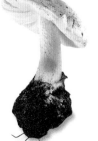

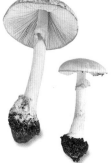

△ Destroying angel.   △ Death cap.

PREVENTING FOOD POISONING

Take these few sensible precautions to reduce the risk of food poisoning.

➤ Follow instructions for defrosting food before cooking.

➤ Use separate chopping boards for raw food such as meat, fish and poultry so they cannot contaminate other food.

➤ Always wash hands thoroughly after using the toilet, before preparing food and after handling raw meat, fish or poultry.

➤ Store raw meat and poultry on the bottom shelf of the refrigerator so it cannot drip on other food.

➤ Tepid cooked food gathers bacteria fast, so store it in the fridge or freeze it.

➤ Cook chicken, pork, burgers, sausages and kebabs slowly and thoroughly, so there is no pink meat left inside.

➤ Be aware that raw eggs, used in recipes like mayonnaise, have a high risk of containing *Salmonella* bacteria.

➤ When visiting countries where the water supply could be dirty, never eat or drink anything that might be contaminated with local water, such as ice in drinks, unpeeled fruit or vegetables, ice-cream or salads (which could have been washed in local water).

➤ When in a part of the world where the water is suspect, clean your teeth with bottled water (or sterilized water) rather than using tap water.

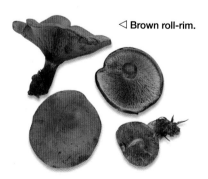
◁ Brown roll-rim.

Managing poisoning in children

SEE ALSO
➤ What is first aid?, p12
➤ Understanding poisoning, p186
➤ Safety in the home, p224

Young children are naturally interested in searching through cupboards and boxes and generally exploring their environment. They will also put anything and everything into their mouths, including mothballs, dishwasher powder and any variety of potentially fatal household products, liquids and powders. Preventing poisoning in children is an essential part of safety in your home. As with all poisoning incidents, find out what has been taken so that the appropriate medical help can be given and keep a close eye on your child.

Children are naturally inquisitive and have no qualms about touching, inhaling or ingesting anything – all pills are sweets, powders are sherbets and liquids are drinks. Parents are often taken by surprise by what is dangerous for young bodies – alcohol is lethal even in tiny quantities, an excess of iron can kill a child and dishwashing powder can corrode their oesophagus (gullet) in seconds.

Poisons are absorbed faster in children than adults, so their effects can be seen fairly quickly. Suspect poisoning in a child if:
- You observe unusual behaviour such as slurred speech, giggling inappropriately, staggering, drowsiness.
- You find a child playing near an empty pill or chemical container.
- You can see scalds, stains or bits of tablet around their mouth.

HOW TO POISON-PROOF YOUR HOME

The best cure is, of course, prevention. Take on board the following advice to ensure your children are never allowed access to potentially deadly poisons.

➤ Never leave unattended glasses full of alcohol around, especially overnight. Children are early risers and may decide to drink up all the dregs while you are sleeping.

➤ Never decant substances from their original containers to empty unlabelled bottles as it may lead to confusion.

➤ Do not use empty food containers such as soft drink bottles to store hazardous substances.

➤ The best place for all potential poisons is out of reach and out of sight in a locked cupboard that is secured with a childproof catch.

➤ Store food and non-food items in separate cupboards.

➤ Make sure all medicine containers have child-resistant lids on them.

➤ Keep a close eye on your visitors, especially grandparents who may have regular medicines to take and may inadvertently leave such pills in an open handbag or overnight bag. Almost all adult medicines can have devastating effects on a child. For example, diabetic pills that lower blood sugar can reduce a child's blood sugar to such an extent that they fall into a coma and die.

FIRST AID FOR ALCOHOL POISONING IN A CHILD

↓

Place a bowl nearby in case they vomit.

↓

If unrousable, start CPR IF they are not breathing and otherwise place in the recovery position.

↓

Call the emergency services and stay with the casualty until the emergency services arrive.

SYMPTOMS OF ALCOHOL POISONING IN CHILDREN

➤ Strong smell of alcohol.
➤ Flushed skin.
➤ Staggering about.
➤ Slurring of speech.
➤ Nausea.
➤ Noisy breathing.

WARNING
Even a small amount of alcohol can be very harmful to a small child.

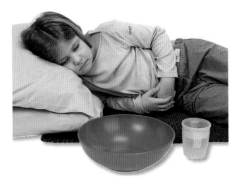

▷ If you suspect alcohol poisoning, place a bowl nearby for any vomit and call the emergency services.

FIRST AID FOR CHEMICAL POISONING IN A CHILD

Try to find out what chemical has been taken. Look for obvious clues nearby.

↓

Do not make the child vomit; the chemical may do more damage on its way back up.

↓

Phone the emergency services immediately, even if the child has no symptoms yet.

↓

If they complain of a sore mouth, moisten the lips only (they should sip/drink nothing).

↓

To soothe burnt lips, keep moistening frequently with water or milk.

FIRST AID FOR FUME INHALATION IN A CHILD

Remove the child from the source of danger, making sure you don't put yourself in danger either.

↓

Check their breathing. If they are not breathing, start resuscitation immediately. If they are breathing, place them in the recovery position until help arrives.

↓

Phone the emergency services.

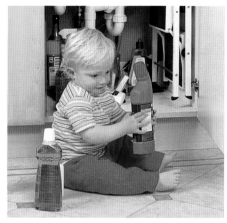

△ All low cupboards should have childproof locks so that household products can be stored safely away from inquisitive children.

FIRST AID FOR DRUG POISONING IN A CHILD

If the child is unconscious, check they are breathing. If breathing seems normal, place them in the recovery position. If they are not breathing, start resuscitation immediately.

↓

Phone the emergency services, who may be able to advise you over the phone.

↓

Look for any signs that the child has swallowed drugs – bits of tablet on the tongue or dye around their mouth.

↓

Try to work out what drug has been taken and how much and how long ago, if possible.

↓

Continue to watch ABC until help arrives. Take the drug container with you to hospital or give to the ambulance crew.

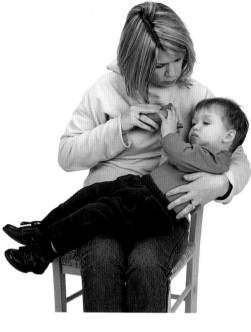

△ Search the child's mouth for any foreign matter. Moisten the lips with water, especially if they are burnt (nothing should be drunk).

FIRST AID FOR PLANT POISONING IN A CHILD

If the child is unconscious, check that they are breathing. If breathing seems normal, place them in the recovery position. If they are not breathing, start resuscitation immediately.

↓

Phone the emergency services or take the child to hospital.

↓

Ask the child what they have eaten.

↓

Use your finger to search the child's mouth and remove any unswallowed pieces of plant – keep these to hand over to medical personnel.

↓

If you know what plant is involved, take a sample with you to the hospital if possible.

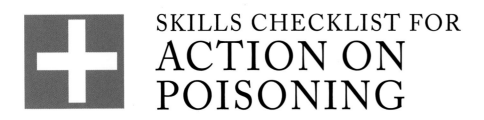

SKILLS CHECKLIST FOR
ACTION ON
POISONING

KEY POINTS

- Never encourage a casualty to vomit back up any poison ☐

- Keep a sample of the suspected poison ☐

- Call the emergency services immediately ☐

SKILLS LEARNED

- Prevention of household poisoning accidents ☐

- How to deal with poisoning in children ☐

- Recognizing the dangers of medicines in excess ☐

- How to deal with food poisoning ☐

- How to cope with illicit drug excess ☐

- How to deal with alcohol poisoning ☐

FIRST-AID KIT

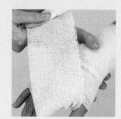

It is immediately reassuring to an injured child or any other casualty if you can produce a well-equipped first-aid kit, and it will probably help you to approach any situation confidently if you have certain essential items to hand. A casualty will certainly feel calmer if you show you can dress and bandage an injury professionally and you know how to apply a sling. However, in an emergency, nothing in a first-aid kit is as important as you and your ability to think on your feet and improvise with materials to hand. Communication with the outside world is also very important, so make best use of telephones, neighbours or passers-by, if you are able to.

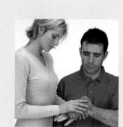

CONTENTS

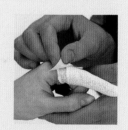

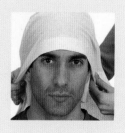

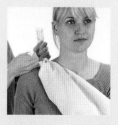

Assembling a first-aid kit

SEE ALSO
➤ What is first aid?, p12
➤ Safety in the home, p224
➤ Travelling safely, p246

A clean and fully equipped first-aid kit in the home, in the car and in the workplace is very important. At home, it should be easily accessible in a kitchen or bathroom cupboard but out of the reach of children. Some items are essential to a first-aid kit but you may find that you'll want to supplement the basic kit with items that you know you use a lot, such as painkillers or antihistamine cream. Such medicines do not form part of the first aid offered in emergencies and should be for personal use only.

As well as making sure that you have a first-aid kit in the home and the car, you should be aware that every workplace and public recreation establishment and so on is legally required to have a first-aid kit on the premises. So an incident at such a location should prompt a call for their kit, which will include items specific for industries or sporting activities with high injury risk, for example, an eye wash kit for chemical splashes. In addition, larger workplaces without rapid access to medical care must have trained first aiders on the premises.

WHAT SHOULD GO IN A KIT FOR PRIVATE USE?

The first-aid kit must be kept clean and dry. A large lunch box is ideal for storage, as it is light, durable and easy to open. The following are essential kit items:

- Adhesive dressings (such as plasters) – a good selection of different sizes, shapes and types, for example waterproof, digit-shaped and fabric-backed. Note that very minor cuts and grazes are often better left uncovered.
- Non-adhesive compress dressings sealed in protective wrappers.

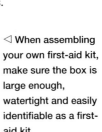

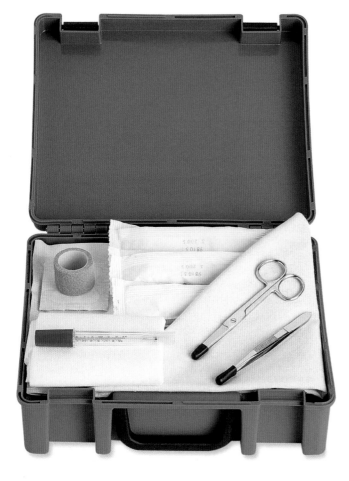

◁ When assembling your own first-aid kit, make sure the box is large enough, watertight and easily identifiable as a first-aid kit.

- Adhesive cloth tape – this is waterproof and can be useful when bandaging areas such as the hands, which often get wet. Some people are allergic to such tape; try to check with them first.
- Antiseptic wipes – for use to clean the skin around a wound. Never use cotton wool on an open wound, as the fluff may stick to, and clog up, the wound.
- Antibiotic ointment.
- Chewable lose dose aspirin (in case of a suspected heart attack).
- Emergency thermal blanket.
- Disposable non-latex gloves (at least 2 pairs) – put on before attending to open wounds, both to ensure that the wound is kept ultra-clean and that your hands are protected.
- A CPR one-way valve face shield, latex-free – a mask or face shield offers protection to you and the casualty if giving mouth-to-mouth.
- Instant cold compress – these gel-filled packs can be warmed up or cooled down. They are useful for easing sprains, bringing down swelling or cooling superficial burns.
- Hydrocortisone ointment.
- Bandages – various sizes and types, especially a triangular bandage (for slings/head wounds), elasticated tubular bandages to be used for injured joints, and roller bandages, for securing dressings and stopping bleeding.
- A digital thermometer to determine body temperature.
- A pair of scissors – choose a sharp pair in which one side is rounded to allow the safe cutting of dressings and clothing (for

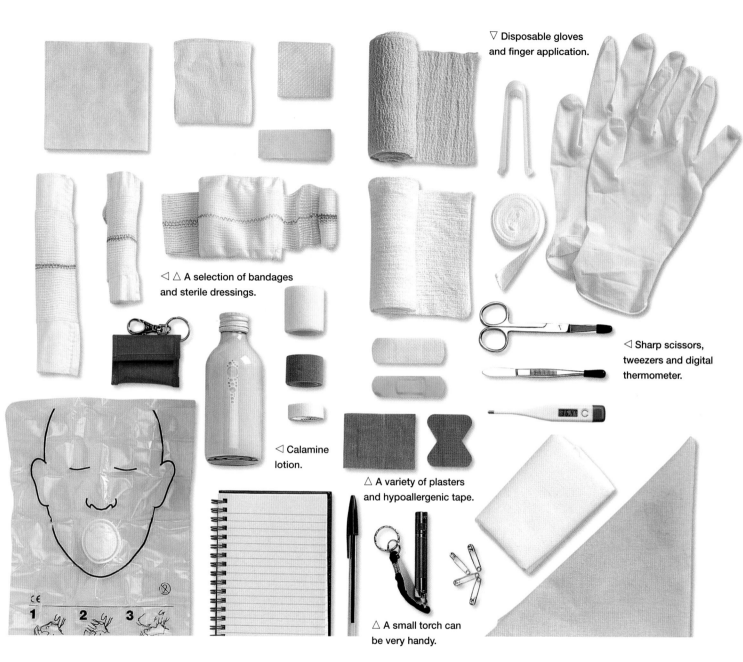

▽ Disposable gloves and finger application.

◁ △ A selection of bandages and sterile dressings.

◁ Calamine lotion.

◁ Sharp scissors, tweezers and digital thermometer.

△ A variety of plasters and hypoallergenic tape.

△ A small torch can be very handy.

△ A face mask for mouth-to-mouth, stored in a small red pouch.

△ A notepad and pen with a list of emergency numbers – and to record your observations.

△ Bandages and safety pins are useful for securing dressings and restricting movement.

example when treating burns or scalds) without the risk of cutting the skin.
- Tweezers – keep some in your kit for removing splinters.
- Safety pins – to fix slings and bandages.
- Emergency first aid guide.

USEFUL FIRST-AID EXTRAS

You may want to add to your kit items such as surgical face masks, painkillers, burn spray or gel dressing, liquid bandage, shrink wrap, wound closure strips (such as Steri-Strips), calamine lotion, antacids, antihistamines, anti-diarrhoea medication or cold and 'flu remedies. It may also be helpful to detail family members' medical history and medications, and to include a list of emergency telephone numbers: for example your doctor, paediatrician, insurance company, pharmacist, nearest

△ These are some of the items you may want to keep in your first-aid kit. Select the items you know you may need and that you feel confident about using.

hospital with an emergency department, neighbours, babysitters and cabs.

In addition , there may be items specific to your activities, such as a flashlight, sunscreen, insect repellent and a tick removal tool for hikers.

Applying dressings and bandages

SEE ALSO

➤ Assembling a
first-aid kit, p198

➤ Applying bandages
1 and 2,
pp202, 204

All first-aiders should be able to produce a makeshift dressing at the scene of an emergency if none is available. Improvising is a key part of giving first aid, and this can apply to bandages, too. Correct methods of bandaging are easy to learn and are invaluable in many first-aid situations. It can take time to become the perfect "bandager", so practise on friends, or on children (when they are well) if you have them. To be effective, bandages should be applied with a certain amount of pressure and be neither too tight nor too loose.

A dressing is any material held over a wound to stop it from bleeding and to protect it from contamination, whereas a bandage is what holds the dressing in place or acts to support a body part.

APPLYING DRESSINGS

There are various types of dressing but common basic guidelines apply to the use of any dressing, whichever type is used.

• If possible, always wear disposable gloves when applying a dressing, except if it's a small adhesive dressing.
• Cleanse any wound with mild soap and water or an antiseptic wipe.

• Apply a small amount of antibiotic cream if appropriate.
• Choose the right size dressing so that it covers all of the wound and its edges.
• Avoid touching the dressing where it will come into contact with the wound; hold it at the sides so that it stays sterile and the risk of infection is less.
• Place the dressing on top of the wound and ensure that it sits over its entire surface and the area immediately surrounding the wound.
• If blood soaks through the dressing, do not try to remove it – place another one on top.

TYPES OF DRESSINGS

Ideally, pre-packed sterile dressings should be used in any incident so that the wound site is free from all germs. However, these dressings are not always to hand and so it's useful to know the other types you can use or how to improvise if you have no first-aid kit whatsoever.

Some different types of dressings include the following:

• Sterile dressings – These dressings are made up from a sterile gauze pad that is covered with a layer of cotton wool and then a bandage. Some sterile dressings come pre-packed and ready to use.
• Adhesive dressings – Also known as plasters, these come in a variety of shapes and sizes (some are specifically designed

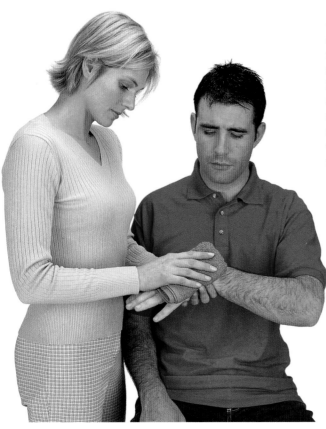

◁ If there aren't any sterile dressings to hand, improvise using a tea towel or similar. If the bleeding continues through this dressing then apply another on top without removing the first one.

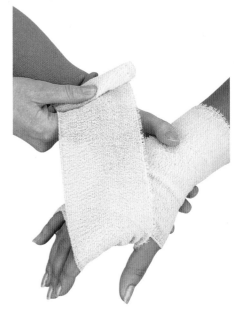

▽ You should aim to wrap a large area of the injured limb in such a way that you are not impeding the casualty's circulation.

to fit a finger or particular body part). Some people have an allergy to certain plasters, so do check with the casualty before you apply one.

- Non-adhesive dressings – These non-fluffy dressings can be applied directly on to a wound and won't stick.

- Makeshift dressings – As is often the case in first-aid situations, improvisation is key. When sterile dressings aren't available, use the cleanest (non-fluffy) material available – tea towels, head scarves or torn-up sheets are all ideal. Sanitary towels make good dressings as they are clean (but not sterile) and bulky.

BANDAGING CORRECTLY

Effective bandaging has several roles – it controls bleeding, aids the return of blood from the wound site, ensures that any dressing stays firmly in place and immobilizes and supports injured limbs. The three basic types of bandage are:

- Roller bandages, for securing dressings and supporting limbs.
- Triangular bandages, for making slings or securing large dressings.
- Tubular bandages, for supporting injured limbs and holding dressings on digits.

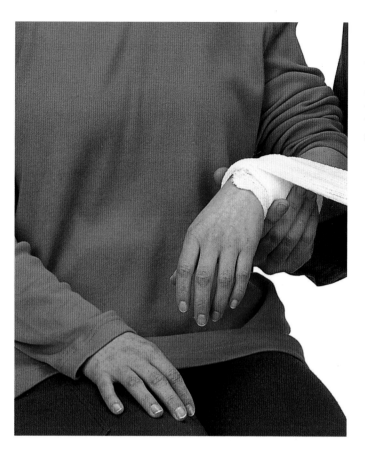

◁ Start from the bottom of the limb and roll the bandage up the arm. Make sure the casualty is comfortable and work from their injured side.

The pressure applied when putting on a bandage is crucial. If a bandage is too tight, fingers or toes will feel cold, the skin will look blue and the limb will be painful. Later on, the skin may look pale and feel cold, and the casualty will tell you that their fingers or toes feel tingly and stiff. Conversely, a loose bandage won't control bleeding or protect a wound site from contamination. Practise makes perfect.

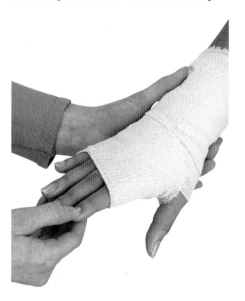

▽ To check that a bandage isn't too tight, press hard on an area downstream of the bandage, a finger in this example. If it takes more than 3 seconds to turn pink again, after being pressed, the bandage needs to be redone more loosely.

THE BASIC RULES OF DRESSING AND BANDAGING

To bandage and apply dressings effectively, follow these simple rules:

DO

➤ Start bandaging from the bottom of a limb and work towards the top.

➤ Bandage firmly; it shouldn't be too loose, but also not so tight that it cuts off the casualty's circulation.

➤ Secure the bandaging with adhesive tape, and guard against loose ends that might get caught when the casualty is being moved.

➤ Use uniform pressure when bandaging, and wrap a large area of the limb, which cuts down the chance of impeding the circulation.

DO NOT

➤ Use an elasticated bandage to hold a dressing in place, as it may be too tight and cut off the blood flow.

➤ Bandage over toes or fingers, unless they are damaged, so that you can check the bandaging is not too tight.

➤ Use the wrong-sized bandage – too big and it will be baggy, too small and it will be potentially too tight.

➤ Fix a dressing with adhesive tape before first asking the casualty if they have an allergy to such tape.

➤ Apply adhesive tape all the way around a limb or a finger or toe as it could cut off the blood flow.

Applying bandages 1

SEE ALSO
➤ Applying dressings and bandages, p200
➤ Applying bandages 2, p204

The only way to become proficient at bandaging is to practise; joints, such as ankles or elbows, can be especially tricky to master. You may find it easiest to watch someone else first and repeat it while you have a chance for some feedback. Make sure that the bandage overlaps on each turn and that you roll it out firmly but not too tightly. If your finished bandage looks floppy within an hour, unwind it and reapply using slightly more pressure. Bandages can become stretched with use but washing quickly restores their elasticity.

The first decision to be made when bandaging is to choose the correct-sized bandage for the affected body part. If it is too small or too big, it won't do its job efficiently and could cause more damage. As a guide, these sizes fit the following body parts: 2.5 cm (1 in) finger; 5 cm (2 in) hand; 7.5–10 cm (3–4 in) arm; and 10–15 cm (4–6 in) leg.

THE BASICS OF BANDAGING

Make the casualty comfortable and offer reassurance. Work in front of the casualty and start on the injured side.

⬇

Make sure the injured part is supported while you're working on it.

⬇

Apply the bandage with a firm and even pressure, neither too tight nor too loose.

⬇

Tie reef knots or secure with tape. Ensure all loose ends are tucked away.

⬇

Check the circulation beyond the bandage and check on any bleeding.

HOW TO APPLY A ROLLER BANDAGE

The tip of a roll of bandage is called the "tail", whereas the roll is called the "head". Keep the head of the bandage uppermost, so that if you drop it, it does not fall on to the ground. Think about how the finished bandage will look before starting.

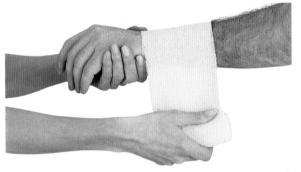

1 Place the tail of the bandage below the injury and work from the inside to the outside, and from the furthermost part to the nearest.

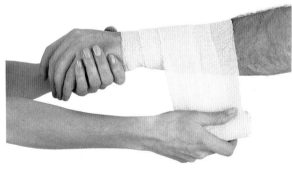

2 Roll the bandage around the limb and start with two overlapping turns. Cover two-thirds of the previous turn with each new one. Finish with two overlapping turns.

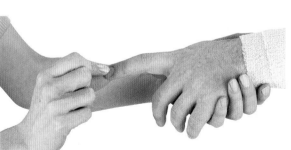

3 Once you've finished, check the circulation; if the bandage is too tight, unroll it and reapply it slightly looser.

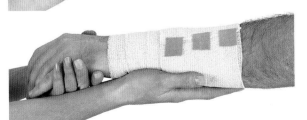

4 Secure the end with pins or adhesive tape or tuck in the ends of the bandage as securely as you can.

BANDAGING A HAND OR FOOT

The bandaging method below for a hand also applies for a foot, although the heel should be kept clear unless injured. When working on a foot, start bandaging at the big toe.

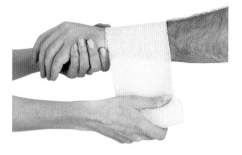

1 Start at the wrist and make two straight turns, working from the inside to the outside of the wrist.

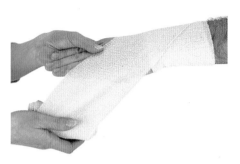

2 From the thumb side of the wrist, take the bandage diagonally across the back of the hand until it is touching the nail of the little finger.

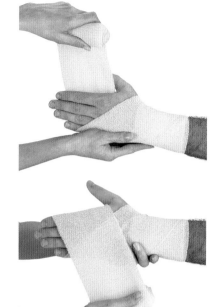
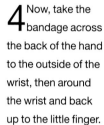

3 Leave the thumb free and take the bandage across the front of the fingers, also keeping the fingertips free.

4 Now, take the bandage across the back of the hand to the outside of the wrist, then around the wrist and back up to the little finger.

5 Repeat these turns, and cover about two-thirds of the previous turn with each new turn.

BANDAGING AN ELBOW OR KNEE JOINT

Bandaging these joints can be tricky, especially if you try to bandage while the joint is fully flexed. So, bandage in a partly flexed position so that it stays in place. For maximum support, these bandages need to be applied using figure-of-eight turns.

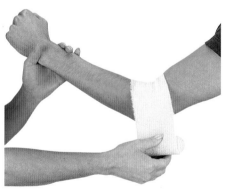

1 Put the tail of the bandage on the inside of the elbow; wind the bandage around the joint twice.

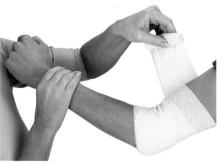

2 Now move the head of the bandage above the joint and wind two turns diagonally, making sure that you have covered half of the previous turn.

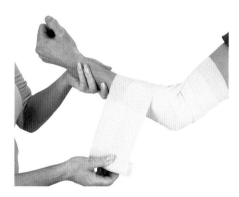

3 Now move the head to below the joint, cover half of the initial straight turns and do two diagonal turns.

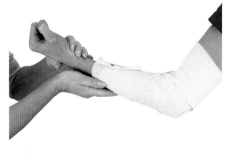

4 Continue doing two diagonal turns above and then below the joint in a figure-of-eight and then finally finish off the bandage with two straight turns.

Applying bandages 2

The head and fingers or toes are probably the trickiest areas to perfect in terms of bandaging technique. Apart from them being difficult areas to make bandages stay in place, they may cause other problems for someone new to bandaging. Tightly wrapped adhesive tape, for example, around a finger can act as a tourniquet. Scalp wounds often bleed profusely and bandages need even but firm pressure to be effective. Here you'll learn how to use a tubular gauze bandage and a triangular bandage, which are included in most first-aid kits.

Tubular bandages come in two types: tubular elasticated bandages for supporting injured joints and tubular gauze for covering a finger or a toe.

Tubular gauze bandages help to staunch the bleeding and also protect a digit from others nearby without impeding its blood flow. If you cannot find a tubular object with which to make the bandage, bend a piece of card in two or, failing that, use a child's sweet tube with the lid removed and bottom punched out.

HOW TO APPLY A TUBULAR BANDAGE TO A FINGER

These elasticated bandages allow sufficient pressure to stop the bleeding but do not impede blood flow. The device shown can be bought from a chemist.

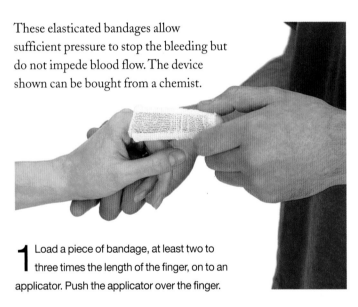

1 Load a piece of bandage, at least two to three times the length of the finger, on to an applicator. Push the applicator over the finger.

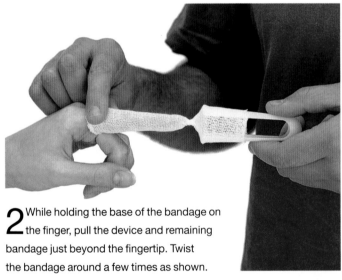

2 While holding the base of the bandage on the finger, pull the device and remaining bandage just beyond the fingertip. Twist the bandage around a few times as shown.

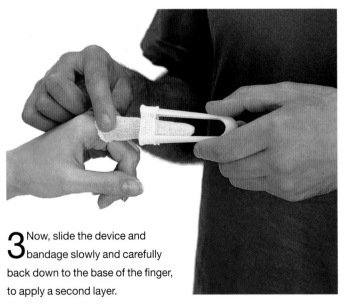

3 Now, slide the device and bandage slowly and carefully back down to the base of the finger, to apply a second layer.

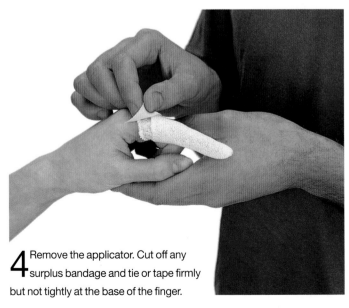

4 Remove the applicator. Cut off any surplus bandage and tie or tape firmly but not tightly at the base of the finger.

HOW TO BANDAGE A HEAD

Initially, apply a gauze wad to a head wound, especially if it is bleeding heavily. The wad helps to apply firm but even pressure across the whole scalp. If blood soaks through the bandage, apply another on top to avoid disturbing any blood clots. A strip bandage could be used, but is harder to keep in place.

1 Apply the triangular bandage with the folded longest edge over the forehead.

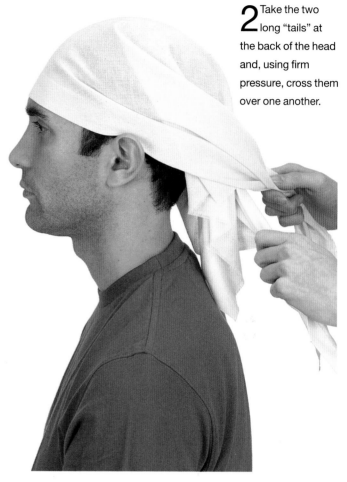

2 Take the two long "tails" at the back of the head and, using firm pressure, cross them over one another.

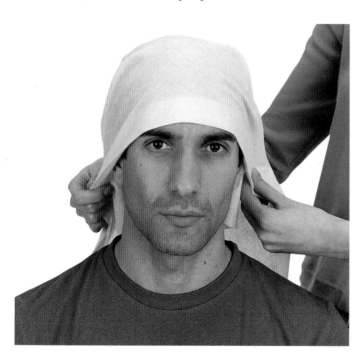

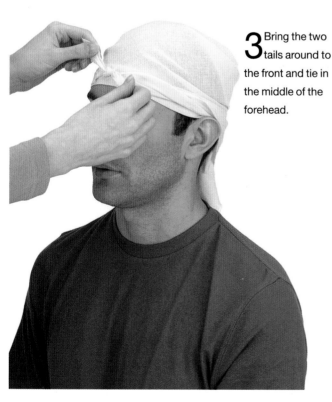

3 Bring the two tails around to the front and tie in the middle of the forehead.

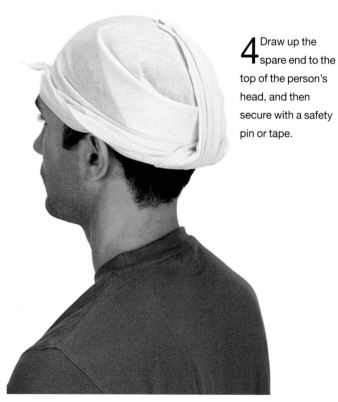

4 Draw up the spare end to the top of the person's head, and then secure with a safety pin or tape.

Fixing slings

SEE ALSO
➤ Wounds and wound healing, p128
➤ Treating infected wounds, p132
➤ Dealing with broken bones, p150

Triangular bandages are first-aid kit staples and most kits will contain quite a few. Usually a large triangular bandage is used for making a sling. If there is not one to hand at the scene of an emergency then you can improvise with the upturned hem of a jacket or shirt, or the sleeve of a shirt or jumper. The important functions of a sling are to support and immobilize an injured part of the body, and, in some cases (called high-arm or elevation slings), to stem bleeding from a wound. Here, you'll learn how to tie both types of arm sling.

Slings usually support the arm and can be classed as either a "broad-arm" sling, which supports the arm horizontally, or a "high-arm" sling, which both supports the limb and helps to reduce swelling and bleeding. High-arm slings also support rib fractures.

HOW TO TIE A HIGH-ARM SLING

This high-arm or elevation sling is used to stop the bleeding in a finger or forearm injury and also helps to reduce pain and prevent further injury by immobilizing the limb. This sling can also be used in burn victims to minimize swelling.

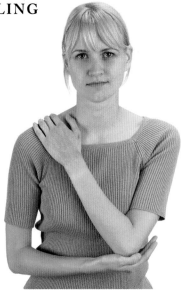

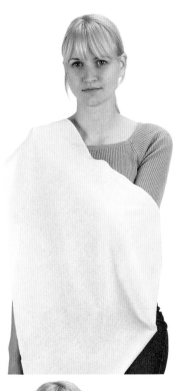

1 Place the injured arm so that the fingers touch the opposite collarbone.

2 Place the triangular bandage to lie over the injured arm with the long edge against the uninjured side and the point to the injured side.

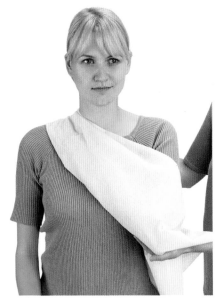

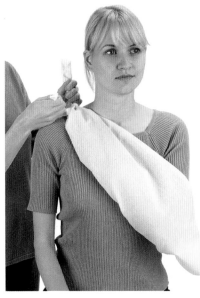

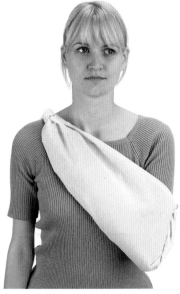

3 Tuck the bandage behind the elbow and forearm. Pass the free end behind the back.

4 At the collarbone, tie the two ends of the bandage together on the uninjured side.

5 To secure the bandage at the elbow, tuck in the fabric or fold and use a safety pin.

FIXING A BROAD-ARM SLING

This type of sling is used for an arm or hand injury, such as a fracture or a sprain. Such a sling immobilizes the limb and can be improvised in many ways.

1 Ask the casualty to support their injured arm so that the hand lies just above the uninjured elbow. Now place the bandage in between the body and arm, so that the straight edge lies on the uninjured side.

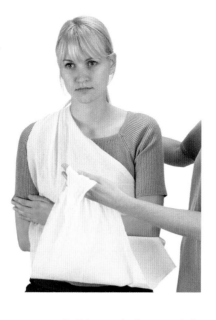

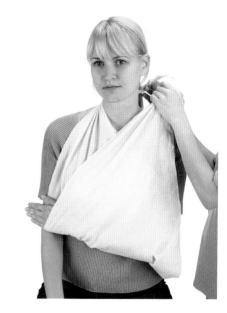

2 Bring up the lower end of the bandage to meet the other end at the shoulder. Tie (or pin) to secure and tuck both ends under the knot.

3 The casualty can let the arm go once you have secured the ends.

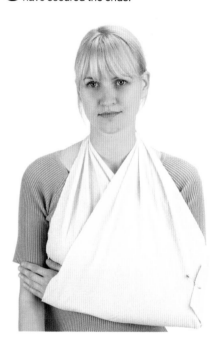

4 Finish the sling by folding over the pointed end of the fabric at the elbow and pinning. This is how the sling should look.

SOME IDEAS FOR IMPROVISING SLINGS

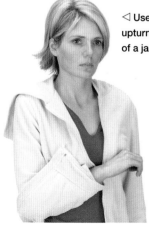

◁ Use the upturned hem of a jacket.

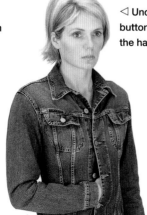

◁ Undo a jacket button and tuck the hand inside.

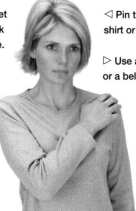

◁ Pin the sleeve of a shirt or jumper.

▷ Use a pair of tights or a belt.

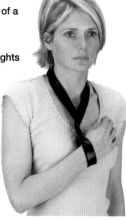

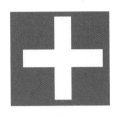

SKILLS CHECKLIST FOR
FIRST-AID KIT

KEY POINTS

- Always have a first-aid kit available at home and in your car ☐

- While a first-aid kit is important the ability to improvise is an essential skill for a first-aider ☐

- Practice your bandaging skills on a friend ☐

SKILLS LEARNED

- How to dress and bandage a wound or injury ☐

- How to improvise dressings and bandages if necessary ☐

- How to bandage an elbow and knee ☐

- How to bandage a finger ☐

- How to cope with scalp bandaging ☐

- How to make slings ☐

14

COMPLEMENTARY THERAPIES

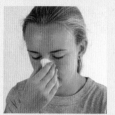

Complementary health therapists believe that their practices encourage the body's natural defences to heal injury – whether that injury be physical or emotional or a combination of the two. Of course, complementary techniques will not be appropriate in emergencies, when conventional medicine is vital. Where they come into their own is in working alongside conventional medicine for more minor complaints, such as cramps, stings and constipation. As with any first-aid treatment, safety must always be your watchword. Only use safe techniques, sterile dressings and medications you feel really well informed about. Always ask for a medical opinion before using complementary therapies on babies and children.

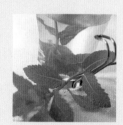

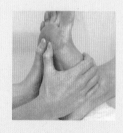

CONTENTS

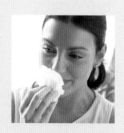

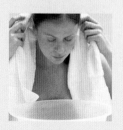

Understanding complementary therapies

SEE ALSO

➤ Complementary first-aid kit, p212

➤ Using complementary therapies 1 and 2, pp214, 216

The complementary therapies frequently referred to when it comes to natural first aid are aromatherapy, herbalism, acupuncture, reflexology and homeopathy. You may find that a number of other therapies – such as Alexander Technique, reiki, massage, colour therapy, meditation or yoga – have a part to play in calming a casualty with minor injuries and in helping them to convalesce. Be sure to seek conventional medical assistance first, and then choose from the many natural therapies to soothe, calm and heal.

It is not that long ago that people had only natural remedies to turn to when dealing with illness or injury. In very recent times, these types of treatment have made a comeback, and new "complementary" approaches have been developed. Many people perceive them to be safer, gentler and more natural than conventional medicines, preferring their holistic approach over modern medicine's perceived emphasis on the disease rather than the person.

Some first-aid scenarios demand life support skills and complementary tactics are not appropriate, but there are many minor cases where alternatives are fine to use. Some of these have been proved effective in clinical trials, while others may not have been formally tested, but are commonly accepted as useful and effective alternatives.

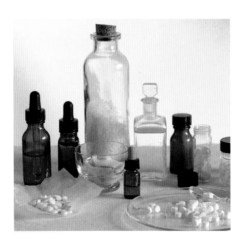

△ A wide range of homeopathic remedies are now widely available at conventional high street pharmacies, where expert help may be on hand to advise about their use.

▽ Herbal remedies can be used for all kinds of conditions, but seek advice before using.

BE SAFE!

➤ **Seek conventional advice first**
Before embarking on a complementary therapy, you should have the casualty checked out by a conventional doctor. In fact, always seek conventional advice whenever considering complementary treatments. This advice applies especially strongly if you have any medical condition at all.

➤ **Use herbal remedies carefully**
Some herbs may interact with certain pharmaceutical drugs. Some interactions may be minor, but others can be life-threatening. For example, St John's Wort, which may help to alleviate mild to moderate depression, can interact with drugs prescribed for other conditions, including the contraceptive pill. Seek medical advice before taking it if you use any other medicines. Herbal remedies and pharmaceutical drugs are not necessarily mutually exclusive, but decisions on taking both at the same time should be left to professionals. The rule is simple: never take herbal remedies at the same time as prescribed medication without consulting your physician.

➤ **Using aromatherapy oils**
Always seek expert help before using these. Many natural oils are potent, and specific ones can be dangerous if taken with certain conditions – pregnant women must be especially careful which oils they use. In most cases, never apply oils directly to skin (lavender and tea tree are notable exceptions), but dilute in a carrier oil. Before applying oils to the skin, always do a patch test.

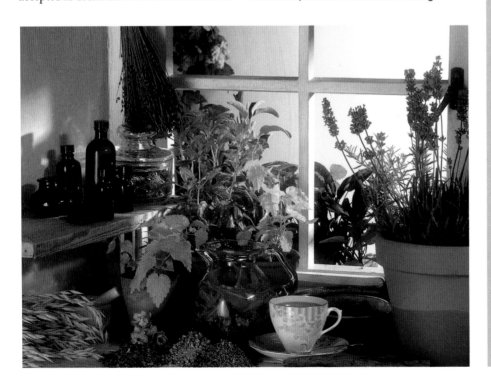

AROMATHERAPY

What is it? This literally means "treatment using scent". The term "aromatherapy" was first used by a French chemist called Gattefosse in 1937. He accidentally discovered the healing powers of essential oils when he burnt his hand and plunged it into a bucket of lavender oil. He was amazed by how quickly and painlessly the burn healed up.

How it works Essential plant oils are used in various ways, including massage, inhalation, baths, cold compresses and vaporizers. The smell of the oils is thought to affect the part of the brain that controls emotions, mood and memory. It may have a calming or an invigorating effect, depending on the aromas used.

Are essential oils harmful? Essential oils should be used with caution in pregnancy and in conditions such as high blood pressure, epilepsy and skin conditions. There may be hypersensitive reactions to sunlight. The oils should never be ingested and always kept out of the way of children.

▽ Steam inhalation of certain aromatic oils can soothe anxiety and tension.

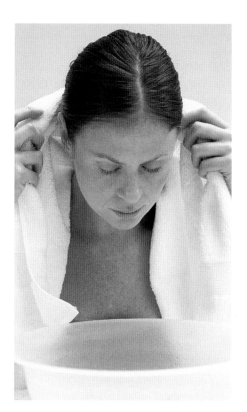

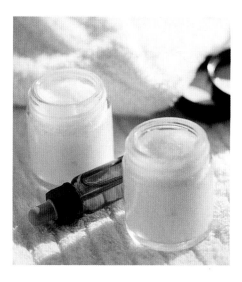

△ Essential oils can be used in many different forms – added to moisturizer, for example.

HERBALISM

Almost all drugs used to be derived from plant parts. Many people like the idea of using herbal remedies, because they feel that they are safer and more natural than conventional drugs.

What is it? Herbal medicine, also known as phytotherapy, is one of the earliest medical systems known and dates back thousands of years. It uses plant-based remedies to treat a variety of symptoms and conditions. It is used by some MDs as well as naturopaths, osteopaths and licensed herbalists.

How are they used? Herbs can be infused, made into tinctures, teas, capsules, creams, compresses and bath products. They may be effective for treating problems such as irritable bowel syndrome, urinary problems and eczema.

ACUPUNCTURE/ACUPRESSURE

An ancient Chinese treatment, used for thousands of years, acupuncture involves the insertion of thin needles under the skin at specific points. The points are located along energy channels or "meridians". Acupressure massages these points instead of using needles. No one is certain how this approach works, but it may increase secretions of the body's natural painkillers – endorphins.

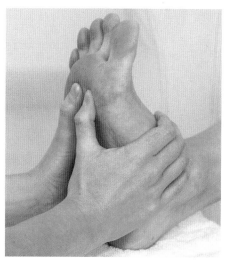

△ Reflexology is claimed to be effective in relieving problems such as back pain.

REFLEXOLOGY

This therapy involves massaging certain areas of the feet and the hands that are believed to correspond to different parts of the body and to specific organs.

HOMEOPATHY

Homeopathy claims to fight disease by treating "like with like". In other words, elements that can cause the symptoms of a particular illness can be used to cure it. However, these elements are used in minute doses, to the point where the prescribed substance is so diluted that it is undetectable.

▽ Try "Rescue remedy" and *Arnica* to help recovery from minor bruises and emotional shock.

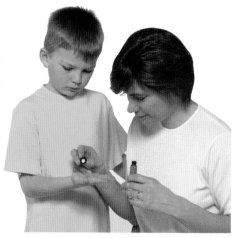

Complementary first-aid kit

SEE ALSO

➤ Understanding complementary therapies, p210

➤ Using therapies 1 and 2, pp214, 216

You can obtain many essential oils and herbs, as well as homeopathic remedies, from high street pharmacies. Choose those that you find appealing or maybe select the remedies that cover most of the common household injuries and the aches and pains that may affect us all from time to time – such as headaches, colds, sore throat, arthritis, insomnia, low mood and anxiety. Always check the expiry dates and bear in mind that it is good to buy in small quantities, until you have established that you find the remedies useful, to avoid wastage.

Recently, a study showed that burning aromatherapy oils on a psychiatric ward had a significantly calming effect on disturbed patients. Different oils, homeopathic remedies and herbs work on different ailments, and you could make up a useful first-aid kit of these to use alongside more conventional remedies.

As with many drugs, there are really only a small number of complementary therapies that are definitely safe in pregnancy. It is a good idea to check with your doctor or obstetrician before trying any therapies – they will be able to advise you on the remedies that may be most useful for you without being toxic to the fetus.

PEPPERMINT

Used as an oil or herb, peppermint has active ingredients that are effective at clearing the upper respiratory tract of mucus, so it is useful as a decongestant in colds and nasal blockage. It is an invigorating herb that can be chosen when you want to feel more awake and alert. Taken as a tea or in capsule form, it is excellent at calming digestive problems, especially trapped wind, heartburn and indigestion. Diluted peppermint oil can also be rubbed into the temples at each side of the forehead and the neck muscles at the top of the spine and around the shoulders to help in the relief of stress headaches.

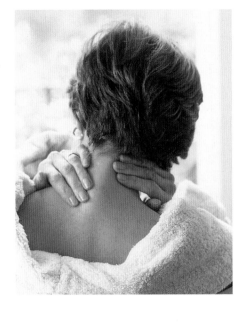

△ Gently massage diluted peppermint oil into the neck muscles to relieve tension headache.

GINGER

This plant is very soothing for digestive disorders and appetite loss. Ginger root is commonly drunk as a tea to ease travel sickness, and it can be used, if advised, to alleviate morning sickness. Effective for muscle spasms and pains, ginger is also useful in rheumatism and arthritis.

CLOVE

Extract of clove is a well-known pain-reliever, and a small amount of clove oil applied to a sore tooth will ease the pain of toothache (note: avoid contact, especially prolonged, with gums or skin, as this can cause some irritation). Clove is also a good insect repellent, so a few drops placed on clothing or bedding will help keep biting insects and mosquitoes away.

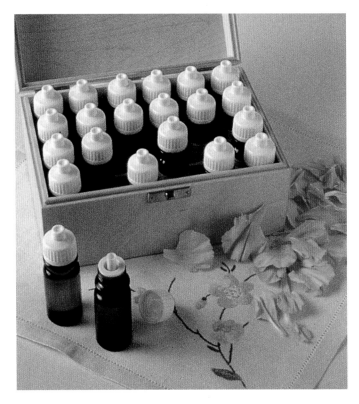

▷ Herbal and homeopathic remedies should be stored away from direct sunlight, in dark glass bottles.

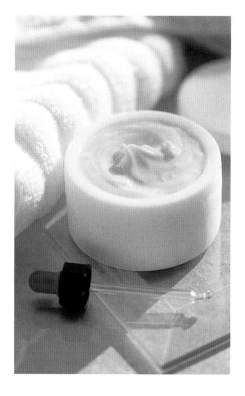

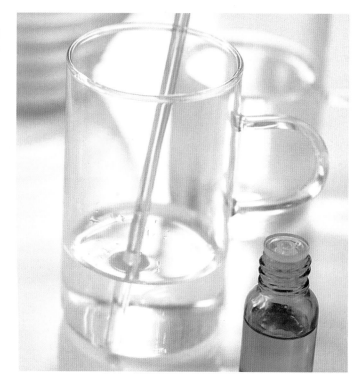

▷ If using oils diluted in water, stir very thoroughly.

ARNICA

This pretty flowering herb is poisonous when taken internally, so should be used only in creams and oils topically, other than as a homeopathic remedy. *Arnica* is useful for bruises, muscle soreness, emotional shock and to promote wound-healing.

LAVENDER

Used as an essential oil, lavender is highly antiseptic and effective when used as a

▽ Sniff a tissue containing a few drops of lavender oil to relieve insomnia.

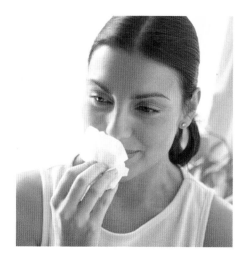

compress for superficial burns, blisters and bites. It can be used to help ease low mood and insomnia – simply add a few drops to a tissue and sniff, or add a few drops to your pillowcase, to help you get off to sleep and enjoy a refreshing rest.

TEA TREE

The essential oil of tea tree is used topically as an antibacterial, antiseptic remedy. Diluted in water, a tea tree spray can ease the pain of a sore throat.

CHAMOMILE

Made up as a tea, chamomile is extremely calming and soothing, and is good for insomnia, low mood and anxiety. A few drops of the oil in a bedtime bath will also aid peaceful sleep.

GERANIUM

This is claimed to be a very effective herb when used to treat wound healing.

CLARY SAGE

This is a useful essential oil for dealing with low mood, anxiety and frayed nerves. It can be added, diluted, to a bath, or dispersed in an oil burner.

SOME OTHER IDEAS FOR YOUR NATURAL KIT

➤ Tincture of *Calendula* (pot marigold) – minor burns and scalds.

➤ Comfrey oil/ointment – bruises and sprains. Never use any oil/ointment on open wounds (it encourages infection).

➤ Witch hazel – insect bites and stings, sprains, bruises, mild sunburn.

▽ Oil from geranium leaves is a calming and cooling remedy, ideal for easing anxieties.

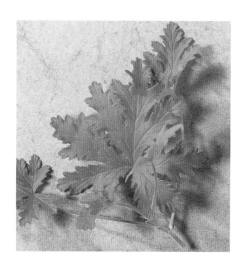

Using complementary therapies 1

SEE ALSO

➤ Refer to index for all other references to these conditions throughout book

Accidents, injuries and trauma may produce a wide range of associated symptoms, ranging from nausea and constipation to cramp. These kinds of symptoms can often be eased by complementary therapies. Psychological after-shock and tension are also natural reactions to injury and accident, and you might find that complementary approaches can be effective in these cases, too. However, always remember that your first priority must be to arrange for conventional medical treatment for an individual's injuries.

NAUSEA AND VOMITING

There are many causes of nausea and vomiting. Most of them will be "self-limiting", which means they will settle without the need for further treatment or investigation. It is recommended that you should seek conventional advice first when tackling health conditions, but mild nausea can usually be treated safely with natural remedies. However, as with diarrhoea, if the symptoms are not settling in 1–2 days and dehydration is developing, or the symptoms are mild but persistent, medical help must be sought.

Herbal remedies An infusion of ginger root may settle nausea. Also try chamomile or black horehound (but always avoid the latter in pregnancy).

Acupuncture/acupressure Use the anti-nausea point that is two thumb widths above the wrist crease, between the two prominent tendons passing to the hand. A therapist can treat this area with a needle, or you can use firm pressure at this point for

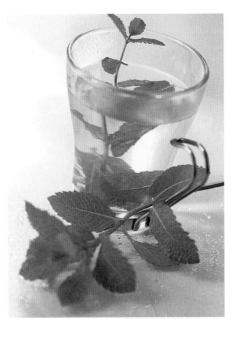

△ A peppermint infusion is a highly effective remedy for nausea and indigestion – and also useful as a general pick-me-up.

one minute. There are also wristbands for sale that exert pressure, and can be used in pregnancy. For travel sickness, press your index finger into the hollow at the back of the jawline for a minute.

Homeopathy *Ipecac* and *Nux Vomica* are said to be useful for nausea. Take up to 12 doses every 2 hours until the symptoms settle.

DIARRHOEA

Herbal remedies Geranium, peppermint and chamomile infusions may help if taken as 45–60 ml/3–4 tbsp of tea three times a day.

Acupressure Use firm pressure four thumb widths above the inside of the ankle just behind the shin bone.

Reflexology Apply pressure to the point for the small intestine (which is located between the arch and the heel of the foot) and then the large intestine points on either side.

Homeopathy *Arsenicum album* is the recommended remedy for diarrhoea.

CONSTIPATION

Aromatherapy Gently massage a diluted mixture of rosemary, marjoram and chamomile into the area around the navel.

Herbal remedies Dandelion roots are a gentle laxative.

Acupressure Place a finger four thumb widths up from the back of the wrist crease. Bend the arm and press the opposite thumb into the outer edge of the elbow crease for a minute, then repeat on the other arm.

Reflexology Use the large intestine pressure point (see picture for exact location). Press firmly and then massage for 10 minutes.

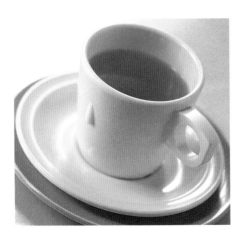

△ Chamomile-containing herbal teas are excellent for soothing anxiety.

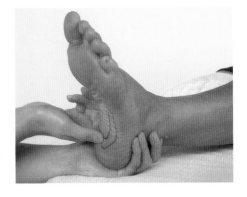

△ A reflexologist is able to massage the large intestine pressure point (the relevant area is drawn on the foot in this photograph) in order to try to relieve constipation.

HEADACHE

Stress and tension, which are commonly associated with the trauma of injuries and accidents, may manifest themselves in different ways. One of the most common is headache. The casualty may complain of tightness in the muscles at the back of the scalp and neck.

Aromatherapy Diluted lavender oil rubbed into the temples is soothing for a tension headache. Inhaling eucalyptus is also very effective for sinus headaches.

Herbal remedies Feverfew may help with a migrainous headache, but should not be taken in pregnancy.

Acupressure Apply pressure to a point between the eyebrows at the bridge of the nose, and to points on either side of the neck at the base of the back of the skull.

Reflexology Press a thumb firmly to the base of the big toe for 10–20 seconds.

Homeopathy *Kali bichromicum* 6c is used to help sinus headache, and *Bryonia* for a general headache.

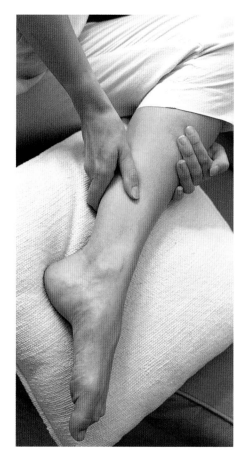

△ Massage cramp with a blend of basil and marjoram diluted in almond oil.

CRAMP

This is when a muscle goes into a painful spasm and feels rock-hard. It occurs most often after exercise, when you are dehydrated, and also often strikes in the middle of the night. Initial measures should involve using the muscle by walking around or stretching and massaging it, and drinking plenty of water every day, at least 2 litres (3 ½ pints).

Aromatherapy Massage with basil and marjoram diluted in almond oil.

Herbal remedies Ginkgo infusion helps ease intractable cramp.

Acupressure Press into the bottom of the calf muscle for 5 minutes.

Homeopathy *Caprum metallicum* tablets may help to ease a cramp-like ache.

▷ Cramp is a common condition that is extremely painful and can happen very suddenly, particularly after exercise.

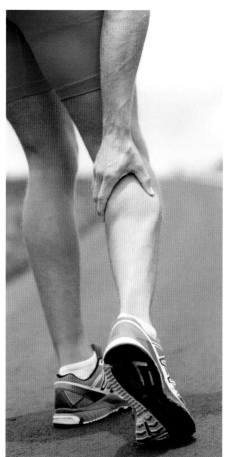

△ Try relieving stress headaches by applying gentle pressure to the area around the temples.

EMOTIONAL SHOCK

Aromatherapy Neroli and lavender oils are known for their relaxing and calming properties.

Herbal remedies Chamomile and lemon balm combine well to make a tea to calm and soothe agitation, and encourage peaceful rest and sleep.

Homeopathy *Arnica* tablets are used for bruising and emotional shock. Arnica can also be used as a topical cream. Aconite may also be helpful for stress and tension.

SOOTHING STRESS AND TENSION

Once any injuries have been treated by a medical practitioner, massage with soothing oils and relaxation exercises can be helpful for easing the stress and tension associated with any accident.

Using complementary therapies 2

SEE ALSO

➤ Refer to index for all other references to these conditions throughout book

Some relatively minor injuries can be treated effectively with one or other of the complementary therapies. There is often a number of options, from which you may choose the one you prefer. For example, to treat bruises you can use *Arnica*, lavender oil or rosemary oil; sunburn can be soothed with lavender oil, *Hypericum* (St John's wort), aloe vera or *Calendula*. "Rescue Remedy" combines five of the Bach flower remedies and can be bought as a tincture or a cream – it is useful for reducing the effects of emotional shock.

There are all kinds of scenarios that respond well to complementary treatments, either used alone or in tandem with conventional first aid treatment. Complementary means exactly that – these treatments are not necessarily an alternative to a more traditional medical approach, and the two approaches should complement each other.

BITES AND STINGS

Aromatherapy Add a few drops of lavender or tea tree oil to a little iced water and apply it to the area. Soak a flannel in the water and place that on the sting, or use cotton wool and apply some of the water every 10 minutes until the pain subsides.

Herbal remedies Fresh onion on an insect bite may take the pain out of the area. Useful herbs for making into an infusion and applying to a burn or sting are chamomile, elderflower or red clover (the latter is also a proven natural alternative to hormone replacement therapy). Fresh leaves of lemon balm, plantain and yellow dock applied to the damaged skin may be soothing and speed up pain relief.

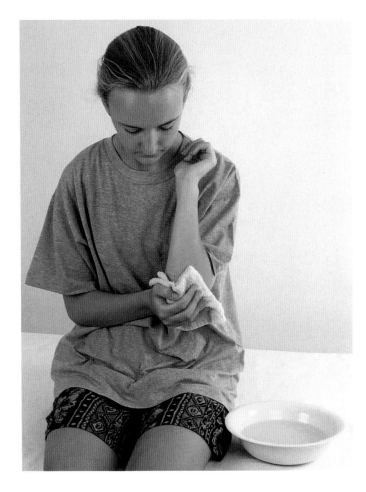

▷ For soothing sore bites and stings, wring a cloth out in iced water or an iced herbal infusion and hold it over the affected area.

BRUISES

Bruising happens because the blood vessels beneath the skin break and the blood escapes. This is usually after a traumatic event, and it can be painful. However, certain people may bruise virtually without injury, perhaps if they are on anticoagulant treatment such as warfarin or have problems with their blood clotting abilities. Anyone who notices an increased bruising tendency should always seek medical help as it may also be a sign of more serious conditions.

Aromatherapy Lavender oil made up as a cold compress may help in reducing swelling and bruising after injury. Diluted rosemary oil massaged into the tissues is also soothing and may speed up healing.

Homeopathy Use *Arnica* on unbroken skin in ointment form or as a bath lotion; the latter is very soothing when suffering from general aching – after an unaccustomed horse ride or aerobics class, for example.

BURNS

Before you do anything to any type of burn or scald you should cool it down. Hold the area under cold running water for at least ten minutes. If the burn is bigger than the palm of the victim's hand, or if the burn is deep or on a baby or small child, they must get medical advice.

Aromatherapy Lavender essential oil is good to help numb the pain of a burn, which can be excruciating. It promotes healing and reduces scarring. Use neat on small areas, on sterile gauze or lint for larger areas.

Herbal remedies Fresh gel from the aloe vera plant is very effective – simply snap off part of a leaf and apply the plant gel directly.

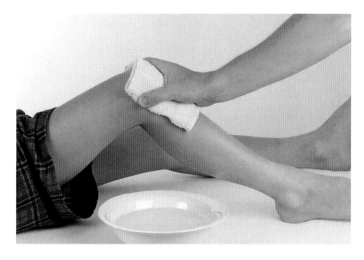

△ Lay the casualty flat to apply a cold compress to sprains and strains.

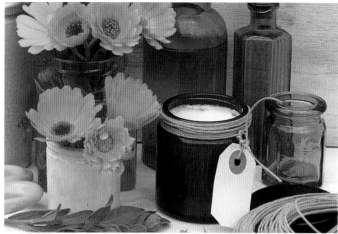

△ *Calendula* (pot marigold) remedies are ideal for healing cuts and grazes.

SPRAINS AND STRAINS

Aromatherapy/herbal remedies It can be useful to add some lavender oil or chamomile to water and store them in a bottle in the fridge so that you have something at hand for soothing sprains and strains. A comfrey or marigold leaf infusion applied ice-cold is also good. Comfrey ointment is effective when applied for a few days after a strain has occurred, or to aching muscles.

Homeopathy Homeopathic remedies include *Arnica*, *Rhus tox.* and *Ruta grav.*

SUNBURN

Aromatherapy For widespread sunburn, add some drops of diluted lavender oil to a lukewarm bath. Lavender oil can also be applied directly to the skin, especially if the sunburn is severe. The blood-red oil of St John's wort and aloe vera juice are highly soothing, cooling and healing.

Homeopathy Homeopathic options include *Cantharis* and *Urtica urens*, especially if the pain of the sunburn is intense and persistent. *Hypericum* or *Calendula* cream is also used.

NOSEBLEED

Aromatherapy A pad of cotton wool soaked in cold water with a few drops of lemon oil added is good at slowing down a nosebleed when placed across the bridge of the nose.

Herbal remedies Cotton wool soaked in an infusion of yarrow and then squeezed at the end of the nose for a few minutes may prove effective in stopping a nosebleed.

CUTS AND GRAZES

Aromatherapy Lavender and tea tree can be used neat on small cuts and scratches, added to a bowl of water for cleaning the wound, or used on a dressing applied over the injury. These oils have a disinfectant effect so may well reduce the chances of infection settling into the wound.

Herbal remedies Witch hazel can be used directly on small wounds or on a dressing, as can tinctures of marigold or myrrh. Comfrey is also a powerful tissue-healer.

Homeopathy A compress of *Hypericum* or *Calendula* can be used direct on dressings, or in ointments once the skin has healed over.

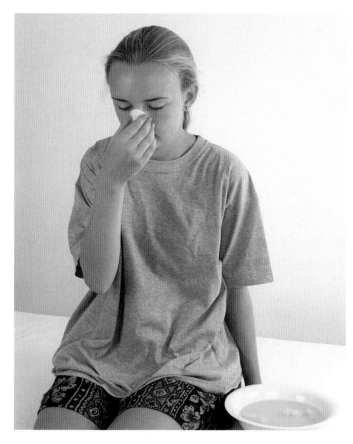

◁ To stop nosebleeds, try applying a pad of cotton wool soaked in a cooled yarrow infusion over the soft part of the nose.

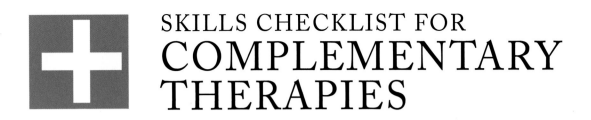

SKILLS CHECKLIST FOR
COMPLEMENTARY THERAPIES

KEY POINTS

- The remedies described in this chapter are intended to be complementary or additional rather than alternatives ☐

- Always seek qualified medical assistance initially ☐

SKILLS LEARNED

- How to treat minor injuries with natural, complementary treatments ☐

- Recognizing that complementary treatments may be effective in the aftermath of injury, trauma or accident, for treating anxiety, insomnia, low mood and stress ☐

- Recognizing that complementary treatments can have side-effects just as conventional medical treatments do ☐

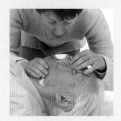

KEEPING SAFE

Safety in the home, safety in the garden and pool, and safety on the road are supremely important considerations in the prevention of accidents. The great majority of accidents are preventable. This chapter looks at the hazards to be encountered both in the home, especially in the kitchen and the bathroom, and outside it. Being aware and taking sensible precautions will help you to minimize the chances of an accident befalling either you or a member of your family. When accidents do occur, coping with them quickly and effectively can do much to mitigate the effects and prevent further injury.

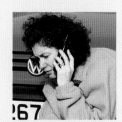

CONTENTS

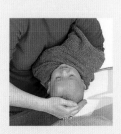

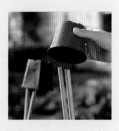

Keeping yourself safe

Most people do not give enough thought to their own safety when they spot someone in danger and in need of assistance. However, you must do everything you can to protect yourself while helping a casualty. Taking time to survey the scene and think through your actions is essential. You should not, for example, rush in to rescue someone from a burning building. Without the necessary training, you are likely to become a casualty yourself and may hinder a rescue operation. It is wiser to wait for the professionals.

The first rule of first aid is not to put yourself in any danger. You may make matters worse if you jump into the scene without first standing back and assessing the situation. You should be aware of your limitations and training. For example, even a strong swimmer should be wary of diving into the water to help someone struggling. You should always consider safer ways to help first, such as throwing in a rope and life ring or an inflatable ball. Rescue attempts often end in a double tragedy that could have been avoided had more time been taken to survey the scene. Always take a few moments to look for danger – there may be flammable chemicals, electric cables or other hazards present, such as traffic in the case of road accidents.

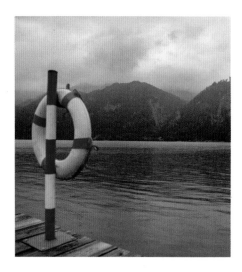

△ Throw a lifebuoy, an inflatable ball or rope to someone who is having difficulties in deep water rather than jumping in yourself.

CARE WITH BODY FLUIDS

Helping a casualty may involve coming into contact with body fluids, such as blood, saliva or vomit. There is virtually no risk of catching HIV or hepatitis from mouth-to-mouth, but this should not lead to complacency.

Generally, HIV needs contact with fresh blood or semen to be dangerous. It is a relatively fragile virus that does not survive outside the body for long. Hepatitis B, on the other hand, can still be active in dried blood, even when it is several days old. It is also possible to contract tuberculosis (TB), meningitis and other infections from body fluids.

To protect yourself, use a mouth shield when giving mouth-to-mouth or do compression-only CPR.

AGGRESSIVENESS

You should never underestimate how violent a person might be, particularly if they appear to be drunk or on drugs. If in any doubt about your own safety, wait for the emergency services to arrive and keep away, especially if you suspect that the person might be carrying a weapon.

Sick people may become aggressive for many reasons, including low blood sugar as a result of diabetes or lack of oxygen. If you are worried about getting hurt, it is best to leave them until someone from the emergency services arrives and is able to give them appropriate treatment.

AVOIDING INFECTION FROM BLOOD AND OTHER BODY FLUIDS

The best way to guard against infection is to avoid the casualty's body fluids altogether. However, if that is not possible, there are several ways to minimize the risk.

➤ Wear a surgical face mask, disposable gloves and wash your hands after contact with blood or other body fluids.

➤ Protect any wounds on your own body from infection by using plasters or bandages to cover them.

➤ Wear plastic goggles or plastic glasses to protect your eyes from splashes.

➤ If body fluids come into contact with your mouth, eyes or nose, wash the area thoroughly for 10 minutes under briskly running water.

➤ If you receive an injury that comes into contact with body fluids, see a doctor. It is possible to detect infection with hepatitis B early on, and to reduce the risk of contracting the disease.

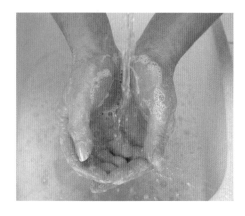

△ Wash your hands thoroughly under running water if you come into contact with body fluids such as blood or semen.

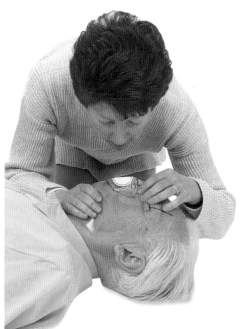

△ Use a mouth shield if you are giving mouth-to-mouth resuscitation.

▷ Be wary of approaching anyone who is drunk or aggressive. You do not know whether they may lash out or if they have a weapon.

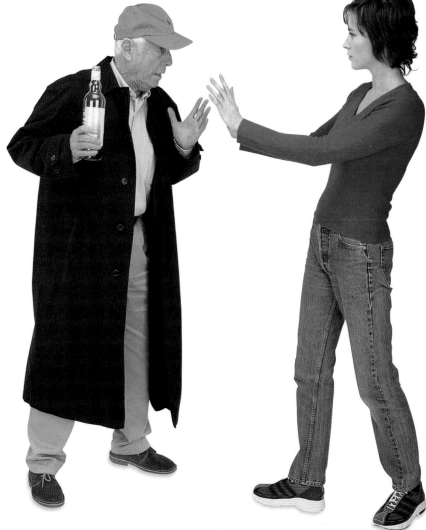

PSYCHOLOGICAL STRESS

It can be exhilarating and rewarding to help someone who is injured or in danger, but it can also be upsetting and disturbing however psychologically strong you are.

You may have witnessed scenes that you find difficult to get out of your mind, even weeks, months or years after the event. You may have disturbing dreams that disrupt your sleep even when you thought you had forgotten the incident. Talking to other people about the event or speaking to a trained counsellor may help you come to terms with the trauma.

Life-threatening emergencies can be frightening affairs, and if death is involved you may feel guilty that you did not do enough to help. You should accept that you may need support to help you to get back to normal.

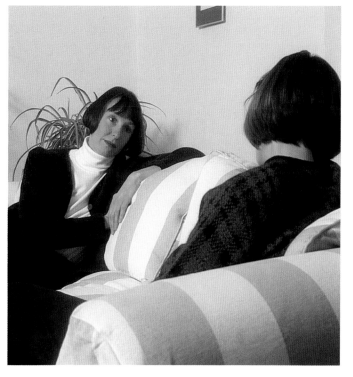

◁ Following a serious accident, bystanders, helpers and paramedics risk developing post-traumatic stress disorder. If you feel agitated or you are sleeping badly after witnessing a trauma, consider seeking help from a psychologist or clinical social worker (CSW) experienced in trauma-focussed psychotherapy. Your family doctor may be able to recommend a therapist.

Safety on the road

SEE ALSO

➤ What is first aid?, p12

➤ Chest compressions, p30

➤ Full Resuscitation sequence (adults), p33

More than half of all road accidents occur within five miles of home – partly because drivers spend most of their time there and perhaps partly because they enter a 'comfort zone' near home and pay less attention to traffic on the road. Most accidents are caused by human error – 95 per cent are somebody's fault, rather than simply an unlucky twist of fate. The best way to avoid accidents is to drive not only safely but also watchfully, so that you can compensate for the mistakes of others on the road.

Roads around the world are becoming increasingly busy. Perhaps surprisingly, most road traffic accidents happen in daylight; less surprisingly however, these often occur in the rush hours: 6–9 a.m. and 3–7 p.m. Rural roads are the most dangerous type of road, partly because they tend to be non-divided and speeding is more common. Average trip duration may be longer in rural areas, increasing the risk of fatigue and inattention. It may take longer to get medical assistance to accident victims and in some areas wild animals such as deer crossing can pose hazards.

Human error underlies most accidents, with speeding the most common behaviour underlying fatal crashes, followed by the influence of alcohol, medication and drugs. Other common contributors to road accidents include failure to stay in the proper lane or give way at crossroads, as well as driver distraction (by mobile phones, talking, eating, adjusting vehicle controls etc), and inexperience or carelessness by young and newly qualified drivers.

Alcohol affects multiple aspects of driving ability – decision-making, self-criticism, balance, coordination, touch, sight, hearing and judgment to name a few. It is best not to drink at all if you are planning on driving rather than trying to stick to a general "safe limit" that may not be safe for a particular individual at all.

Inexperienced and young drivers, especially men, often drive without enough thought for road safety or their responsibility as drivers. This is why young

> **WARNING**
> Restrictions on mobile phone use when driving vary from country to country but even hands-free use poses a significant increased risk of distracted driving and subsequent collision.

drivers can be a hazard on the road and may have to pay increased premiums for their motor vehicle insurance.

Older drivers can be a danger to themselves and others if their eyesight or reaction speeds are failing, particularly if they do not have any insight into the problem. Lack of concentration caused by chatting to others in the car, turning to reprimand children or talking on a phone can also cause an accident.

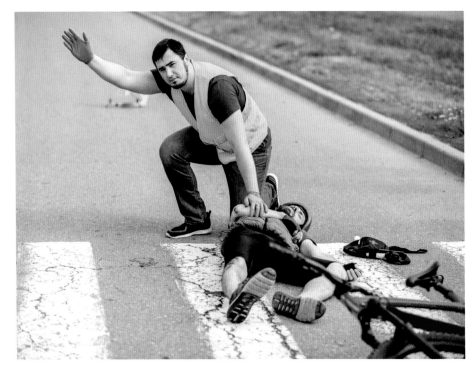

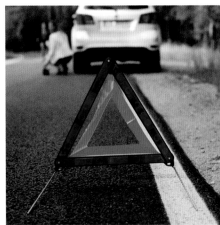

△ Always carry a reflective highway warning triangle in your vehicle. Place this near the stationary vehicle to warn approaching drivers of an accident.

◁ Make sure that the casualty is safe – but move them only if absolutely necessary – then call the emergency services for help.

Tiredness is a major killer. Its incidence is probably underestimated because no one can know the exact details of what has gone on before a fatal car crash. Planning regular breaks, being aware of times when you are likely to feel drowsy (for example, just after lunch or between the hours of 2 a.m. and 6 a.m.) and stopping for a nap or a coffee if tiredness hits can all help to prevent a tragedy.

Motorways are particularly hazardous because the monotony of driving on long, straight roads and the lack of gear changing can cause the driver to feel tired or be inattentive. But fatigue and lack of concentration can also cause accidents on urban and suburban roads just as easily. Most road accidents occur within two miles of the driver's own home.

WHAT TO DO IN A TRAFFIC ACCIDENT

If you witness a road accident, be aware that stopping could jeopardize your own and others' safety. Check all your mirrors before pulling up at the scene. Stay calm and ensure that your vehicle is visible and that the accident scene is protected from oncoming traffic. Switch on your hazard lights as soon as you have stopped.

If the accident happens on a bend, warn approaching drivers by using a highway warning triangle or asking another driver to signal to vehicles behind. Watch out for broken glass and metal. Turn off your ignition, make sure that your handbrake is on and that your car is in park.

On motorways, the speed that vehicles travel may well make stopping to help too

FIRST AID FOR ROAD TRAFFIC CASUALTIES

People are often trapped in cars after accidents. This should not stop you from initiating first-aid measures. You can still protect and open the airway on a casualty in the upright position.

Make the area safe. Move people to safety if possible. But do not move anyone who is injured unless they are in further danger.

Telephone the emergency services with precise details of your location.

Stop heavy bleeding.

Instigate CPR if needed.

hazardous. If this is the case, drive on and use a telephone to summon help as soon as it is safe to do so.

TO REDUCE THE RISK OF FIRE

Turn off the damaged car's engine if you can do so safely. Stop people from smoking at the scene, and if possible cover any fuel spillage with soil or sand.

▷ When dealing with any roadside casualty, assume that there may be a neck/spinal injury and handle with great care. Wherever possible, treat the casualty in the position found.

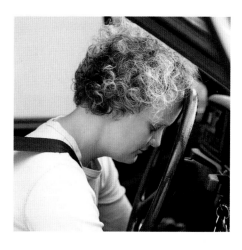

△ A casualty slumped forward in the driver's seat should be moved so their airway is opened, taking great care if spinal injury is a possibility.

▽ To clear the airway of a casualty who is still in the car, tilt their jaw slightly upwards and remove any blood or vomit. Then use the resuscitation techniques.

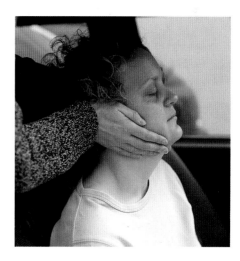

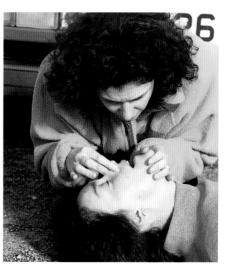

Safety in the home

One in three of all accidents happen in our own homes, the place where we feel safest and at our most comfortable. Our houses are filled with hazards – from faulty electrical appliances to ill-fitting carpets or sticking-out nails in the floorboards. Even a hot pan of soup can cause a serious injury. Most of these accidents are preventable, so making our homes safe must be a prime consideration. The majority of home accidents involve children. So, if you have children or if children may visit your house, home safety is all the more important.

Most of us love our homes, and we feel secure and safe when we are in them. However, although we may feel protected from the dangers of the outside world, our home environments are actually filled with potential hazards.

Domestic accidents are what keep the country's accident and emergency departments busy. On average, more people are killed every week in domestic accidents than die in road traffic accidents. A lot of these accidents are due to a combination of carelessness, ignorance and human frailty – and most of them are preventable.

HOME HAZARDS

Almost anything has the potential to be a hazard. For example, accidents suffered by older people are often a result of wearing footwear that is loose, worn or has inadequate grip. Trousers are another unsuspected hazard, especially people who are older or less physically able. Simply sitting down before attempting to put on a pair of trousers cuts down the chance of an accident. Naked feet are also vulnerable – stepping on broken glass or dropping something on your foot can cause a nasty injury.

◁ Loose area rugs are a common cause of bad falls in the home. Half of all accidental deaths in the home are the result of a fall.

△ Sit down to put on trousers, pants, tights and socks. Standing up while getting dressed can lead to a clumsy fall, especially if you are older or have impaired mobility.

AVOIDING ACCIDENTS
Most accidents can be prevented by taking a few simple precautions.

➤ Don't leave toys lying around.

➤ Don't leave plastic bags within easy reach of children.

➤ Don't smoke in bed.

➤ Don't leave shoes in people's way.

➤ Don't leave flexes trailing or hanging.

➤ Don't allow pets to play on the stairs.

➤ Don't ever put a mat at the top or bottom of stairs.

➤ Don't place anything on a table with an overhanging cloth if you have children.

➤ Don't hang a mirror or toys over a fire.

➤ Don't put plants on the television – it is hazardous when you water them.

➤ Repair or throw away rickety ladders.

A TIDY HOME
Messy houses are without a doubt more dangerous than immaculate ones. Falls – the number one killer in the home – are much more likely to occur if the floor is covered with clutter. Glossy magazines strewn across a sitting room floor can be as slippery as a sheet of ice, and a bean bag in a hallway is difficult not to trip over. Children's toys left scattered across the floor are another major source of accidents.

Keeping a house clear of hazards is obviously a good idea, but this can be difficult when you are busy. The best policy

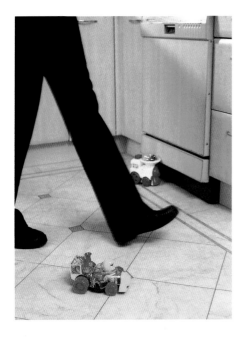

◁ Never leave toys or shoes lying around on the floor because they are a common cause of falls.

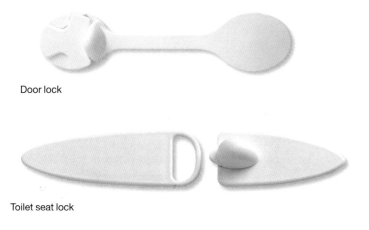

▷ Protect toddlers from falling down stairs by fitting gates at the top and bottom of each flight.

is to have a place for everything and to make sure that all walkways are kept as free of clutter as possible.

SAFE STAIRWAYS

It is particularly important to keep the stairs absolutely clear. Leaving objects on the stairs to be taken up (or down) later on, when you get around to it, is a major hazard. A vacuum cleaner left at the top of the stairs while you are dusting a room, for example, is easily tripped over.

Stair carpets wear out quickly and may develop lethal holes or tags. Repair any damage as soon as possible. Fitting stair gates helps to protect children from falls. These gates need to be at the top and bottom of the stairs.

PREVENTING FIRE HAZARDS

Cracked plugs, loose flexes, old wiring, furniture placed too close to the fire and unguarded fires are all common factors in house fires. Fire is one of the most serious hazards in the home, and yet one of the most preventable. Smoke alarms cut deaths from fires by 60–80 per cent, but even people who install smoke detectors often fail to maintain them by ensuring the batteries they contain are in working order.

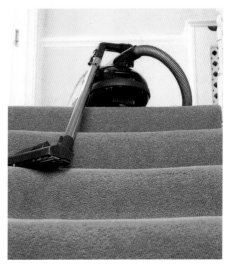

△ Keep the stairs free of appliances, toys and pets to reduce the chance of an accidental fall.

Door lock

Toilet seat lock

△ Child-safety gadgets, such as door locks, toilet seat locks and table corners, are a worthwhile investment for your home.

Table corner protectors

MOST COMMON CAUSES OF ACCIDENTS IN THE HOME

➤ Falls.

➤ Poisonings.

➤ Suffocation.

➤ Drowning.

➤ Inadequate railings and banisters.

➤ Unsafe storage of medication.

➤ Water heaters set too high.

➤ Firearms improperly stored or locked up.

Safety in the kitchen

SEE ALSO
➤ Safety in the home, p224
➤ Dealing with fire, p232
➤ Avoiding electrical accidents, p233

Hundreds of thousands of accidents occur in kitchens every year. This is not surprising since many of us spend a lot of time in the kitchen, where we come into contact with many potential hazards from sharp knives to hot surfaces and electrical appliances. The kitchen is also a place where we use both water and electricity, which must be kept separate. As well as making the kitchen as safe as possible, you should keep a fire extinguisher or a fire blanket and a sturdy pair of oven gloves always within reach, in case an accident does occur.

A few simple precautions taken when planning and designing a kitchen will prevent a lot of the problems that occur in this part of the house. In addition, laying down some basic kitchen rules may serve a useful purpose in protecting you and other house-dwellers from avoidable accidents.

CLEAR UP CLUTTER

It is impossible to stop children bringing toys into the kitchen, but having to dodge dolls, small metal cars or a farmyard on your way to the sink is an obvious and avoidable hazard. Take special care to clear toys from the floor.

Likewise, keep counters and tabletops clear of appliances unless they are in daily use. Even then, it may be much safer to put them away.

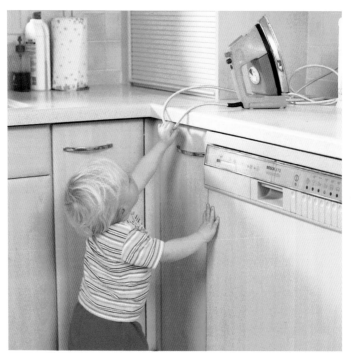

◁ Ensure that flexes and cables are kept to the back of kitchen worktops to prevent a child from pulling down a heavy appliance.

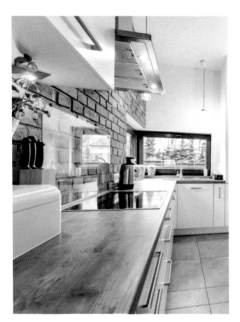

△ Keep surfaces clear of clutter to prevent heavy items being knocked onto the floor.

GUARD AGAINST BURNS

• Toddlers are at a perfect height for grabbing and yanking things off kitchen surfaces. If what they reach for is attached to a coffee maker or an iron, they could be badly hurt. Put irons away when you have finished with them, and never leave an iron unattended on the ironing board.

• Remember that tablecloths have dangling edges that are very tempting to small children wandering past.

• Use mugs for hot drinks. As civilized as it is to drink out of cups and saucers, they are much more likely to be tipped over than mugs.

• Don't try to drink your coffee or tea with a small child in your lap; they may wriggle and cause you to spill it.

• Make a habit of always using the back rings on the cooktop, and of turning the handles of pots and pans away from the edge of the stove.

• Oven doors can get very hot. The time around opening the oven door and getting the food out can be an especially dangerous one. Your attention may be on ensuring that you get the food on to the kitchen surface in one piece, and not on the small child heading for the oven.

• Burning oil is one of the biggest hazards in a kitchen. If you deep-fat fry a lot, you should seriously consider buying an electric fryer.

• Leaving the gas on and unlit for more than 10 to 15 seconds can result in a fireball, which will burn you and whoever is beside or near you. If you can smell gas, but cannot see anything left on that is causing it, get out of the house immediately and call the emergency number for your local gas supplier. They are available 24 hours a day.

- Putting a shelf above your stove is never a good idea. As you stretch over the stove to reach it, you may burn yourself. If the shelf is made of wood or contains flammable objects, it will also increase your chances of setting the kitchen on fire.
- Scalding can occur from hot steam as well. Take care lifting lids from hot food.

PREVENT SKIDS AND FALLS

- Try to mop floors in the evenings when everyone is settled and out of the kitchen.
- Keep drawers and doors closed when not in use – when open, they are an obstacle.
- Hook-on high chairs that screw on to kitchen tables are dangerous. Avoid them.
- Always wipe up immediately any grease and food spills, and wipe the patch with a dry cloth afterwards.
- Keep the floor clear of obstacles.

MINIMIZE HAZARDS

- Never leave any electrical wiring exposed; if cords are damaged, worn, cracked or corroded, stop using the appliance until the wiring is repaired.

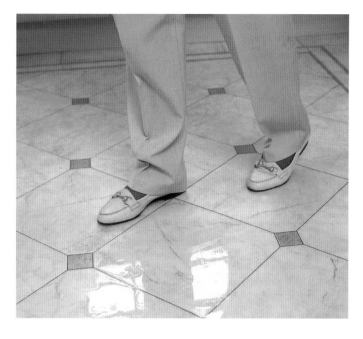

◁ A wet floor can be as slippery as an ice rink – and a fall could put out someone's back for weeks.

- Most people store their bleach, cleaning fluids and dishwasher powder under the sink. Cupboard locks are simple to fit and prevent a child gaining access to these harmful substances.
- Lacerations from careless chopping account for a lot of kitchen injuries. Keep knives sharp as blunt ones are more likely to slip.
- Use a chopping board and cut with all your fingers above the blade of the knife.
- Do not use broken crockery and glasses; throw them away.

- Beware of searching for broken glass in a sink full of water. Let the water drain out and then clear up the glass.
- Store heavy pans or equipment at waist height to avoid straining your back when reaching for them.
- Store plastic bags, knives and matches out of sight and reach of children.
- Don't leave the kitchen with pots and pans cooking on the stove. Be sure to turn burners off after cooking.
- Be aware that electric hobs will retain heat after you have turned the rings off.

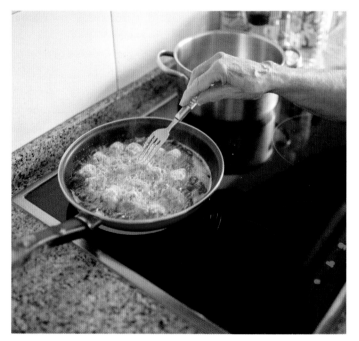

◁ Use the back burners in preference to the front ones and turn handles away from the edge.

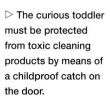

▷ The curious toddler must be protected from toxic cleaning products by means of a childproof catch on the door.

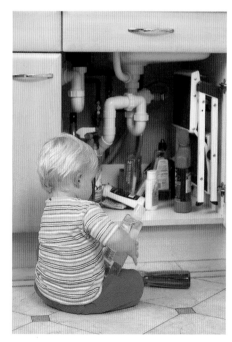

Safety in the bathroom

SEE ALSO
➤ Dealing with shock, p68
➤ Safety in the home, p224
➤ Avoiding electrical accidents, p233

The bathroom can be the most dangerous room in the house, with the most frequent injuries occurring while bathing, showering and getting in and out of the tub or shower. This is a common cause of falls for every member of the household but particularly among the elderly, but these can be minimized by choosing a bath with side grips and using non-slip mats on the bath base, in the shower and on the floor. Children love bathtime but need to be supervised at all times – leaving them alone in the bath could have fatal results.

Over 80 percent of bathroom injuries are caused by slips and falls, perhaps not surprising given wet, slippery hard surfaces. More than a third of people over age 65 slip and fall each year, and 80 per cent of those falls occur in the bathroom. The risk can be reduced by having grab bars installed in the bath and shower and on adjacent walls, using non-slip rubber mats and maintaining good bathroom illumination. Those who are frail should wear an emergency alarm to enable them to summon help in the event of an accident.

BABIES AND YOUNG CHILDREN

Children can drown in just a few inches of water, so babies and children up to the age of 5 years should always be supervised in the bath by an adult. Never leave a small child, not even for a moment – if you cannot ignore an interruption such as a doorbell, take the child with you to answer it. Always close the lavatory lid, and fit a child-proof lid lock so a toddler cannot try to play in the water and fall in.

If a small child could gain independent access to a bathroom, install a latch on the outside of the door well above child height. Make sure that any lock on the door can be opened from the outside, so that children cannot lock themselves in the bathroom.

Young babies should always be bathed in a baby bath or on a specially shaped foam insert for a normal bath. For toddlers and older children, make sure you do not overfill the bath and avoid using slippery bath foams. It is essential that you test the temperature of the water before the baby or child is immersed. For a baby, use your elbow – the water should feel just warm.

Medicines left within reach of young children are also a major hazard. All medication should be kept in a medicine cabinet – this is particularly important if children live in the house or are likely to come to visit. The cabinet should be screwed to a wall, out of the reach of children.

SAFETY IN THE BATHROOM

➤ Turn down the hot water heater to no more than 48.9°C (128°F).

➤ Any electrical appliances used in the bathroom, particularly hair dryers and razors, should be unplugged after use and stored in a cabinet with a safety lock.

➤ Have a non-slip floor. Avoid using rugs and mats in the bathroom.

➤ Make sure bathroom wall sockets have ground-fault circuit interrupters to reduce the risk of electric shock if an appliance falls into the water in the sink or bath.

TEENAGERS

Favourite teenage pursuits often include soaking in the bath for several hours at a time, and bathing by candlelight and while listening to music. Make sure they know the dangers of using electrical equipment in the bathroom – water is a great conductor of electricity, so electric shocks in the bath are usually fatal.

Teenagers should also be made aware that falling asleep in the bath or bathing after they have consumed alcohol or illegal drugs is potentially very dangerous.

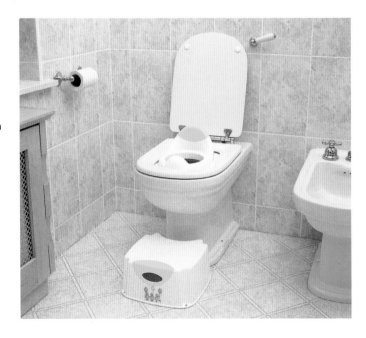

▷ The bathroom should be kept completely clear of obstacles. Invest in special lavatory stools and seats for infants and toddlers so that they can learn to use the toilet without any danger of accidents.

BATHING A BABY

Until your baby starts to demand the right to sit up and play, this is the way to hold them safely in the bath so that they cannot slip or roll over. Always remember to check that the water is not too hot before you begin bathing.

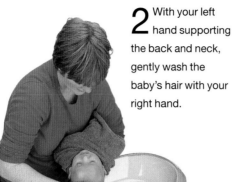

1 Hold the baby cradled in your left arm (right arm if left-handed).

2 With your left hand supporting the back and neck, gently wash the baby's hair with your right hand.

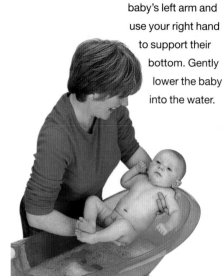

3 Hold high up under the baby's left arm and use your right hand to support their bottom. Gently lower the baby into the water.

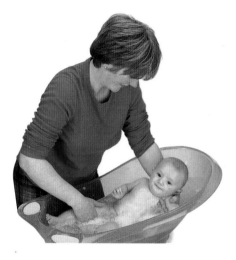

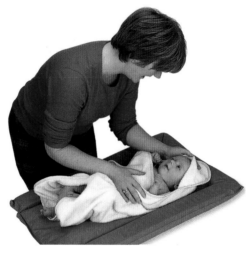

4 Use your right hand to wash, while continuing to keep a firm grip of the baby with your left hand.

5 Once you've finished bathing the baby, wrap their head and body in a towel and dry thoroughly.

TIPS FOR BATHING BABIES

➤ Never leave a baby (or child) unattended in the bath.

➤ Be wary of leaving bathtime to someone who is not familiar with bathing children. Drowning accidents happen most often when the bathing is carried out by someone who does not realize the dangers.

➤ Even if the baby is in a baby bath seat, do not leave them unattended.

➤ Ignore a ringing telephone or doorbell – or get your child out of the bath before you answer it.

TIPS FOR BATHING CHILDREN

➤ Always run the cold water into the bath before the hot. This avoids any risk of the child scalding themselves if they get into the water unaided.

➤ Never leave a step or chair near or next to the bath. Toddlers are fearless, and if they see a toy floating invitingly on the surface of the water they will reach for it.

➤ Don't ask an older child to watch your toddler in the bath. They are unlikely to exercise the same care as an adult.

➤ Don't give children baths in shifts if it means leaving in the bath water with no adult in attendance. Empty the bath while you put small children to bed, and refill it for the older children later.

➤ Be aware that a razor looks like a toothbrush to a toddler, so they might try to use it like one. Keep all sharp objects out of their way.

➤ Bathroom doors should be impossible for a child to lock. The easiest way to achieve this is to place the lock high up out of small children's reach.

Safety in the garden

SEE ALSO
➤ Drowning: what to do, p60
➤ BURNS AND SCALDS, p173
➤ Avoiding electrical accidents, p233

The garden can be an oasis of calm in a busy life. However, pools, bonfires, barbecues, and even plants can all present hazards, particularly if children are around. To ensure your garden is a safe haven for everyone, you'll need to take a few precautions. Choose water features that are child-friendly, fence off a swimming pool, and make sure that paths are easy to negotiate. Check that children and pets are out of the way before you start to mow, and store garden tools and implements in a locked shed together with all garden chemicals.

A little forward planning and common sense will go a long way towards preventing accidents in the garden. Many accidents happen when a child or older person is visiting a garden that has not been made safe for them. Small children, including those from neighbouring houses, often go wandering. Your elegant ornamental pond with its shimmering goldfish may be a fatal attraction for them.

CARE WITH CHEMICALS

Lock away garden chemicals in a dark, dry and cool place, out of reach of children and animals. Follow the instructions for use exactly and do not decant chemicals into other bottles; keep them in their original containers so you know what they are. Minimize chemicals in the garden: for example, rather than using slug pellets, use environmentally-friendly methods such as dishes of beer sunk into the soil.

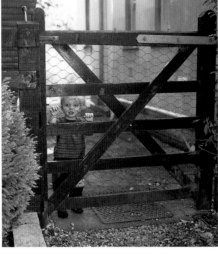

WATER SAFETY

Residential swimming pools are a major hazard for children. A child can drown in the time it takes to answer the phone. All swimming pools in houses with children should be completely enclosed by child-proof fences with gate latches set well

◁ Do not underestimate the climbing abilities of a toddler; this type of gate has been designed to keep out horses not children.

above a child's reach. Even so, maintain constant vigilance – in one survey, most child drowning victims were not known to be in the pool area; most were being supervised by one or both parents at the time, and most were missing from sight for less than five minutes before being discovered. Don't forget pools at friends' and relatives' houses, which account for around one third of submersion incidents.

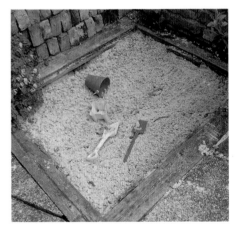

▷▽ A pond can be converted into a sandpit to provide children with an extra play area. When not in use, a sturdy cover will help to keep the sand clean.

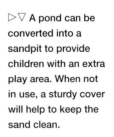

◁ Children are curious to explore their environment through taste and touch. A pond is particularly inviting – but is a potentially fatal hazard.

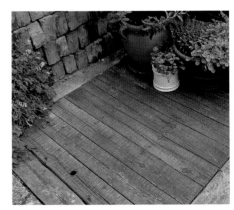

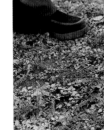

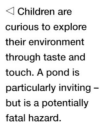

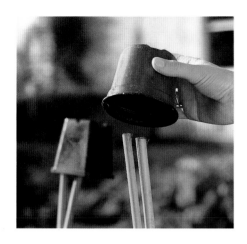

△ Place plastic containers or flowerpots on top of your garden canes, to protect your eyes when you are bending down near them.

ELECTRICITY IN THE GARDEN

- All electric garden tools should be plugged into residual current circuit breakers, so that the current switches off instantly if there is an accident.
- When using electric tools, keep the cable over your shoulder and well away from lawnmower blades and hedge trimmers.
- Keep children out of the garden when you are mowing the lawn or using anything electrical in the garden.
- Water conducts electricity, so great care should be taken when using the two together in a water feature. Many of the pumps available for water features are completely sealed and will automatically switch off if the system fails in any way.
- Exterior lights are designed to be used safely in the garden. If you are unsure, get an electrician to install or check them.

USING LADDERS SAFELY

Accidents on ladders are common but almost entirely avoidable. Make sure that all the rungs are safe before climbing up a ladder. Do not place it so that you have to lean over or stretch up to do the job – move the ladder or use a taller one if necessary. When pruning trees, use two ladders with a plank between them. If you are using a ladder up against the side of the house, ask someone to stand at the bottom to secure it; or if it is a long job, put up scaffolding.

MAKING YOUR YARD SAFE

➤ Steps should be well lit. They should have a handrail if older people or those with impaired mobility are to use them.

➤ Moss gathers on patios and can be slippery. Wash surfaces with diluted bleach to get rid of it.

➤ Nylon line trimmers throw up stones and other potentially dangerous things, including irritants from plant sap. Wear goggles, long-sleeved shirts and trousers when using them.

➤ Get into the habit of wearing heavy boots and thick gloves when you are working in the yard.

➤ To stop canes from poking your eyes, place film canisters, plastic bottles or flowerpots over the top of them.

➤ Keep all yard tools tidy and store them in a locked shed. Lock away petrol, kerosene and chemicals.

➤ Ensure that a clothesline is not positioned at children's neck level.

CHILDREN AND PLANTS

Few children die from eating poisonous yard plants. However, they can become ill with stomachache and diarrhoea. It is best to discourage young children from eating any flowers, fruit or foliage, rather than teach them which ones to avoid.

Certain toxic plants are best kept out of the yard altogether since they are very poisonous in small amounts. These include laburnum, foxgloves, monkshood, bittersweet nightshade and deadly nightshade. Others, such as yew, could be fenced off. Cut back trailing plants, such as thorny brambles and roses, if they could catch a child across their face.

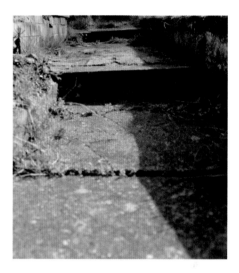

△ Uneven and weed-strewn paths could lead to an senior person falling in the garden.

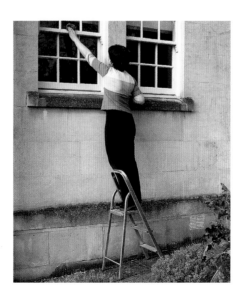

△ The golden rule of DIY safety is to be on top of the job – these steps are too low.

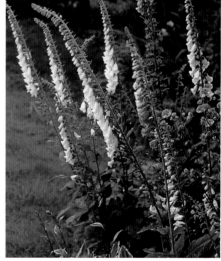

△ Foxgloves are poisonous and have no place in a yard where young children play.

Dealing with fire

SEE ALSO
➤ Tackling fume inhalation, p58
➤ BURNS AND SCALDS, p173
➤ Avoiding electrical accidents, p233

Fires in buildings produce invisible toxic fumes that kill in a few minutes. It is the suffocating effect of these as much as the flames that kill. No one should enter a burning building unless they are trained to do so. Oxygen feeds the flames, and if a door is opened into a burning room, the effect will be a massive explosion. Even a small amount of smoke should be a warning to keep out. Fire may be hidden behind walls, under floors and above ceilings. The most useful thing an untrained witness to a fire can do is to call the local fire department.

An untrained person is easily able to put out small fires, such as one in a chip pan (see Warning box) or in a wastepaper basket. However, once fire starts to spread, expert help is needed and the best thing you can do is to get away from the flames.

FIRE IN A BUILDING

- Try to stay calm, and if you are at work or in a public building follow the evacuation protocol. Walk to the nearest fire exit quickly and calmly. Do not go back for a bag, coat or any other possessions.
- Don't use elevators. Some have heat-activated panels that prevent them stopping at the fire floor, but if the electricity fails you may be trapped in the elevator. The elevator shaft can act like a chimney, sucking up flames and fumes.
- If you find yourself in smoke, stay close to the floor. If possible, cover your mouth and nose with a damp cloth or towel.

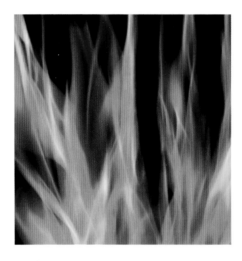

△ Fire is unpredictable and you should not underestimate how quickly it can spread.

- Close doors on the fire as you leave the building, thus starving it of oxygen.
- Never open a door that feels hot or has hot door handles – this suggests that there is a fire raging behind.
- If you cannot find an escape route, find a fire-free room with a window, shut the door, open the window and shout for help. Keep close to the floor.
- Don't turn on a light even if it is dark, since this may cause an explosion.
- Breathing in toxic fumes quickly leads to disorientation and confusion. If you have to enter a smoky area keep to the walls to guide you in and out.
- Remember that children may hide away from fumes in places such as wardrobes and cupboards.

What to do when clothing is on fire

Remember to STOP, DROP and ROLL. STOP the victim from running around as

WARNING
Deep-frying pans are a very common cause of fires in the kitchen. Never put water anywhere near a burning oil pan. Water will feed the flames and cause a massive flare-up. Cover the flames with a pan lid or blanket to deprive them of the oxygen they need.

this fans the flames. DROP them to the ground. Having them lie horizontally stops the flames rising to their face. ROLL them on the ground to put out the flames, ideally after wrapping them in non-flammable material such as that of curtains or a winter coat.

Once the flames are extinguished, you should assess the victim's airway, breathing and circulation. Start resuscitating if necessary. Carry out first aid on burns.

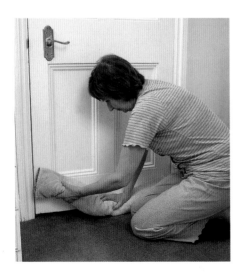

△ Blocking a door helps to keep fumes out of the room you are in and may deprive a fire of oxygen.

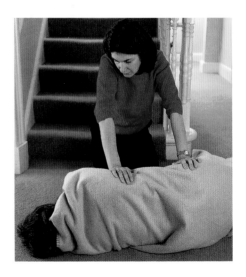

△ Stop, drop and roll someone whose clothing is on fire. Place them in the recovery position.

Avoiding electrical accidents

The danger of electricity is that it surrounds us in our everyday lives, and it is easy to become complacent about it. The cracked plug on the iron, the bare wires on the vacuum flex, and the gaping sockets left uncovered with a toddler in the house are all electric shocks waiting to happen. Electricity harms because it can cause the heart to beat irregularly and then stop; the muscles, nerves and blood vessels to fry; and the skin to burn. One-third of all victims of electrical accidents are children, and 20 per cent of these children die as a result.

One of the main causes of electric shock is contact with faulty electrical appliances or exposed wiring. The most common causes are young children poking sharp metal objects such as forks into unguarded sockets or appliances, or chewing on electrical cords.

ELECTRICAL INJURIES

The severity of an injury due to electricity depends on several factors:

- How long the victim is in contact with the electric current – the longer the contact, the greater the damage.
- If the skin is wet then it will cause a greater current to flow through.
- The path of the current is also important. If the current flows through the heart it is likely to be fatal.
- The type of current – alternating Current (AC) is used in mains electricity and power cables, because it allows greater amounts of electricity to be sent down the power lines. It is more likely to cause cardiac arrest at lower voltages than Direct Current (DC), which is what batteries produce. AC may also cause muscle spasms, with the result that the victim cannot let go of the electrical source.
- The size of the current – overhead power cables and lightning are more damaging than mains electricity and batteries.

ELECTRICAL ACCIDENTS

Never touch someone who is still in contact with a live circuit, as you may be electrocuted too. Turn the power off at the breaker box if you can, or unplug the appliance at the socket.

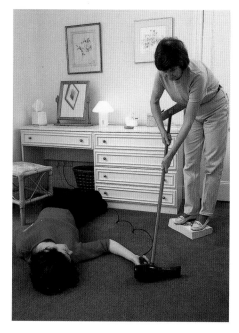

△ Separate a casualty from the source of electricity using a wooden or plastic object while standing on a non-conducting surface.

If you cannot turn off the power at source or unplug the appliance, try to separate the victim from the power using a non-conducting object, such as a wooden or plastic broom handle or chair or a rubber doormat. To protect yourself further, try to do this while standing on something dry and non-conducting such as a pile of dry newspapers, a thick book, a rubber floor mat or a board.

If the source is a high-voltage current from a power line, be aware that the currents can flash or arc, jumping a considerable distance. Call an ambulance and do not approach the casualty until the power lines are off. Once they are free of the current, check if the casualty is breathing. If not, begin CPR.

Treating the casualty

Once you have excluded any further danger to yourself, approach the victim and assess them. If you are alone, call the emergency services now. Otherwise get someone else to do it for you.

If the casualty is not breathing, call an ambulance and begin resuscitation using chest compressions.

Be aware that if the person has fallen or been thrown as a result of the shock, they may have cervical spine damage. If the casualty is a child, the shock itself may have caused a spinal fracture. Avoid moving the head and neck if you can, particularly if they are unconscious.

Be alert to other injuries if they have been thrown, and splint if necessary. If they have obvious burns, remove any clothing and rinse the burn under cool, running water. Apply a sterile dressing.

Any child who has received a shock should be assessed urgently by a pediatrician as there may be internal organ damage that is not obvious.

PREVENTING ACCIDENTS

➤ Never attempt to use electrical appliances when you are wet, or if there is any water on crucial parts of the appliances.

➤ Teach children about electrical dangers.

➤ Never place an electric socket or switch less than 30cm (ft) away from a water source.

➤ Throw away old, faulty appliances.

Safe home for infants

SEE ALSO
➤ Safety in the kitchen, p226
➤ Safety in the bathroom, p228
➤ Safety in the garden, p230

When safety-proofing your home for a new baby, be at your most paranoid and suspicious. Accidents happen in seconds, and most of them are preventable. It helps if you crawl around at your baby's level, seeing what looks interesting, what dangles enticingly, and what might be eaten, opened, poked or climbed. But remember that children grow fast, and their safety needs change just as quickly. In trying to make your home safe, you must be prepared to keep re-evaluating the potential hazards in the light of your child's development.

There is a wide range of dangers for babies and young children in the home, and they will vary depending on the child's age. For example, an 18-month-old may have neither the interest nor the dexterity to do any damage with your lighter, whereas a 2-year-old could burn the house down. Don't forget that an older child could potentially harm a baby, and their age and sense of mischief should be taken into account. Another possible hazard is a grandparent or person who is not tuned into children – they may keep medication where a child can reach it or forget to empty the bath. It is wise to be vigilant when visiting friends and family as their home could prove treacherous to babies and young children.

CHILDHOOD ACCIDENTS

Research has shown that accidents involving children happen more often when there are more than two adults in the house, probably because the carers are distracted by their guests. Try to get a child used to a playpen at a young age, so that you can use this to keep them safe when your attention is elsewhere.

Protection from falls and crushing
• Avoid using baby walkers – the baby may walk off steps or into burning fireplaces.
• Use stair gates at the top and bottom of stairs. For older children, make sure all stairs have handrails and are well lit.
• Keep beds, chests and toy boxes away from windows, and make sure all windows have locks on them.
• If using a high chair, make sure it is appropriate to the child's age and they are securely strapped in.
• Make sure that bookshelves and other pieces of furniture are screwed to the wall in case your infant tries to climb up them.
• Place safety catches on toy boxes or the lid may crush their fingers.

Avoiding poisoning and choking
• Lock up all potential poisons and do not take medicines in front of children.
• Remember that some plants are toxic.
• Avoid toys with buttons, eyes or other small parts that could be pulled off.
• Make sure blinds and curtains are child safe, with no hanging loops or cords.

Preventing burns and drowning
• Put away hairdryers, irons, and toasters when not in use.
• Use the back burners on your cooktop or

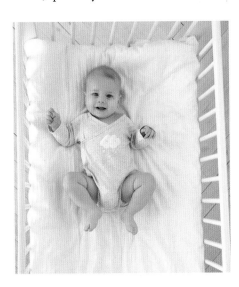

◁ Choose a modern, well-made cot with a well-fitted mattress and high sides.

COT (CRIB) SAFETY
Make sure that your baby's cot is a safe place for them to sleep.

➤ The cot rails should be no more than 6cm (2³⁄₈ in) apart.

➤ Do not use an old-fashioned cot with drop sides – malfunction can lead to suffocation.

➤ The mattress should be the correct size for the cot, with no gaps.

➤ Avoid blankets that have loose tassels, fringes, or ribbons as a baby may get tangled in them.

➤ Do not place the cot next to a radiator, in a draughty place or near any hanging cords or drapes.

➤ Avoid any soft, squashy articles such as pillows or pacifiers and do not let a baby under 12 months sleep with a soft toy.

➤ You should not use a pillow until the infant has transitioned to a proper bed.

➤ Place your baby at the bottom of the cot so that there is no danger of them wriggling down and underneath the covers on top of them.

range and turn handles towards the back.
• Cover all electric outlets.
• Use a fixed fireguard in front of the fire.
• Fill the bath tub with cold water first before adding the hot. Double-check the temperature with your elbow.
• Do not leave a child alone in the bath tub.
• Cover fish-tanks with a fixed top.
• Cover hot pipes and radiators.
• Keep all matches and lighters out of reach.

Avoiding sudden infant death syndrome

SEE ALSO
➤ Resuscitating a baby or child, p46
➤ Recognizing childhood illness, p110

Most of these deaths occur without warning while the baby is asleep, with no outward signs of suffering. Any death of a child is a tragedy for the parents, but those due to sudden infant death syndrome (SIDS) can be particularly traumatic because they are unexpected and sudden. SIDS, formerly known as cot or crib death, is the otherwise unexplained death of a baby under 12 months. It is most likely to occur in babies aged between 1 and 4 months. Nobody knows exactly why it happens, but there are certain risk factors that make it more likely.

There are many theories about why SIDS occurs, but the exact causes are still unknown. Some of the known risk factors, such as smoking around the baby, can be avoided; but unfortunately others, such as prematurity and poverty, cannot. SIDS is known to be more common in the winter months and in male babies. However, there is still much you can do to help keep your newborn safe.

REDUCING THE RISK

- Always place babies on their back to sleep, with their feet at the foot of the cot, basket or pram and their head uncovered. Babies are at 13 times the risk of sudden death if they lie on their front. They are no more likely to choke if they sleep on their backs, but may overheat if they lie prone.
- Never put a baby to bed with a hat on, as losing excess heat through their head is an important cooling mechanism.
- Breastfeeding for at least two months halves the risk of SIDS.

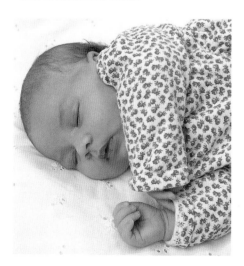

◁ A baby should initially be placed on their back to sleep, but as they get older it is quite normal for them to move on to their side as they nap.

- Do not smoke while pregnant or if you have a baby. Do not allow anyone to smoke anywhere near the baby, and avoid taking the baby into smoky areas.
- Do not overheat the baby. Try to keep the bedroom at about 16–20°C (60–68°F). Avoid heaters, hot-water bottles, placing the baby in direct sunshine to sleep and electric blankets. If the baby's stomach feels hot to touch or they are sweating, take off the blankets. If they have a fever, take off blankets.
- Avoid sleeping in the same bed with a baby, especially if you smoke, have drunk alcohol, are excessively tired or have taken sedatives. Keep the baby's cot in your bedroom until they are at least 6 months old and can roll both ways on their own.
- Do not use duvets or pillows until a baby is over 1 year old.
- Using a pacifier may reduce the risk of SIDS. For breastfed infants, do not offer a pacifier until the baby has learned to feed.
- Make sure everyone involved in the care of your baby is aware of these important recommendations to help prevent SIDS.

BREATHING MONITORS

Some parents buy breathing monitors for their babies which sound an alarm if the monitor detects no movement. These have not been shown to prevent SIDS, but they do create anxiety in the parents as they are prone to false alarms and may go off

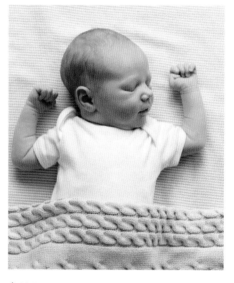

△ Make sure that your baby does not get overheated when asleep; don't use too many blankets, keep the room cool and do not cover their head.

several times in a night. The same applies to the new generation of wearable baby monitors, which may lead to unnecessary tests on the infant.

WARNING

You should seek urgent medical attention or call 911 if the baby:

➤ Stops breathing or turns blue.

➤ Is unresponsive and shows no awareness of what is going on.

➤ Has glazed eyes and does not focus on anything.

➤ Cannot be woken up.

➤ Has a fit.

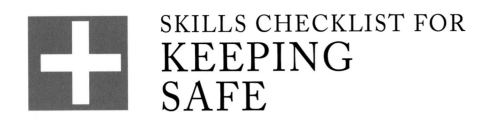

SKILLS CHECKLIST FOR
KEEPING SAFE

KEY POINTS

- Most road accidents occur within two miles of the driver's own home ☐

- Keep your stairway clear ☐

- The kitchen and bathroom are the most hazardous rooms in your home ☐

- Never leave a young child unattended in the bath – even for a moment ☐

SKILLS LEARNED

- Making your kitchen a safe place to be ☐

- How to bathe babies and children ☐

- Using common sense to make your garden a less hazardous place ☐

- Putting out a deep-fat fire ☐

- STOP, DROP and ROLL to put out burning clothing ☐

- Making your home safe for babies and young children ☐

16

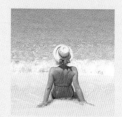

OUTDOOR SAFETY

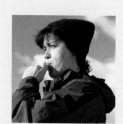

Outdoor pursuits offer a wide variety of hazards for which the sensible person must be fully prepared and properly informed. Appropriate clothing, footwear and equipment, together with a basic first-aid kit, are essential to enjoy your chosen sport or activity without unnecessary risk. Always be on the alert for changing environmental conditions (such as weather and tides) and for warning notices by seas, rivers and lakes. When travelling, be as informed as possible about your surroundings and about issues such as the safety of local drinking water and where to contact a doctor who speaks your language.

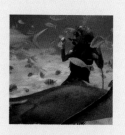

CONTENTS

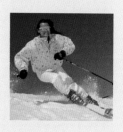

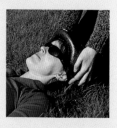

Safety in sport

SEE ALSO

➤ What is first aid?, p12

➤ Managing heat and cold disorders, p106

➤ Assembling a first-aid kit, p198

The thrills of outdoor sports are great, but sometimes the risks can be even greater. Being aware of potential risks is vital and taking appropriate actions to avoid accidents in the first place is a much better approach than just learning how to deal with an emergency. Safety is the key word, and this doesn't take away all the fun. So, if you're undertaking an outdoor sport in a new location, be prepared – even find out where the nearest hospital is. On the subject of having fun, it goes without saying that alcohol and sporting pursuits never mix.

Adventure sports have never been as popular or as accessible as they are today, each new one a little more dangerous and thrilling than the last – whitewater rafting, bungee jumping and abseiling down mountains are all possible, even for the novice. But all such activities have strict safety guidelines and provisions to ensure your safety at all times.

Even though some outdoor sports require a certain level of training, it is surprising that many people embark on outdoor pursuits, such as mountain or hill climbing, with little or no training and little or no thought to safety issues at all. It's a good idea when setting out on an outdoor activity to be prepared for the worst-case scenario – in that way, you'll be alert to potential hazards and be able to avoid them, if possible, and if not, then be best placed to deal with them.

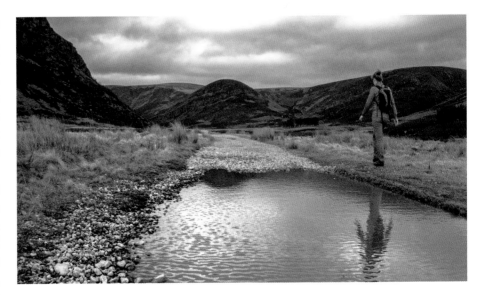

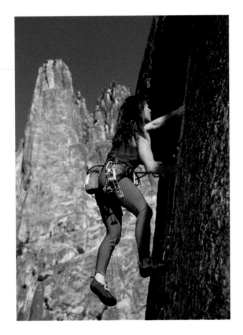

HIDDEN PERILS

It is not always amateurs that come to grief, but inexperience and ignorance of a sport's risks and dangers inevitably increase the chances of mishaps and accidents. Most problems can be traced back to poor training, a lack of fitness or poorly maintained equipment. While a certain amount of risk adds to the enjoyment and attraction of some sports, prevention of accidents through awareness of the safety aspects is the best course of action when considering engaging in any outdoor pursuit. Initial training is a good way to find out about risks, and practising with experienced people reinforces this.

◁ Never climb alone. Climbing as part of a team means that a rescue and first aid can be easily organized if necessary.

▷ Weather at sea is notoriously changeable. Be sure to carry flares, a cellphone and warm clothing and always wear a life jacket.

△ Weather can change without warning so be prepared with waterproofs and extra layers.

UNPREDICTABLE WEATHER

All outdoor pursuits have one thing in common – exposure to the elements. Weather in cities and towns is often a minor irritation that happens high above the rooftops, but in isolated situations a sudden and unexpected change in the weather can make the difference between

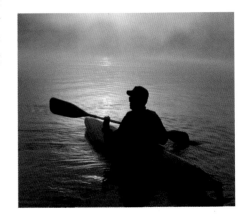

life and death if you are unprepared. Certain areas of the world are renowned for their sudden and unpredictable changes in weather, but it's a good idea to be prepared for the worst wherever you are and whatever you are doing.

PEER PRESSURE

Although it is certainly safer to perform many outdoor sports in a group, there is sometimes a herd mentality at work in group activities, particularly when there is a physical challenge such as climbing up a mountain. It's easy to be spurred on by the group to do things that you know are unwise and possibly beyond your level of skill and stamina. In such circumstances, try to hold on to your common sense and resist the urge to undertake a challenge to be "part of the group". You'll probably know instinctively if an activity is one step beyond your capabilities or confidence.

It is also worth remembering that many people view extreme sports as the ultimate challenge, a way of proving something to themselves and others. They may not be willing or able to accept their limitations until it is too late and they are in trouble.

FIRST AID – BACK TO BASICS

All of the principles of first aid are as applicable out in the wilds of a windswept mountain as they are in a domestic or workplace setting. The main difference is that the victim may be isolated and a long

▽ Check that adventure sports organizers are qualified and experienced before you set out on an activity with them.

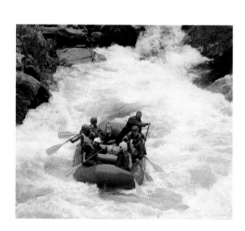

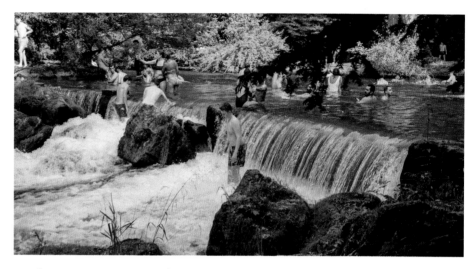

△ On hot days it is tempting to cool off at a popular swimming spot but you should consider the dangers of swimming in strong, flowing water.

way from any rescue centre or hospital, and may have to wait some time for treatment in the case of illness or accidental injury.

Keeping a clear head (and making sensible, safe decisions) is just as important as knowing the correct first-aid approach for a particular condition. Applying the perfect leg splint, for example, is a useless skill if you then abandon the casualty with no or little protection against the elements and/or equipment to continue to call for help while you go for assistance.

Try to remember that first aid is often about knowing what not to do, just as much as it is about knowing what to do.

A BASIC SURVIVAL FIRST-AID KIT

Whatever your choice of outdoor activity, always carry a basic first-aid kit with you. A suitable kit need not be heavy or widely comprehensive but should contain the following items:

➤ Plasters in various sizes.

➤ Sterile dressings and bandages in various sizes.

➤ Surgical tape.

➤ Sterile wipes or alcohol spray.

➤ Wound closure strips.

➤ Antibiotic ointment.

➤ Scissors and tweezers.

➤ A lightweight foil survival blanket.

➤ A mobile phone.

➤ A first aid guide.

➤ A compass, whistle, torch and folding lock blade knife are other advisable items.

Depending on your destination, bug repellent and a tick removal tool may be helpful.

For long trips in remote areas, add a signalling mirror, flares, a fire starter, fishing kit, water filter and purification tablets, clean plastic bags (to collect water from trees), emergency candles, lighter and waterproof matches, snare wire, a paracord bracelet, glow sticks, bouillon packets, energy bars or hard candy.

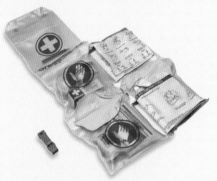

△ A basic first-aid kit is an essential part of any outdoor-based pursuit.

Safety in land sports

SEE ALSO
➤ What is first aid?, p12
➤ Dealing with shock, p68
➤ Dealing with broken bones, p150

Mountaineering, walking, trekking and cycling all have their hazards as well as presenting exciting and tremendous challenges. As well as being alert to potential dangers of the activity itself, remember to be aware of the possibility of changes in your environment and the havoc these can wreak – sunburn, heat stroke and frostbite, to name a few. Always carry maps of the area you're exploring and make sure you're well equipped regarding footwear and clothing. Also, tell someone where you're going and never go alone – there's safety in numbers.

Like many people, you probably love to escape civilization once in a while. Putting on a pair of walking boots or getting on a bike are two of the most accessible and popular leisure activities. What's more, they are also fantastic ways of getting fit.

But any outdoor activity comes with its own hazards and it's a good idea to know what these are so that you can avoid them or, in the worst cases, have some idea what first aid you might need to give.

CYCLING IN SAFETY

Almost 75 per cent of cyclists killed in accidents die from injuries to the head. So no wonder safety pundits recommend that all cyclists – whether in cities or the countryside – wear a cycle helmet. Such safety helmets reduce the chances of death from a head injury by 65 per cent.

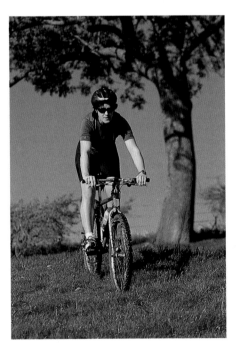

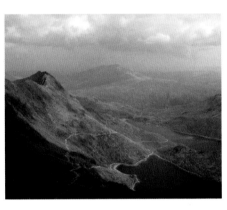

On the roads, most cycling accidents happen at junctions, but cycle-related injuries don't just happen on roads. With the ever-increasing popularity of mountain biking, a growing number of accidents take place on hills well away from traffic. As with other pursuits, it is important not to push yourself too far too soon, and to always cycle as part of a group. Make sure at least one person has a first-aid kit and a cellphone. Many mountain bikers carry water reservoir rucksacks on their back. Having plenty of water is vital to avoid dehydration – a condition that could lead to dizziness and fatigue.

Common causes of biking accidents are:
• Collision with a motor vehicle
• Wet surfaces, leading to loss of control (wet bike brakes).
• Travelling too fast downhill or around corners.
• Mechanical bike failure.
• Hitting an animal or pedestrian.

◁ Always wear a well-fitting helmet and appropriate footwear for safety's sake. And a padded pair of shorts will cushion your ride.

◁ When walking in mountainous regions be sure to leave your route details with someone you can trust and let them know when you are back.

HAZARDS WHEN WALKING

Most of the following hazards are avoidable by being aware and taking adequate precautions before you set out on a trek.

Blisters

Some people are prone to getting blisters, but commonly they develop in those with ill-fitting boots and in those who don't undertake such walking very often. Make sure your boots are comfortable, that you wear socks that wick moisture away from your foot, and that your boots are neither too loose nor too tight. A piece of duct tape or surgical tape can help to prevent a blister forming on areas that rub. If you do get a blister, cover it with a dressing; don't pop it unless it is large, painful or likely to be further under pressure. If you do need to burst a blister, use an antiseptic wipe first, use a sterile needle and apply antibiotic cream under the dressing afterwards.

Heat exhaustion

To avoid heat exhaustion, make an early start when hiking so that most of the walk is done in the cool of the morning.

Hypothermia

Walking in cold conditions requires a serious approach to the risks of such extreme low temperatures. If a person appears confused, quiet or is stumbling a lot, they could have hypothermia. In such

▷ Prevent a casualty with hypothermia from losing more heat and rewarm them slowly.

instances, get them into some shelter, remove any wet clothing and wrap them in spare dry clothes or a sleeping bag. Give them something warm to drink, avoiding caffeine- and alcohol-containing drinks.

Sunburn

Always wear at least 15SPF sunscreen, and sunblock on the lips and eye area. Remember to reapply every few hours

Potentially dangerous wildlife

If you are going to an area with potentially dangerous animals, never hike alone and don't let small children wander ahead. Don't leave food packs unattended, and if you're hunting or fishing don't pitch camp near to where you have processed your catch. Pack a bear spray and snake bite kit where appropriate. Wear snake-proof

FIRST AID FOR A SNAKE BITE OR SCORPION STING

➤ Wash the area with soap and water to remove as much venom as possible.

➤ Keep the affected part below the level of the heart if you can.

➤ If the bite or sting is on a hand or arm, remove rings and watches in case of swelling.

➤ Wrap a bandage tightly around an affected limb, 5–10cm (2–4in) above the puncture point; the idea is to make it tight enough to reduce the spread of venom but not so tight that it stops circulation altogether.

➤ If you have one, a snake bite kit can help to draw venom out of the wound. Do not cut or suck the wound and don't apply ice.

➤ Call for help and try to keep the victim calm and still to avoid increasing the circulation of venom.

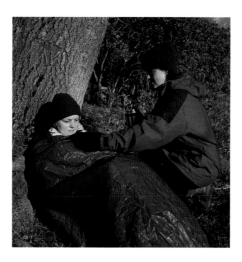

boots and avoid tall grass if you can. Carry a stick and never put your hand into a dark crevasse without first checking that there's nothing lurking in there. Remember that snakes can climb trees. Avoid pitching camp near overhanging branches, logs, grassland or rocky outposts, and make sure to zip up the tent tightly. Keep boots covered inside the tent and always put them on before you venture outside. Check yourself for ticks and remove them carefully (see page 105).

If you are in crocodile or alligator territory, treat any body of water as potentially infested; don't swim or wade and stay at least 5m (16ft) away from the water's edge. Keep children and dogs even farther away. Camp at least 50m (160ft) away, preferably on higher ground. Don't hang over the edge of boats, and use a landing net to retrieve or release fish.

MOUNTAINEERING SAFETY

Mountains should be treated with great respect. Demanding climbing combined with unpredictable weather can mean accidents are more likely. Any mountain rescue can be difficult, especially when changing weather causes a loss of visibility and plummeting temperatures.

In cases of serious injury or in severe cold, use a mobile phone to alert the mountain rescue team; or send one or two people from your party to get help. If you

▷ Acknowledge a distress signal by blasting three times, repeating after 1 minute.

SIGNS AND SYMPTOMS OF MOUNTAIN SICKNESS

This serious problem can hit anyone above 2,400m (8,000ft). It is usually caused by ascending too fast and is due to reduced atmospheric pressure and oxygen levels at high altitudes. It can be fatal if urgent action is not taken. Early symptoms include increasing fatigue, breathlessness that is unrelieved by rest, headache and vomiting.

If the person continues to climb, they may develop:

➤ Confusion, unsteadiness and lassitude.

➤ Pulmonary oedema, in which the lungs fill with fluid.

➤ Cerebral oedema, in which the brain swells.

The golden rule is that if the mild symptoms do not settle after a day of rest and plentiful fluids or if they worsen, the person must descend at least 1,600ft (500m) until they recover.

have to leave an injured person, protect them from the elements, leave them a flashlight and whistle, food and water if possible, mark the site and note local landmarks. Know how to transmit a distress signal: three successive whistle blasts, light flashes, gun shots etc., repeated after 1-minute pauses, or three fires, groups of rocks for visibility from afar or from the air.

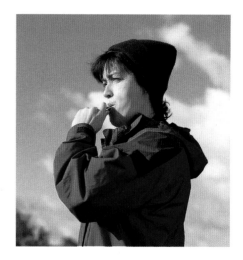

Safety in water sports

SEE ALSO

➤ Understanding resuscitation, p26
➤ Drowning: what to do, p60
➤ Managing heat and cold disorders, p106

Splashing about at the seaside, zooming about on jet-skis or windsurfers or skimming the waves in a motorboat are just a few of the ways we enjoy the water. Like other sports, all water sports come with their own hazards and a watery environment poses its own unique risks too. To be safe in the water, you must be a proficient swimmer and be aware of the power of the sea and the dangers of animals and plants that live beneath the water's surface. Also, bear in mind that many water-related accidents happen when people have been drinking.

Both salty and fresh water areas provide chances for recreational activities. Like any outdoor pursuit, water sports should be treated with great respect. It is vital to be aware at the outset of the possible hazards involved – many people underestimate water-related dangers.

Bodies lose heat more quickly in the water than on land, even in warm tropical waters, so it's advisable to wear a wet suit for sports such as scuba diving or windsurfing. A full wet suit, or what's called a dry suit, with head and hand gear is required during the colder months.

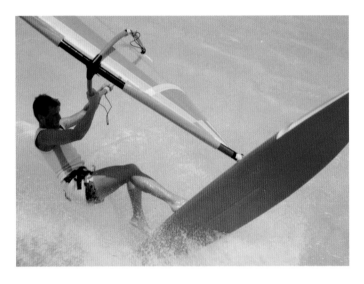

◁ Windsurfers should beware of spring tides and rip tides pushing them far out of their depth.

WEATHER AND THE WATER

Water skiing on all but the calmest waters is ill-advised, but sailing in high winds and choppy seas is what experienced sailors thrive on (although it is not advisable for a novice). Always check the weather forecast to ensure that it suits your plans and that you are prepared. Sunglasses are vital in most water sports as the water increases the sun's glare which can burn the eyes' cornea, causing temporary or even permanent damage. Don't forget that you can still get sunburn even when you are in the water so it is vital to wear waterproof sunscreen lotion and replenish it regularly.

◁ It is always safer to swim on a beach patrolled by qualified lifeguards.
▽ Children should always be supervised when near the water's edge.

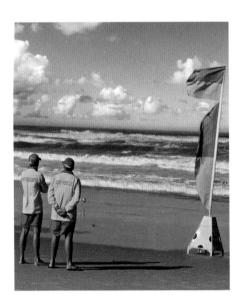

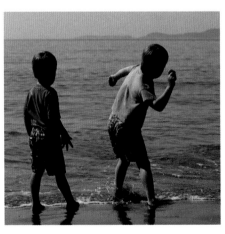

SWIMMING SAFELY IN THE SEA

Some beaches are patrolled by lifeguards and are safer than others. These beaches are usually marked by flags and sealed by joined floats to keep watercraft out of the area. If conditions are dangerous, the lifeguards will fly a warning flag. It's good practice to check the colour of the flag flying before setting off for the water. Know what the different flags mean.

• Yellow flag – Swim with care.
• Red/yellow flag – Lifeguards are on patrol and you should bathe only in the area between the flags.
• Red flag – Dangerous to bathe - great care should be taken. You should not enter the water.
• Red/Red flag - water is closed.
• Black/white check flag – Area is zoned for surfboards and it is not safe for swimmers.
• Yellow/black circle – Surfboards and other non-powered waterboards are not allowed in the area.

Any child under 12, should be supervised near the water's edge, especially if wading or swimming. Keep clear of rocks when swimming and keep an eye out for animals in the water such as sea urchins and jellyfish. In tropical waters, avoid swimming near the beautiful but dangerously sharp coral.

TIDES AND RIP TIDES

A large part of the sea's danger lies in the tides. Sands seemingly miles away from the shore can be covered by an incoming tide in seconds. Rip tides are narrow bands of current that create a powerful force in the water, often pulling swimmers or surfers out to sea. Swimming against these forces is pointless; it rapidly leads to exhaustion and the risk of drowning. The simplest way to safety is to work out the direction the rip tide is taking you and swim at right angles (90°) to this for about 10–20 m (33–64 ft), and then swim towards the shore.

SCUBA DIVING

Anyone taking part in scuba diving has to undergo rigorous training in the use of equipment, signalling between divers and how diving affects the body. Even so, accidents can happen, such as near drowning, decompression ("the bends") and ruptured eardrum and/or lung.

▽ During any water activity, and even in still water, it is important for everyone to wear a lifejacket, young and old alike.

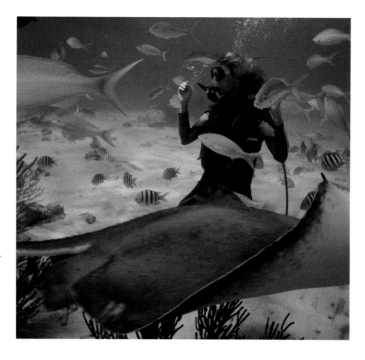

◁ The world beneath the ocean's surface can be exciting to explore, but you should be aware of potential dangers. For example, if coral grazes the skin it can lead to infection.

HAZARDS IN FRESH WATER

Most water-related accidents involve swimming in strong currents or cold water. Ponds, rivers, lakes and reservoirs can be extremely cold and pose a serious threat to life from drowning and hypothermia.

Deep rivers and lakes often have dangerous debris hidden beneath the surface. Pollution can cause skin reactions and infections such as Weil's disease. Getting in and out of the water can be tricky, and slimy banks with reeds and grasses can be hazardous.

▽ Avoid fast-flowing water and be aware that sharp branches and other hazards may be hidden in deep water.

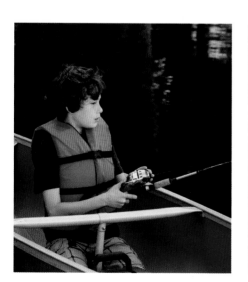

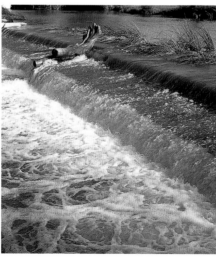

MAKING A WATER RESCUE

Giving first aid while in the water is extremely difficult, so unless you have proper training get the casualty to dry land before resuscitating them.

Avoid getting into the water: use a branch to pull them out or throw a float.

Once out of the water, protect them from the wind and lay them on their back.

Open their airway and check breathing. Be prepared to start resuscitation.

Remove any wet clothing and wrap in warm blankets to avoid hypothermia.

Safety in snow sports

SEE ALSO
➤ Managing heat and cold disorders, p106
➤ Handling lower-leg injuries, p164
➤ Managing sprains and strains, p168

Having a good attitude towards safety will mean that snow sports are enjoyable rather than dangerous. Your first considerations should be clothing and footwear. Make sure you've got enough warm layers on and a waterproof jacket. A hat will keep you cosy as a huge amount of heat is normally lost through your head. Gloves are a must, as are ski goggles or sunglasses. Boots need a good grip and should be roomy enough for thick, warm socks. Once properly kitted out, you can concentrate on having fun in the snow.

People unaccustomed to snow often improvise a sled from plastic bags, trays, crates or even cardboard and, not surprisingly, sometimes sustain injuries, from sprained ankles to fractured limbs or head injuries.

With the increasing popularity of snow sport holidays, such injuries are becoming more common as people spend only a week a year on the slopes and underestimate the level of fitness and skill required.

AVOID INJURIES ON THE SLOPES

• Ski in control. Some people seem to delight in skiing or snowboarding on slopes beyond their level, but they risk injuring others as well as themselves.
• Train beforehand. Snowboarding and skiing are arduous sports. Make sure you build stamina, strengthen leg muscles and improve flexibility before you go.

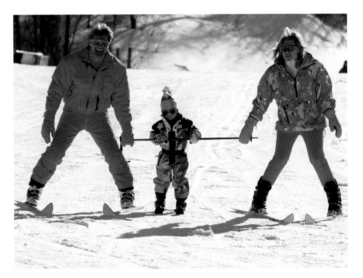

◁ Help your child to learn properly on lower slopes before taking them on steeper slopes.

• Use properly maintained equipment. Wearing someone else's ski boots and an old pair of skis is just asking for trouble.
• Stop as soon as you feel tired or cold, because this is when injuries happen.

If you fall while skiing, do not try to get up until you have stopped sliding. Ski patrols regularly check the slopes and are trained in first aid. To warn others that you are injured, get someone to plant your skis in an X pattern just uphill from where you're lying. Stay calm until help arrives.

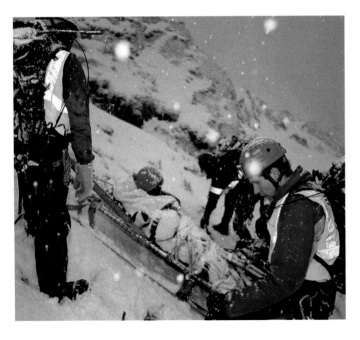

◁ This mountain rescue team have wrapped the casualty in a waterproof covering to protect him from the cold. The team paramedic assesses the injuries before they transport the casualty down the mountain.

SIGNS AND SYMPTOMS OF FROSTBITE

➤ The affected area of skin goes white and feels cold and painful. After a while it may develop into pins and needles.

➤ Sensation is gradually lost and the skin feels numb. The colour changes from white to blotchy.

➤ The skin and underlying tissue start to feel hard and stiff.

➤ The affected skin turns red or blue and blisters may develop.

In severe frostbite the skin turns black as gangrene sets in and the tissues die.

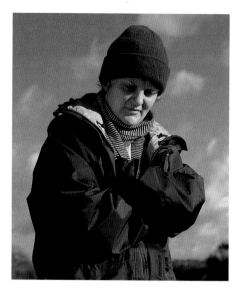

◁ If you suspect you have frost-bitten fingers, warm your hands under your armpits.

DEALING WITH FROSTBITE

In temperatures below freezing, the body diverts blood to the vital organs and away from the ears, nose, hands and feet. If tissues freeze, the condition is known as frostbite. Freezing temperatures or cold and windy conditions can cause frostbite, which often occurs with hypothermia.

If you suspect someone has frostbite, it is essential that you try to warm them up slowly and arrange to get them to hospital.

- Initially, get them out of the cold, replace any wet clothes and warm their hands by placing in your hands or lap or under their armpits, after gently removing rings and any other constricting objects.
- Once in the warm, put the frostbitten part in a sink or bowl of warm (never hot) water and dry it without rubbing.
- Elevate the affected limbs and support them to reduce any tissue swelling.
- Arrange transport to hospital.

COMMON INJURIES

Propelling yourself at high speed down the rough terrain of a mountainside is bound to entail the risk of falling. Most injuries on the slopes are sprains and strains, and so you should follow the RICE (rest, ice, compression, elevation) first-aid guidelines.

Knee injury

There are several ligaments in the knee. The one that is most commonly damaged in skiing is the anterior cruciate ligament.

If a skier straightens their leg at the knee, often while still in motion, and a ski edge catches their knee twists nastily. The knee does not always swell, but it is extremely painful and may give way suddenly.

Skier's thumb

If the thumb becomes jammed by the ski poles in a fall, a small ligament in the lower part of the thumb (the ulnar collateral ligament) may become sprained or even completely ruptured.

Snowboarder's wrist

Injuries to the wrist and bones in the hand are common in snowboarding where people use their hand to steady themselves and land on it outstretched.

SNOW BLINDNESS

The sun reflects off the snow, thus doubling its harmful effects. Without sunglasses or ski goggles, the sun may burn the layer of cells covering the eyeball (the cornea). This causes temporary blindness and great pain. As a first-aider, cover their eyes and get them to medical help.

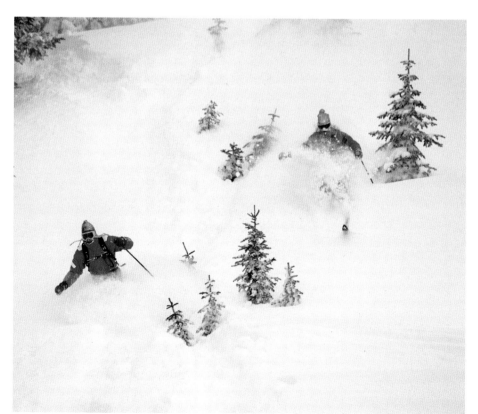

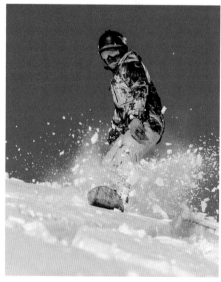

△ Novice snowboarders are at a greater risk of wrist fractures due to frequent falls.

◁ Skiing off-piste is the ultimate challenge, but carry an avalanche transceiver and mobile phone in case of snow drifts or avalanches. Collapsible probes and shovels are also recommended.

Travelling safely

SEE ALSO
➤ Dealing with vomiting and diarrhoea, p115
➤ Tackling sunburn, p183
➤ Keeping yourself safe, p220

Whether you are going to Florida or Fiji, it pays to prepare for the trip. As airfares become cheaper, people travel to more and more exotic destinations. With far-flung places come new and sometimes deadly hazards. But, by following a few simple guidelines, you can ensure that your trip will be as safe as possible. Even the journey can be hazardous – so stretch your legs, drink plenty of water and avoid alcohol. And don't forget to take out travel insurance; if you do have an accident abroad it is vital for prompt medical assistance.

If you are heading somewhere off your usual beaten track, it's advisable to visit your family doctor for travel advice at least eight weeks before going away. You may need to have certain immunizations or start a course of antimalarial tablets in advance of your departure date.

DO YOU NEED ANY JABS?

Immunization offers protection against particular diseases. Common conditions to be immunized against include hepatitis A and typhoid. Some immunizations, such as that against yellow fever, are mandatory in some places, and a certificate dated with the time and place of immunization is an entry requirement for some countries.

Even if you're heading for places in North America, Europe, Australia, or New Zealand, it is sensible to be up-to-date on tetanus and polio immunizations. Which immunizations are needed for which

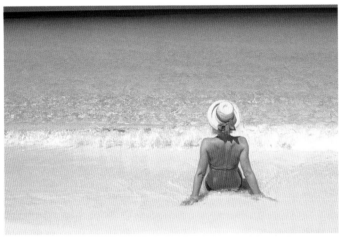

◁ The sun's rays are intensified as they are reflected off the water. Protect yourself by wearing a wide-brimmed hat, sunscreen and sunglasses.

countries varies between countries and over time, so always check in plenty of time before your trip.

TRAVELLER'S DIARRHOEA

This common condition usually strikes in the first two weeks of a visit; most often it's due to bacteria or viruses in the food and/or local water. Follow these simple prevention tips and you will stand a good chance of avoiding the problem:

• Wash hands before you eat anything.
• Wash all fruit, vegetables and salad leaves in purified or bottled water, and peel fruit and vegetables if possible.
• Avoid eating undercooked shellfish, meat and fish.
• Buy bottled water or purify local water using iodine, puritabs or a water-purifying pump.
• Avoid street food vendors and any uncooked foods or cold drinks that may have been in contact with local water (and therefore possibly loaded with germs) – drinks with ice cubes, ice cream, salads, fresh fruit and vegetables.
• Use bottled water (check the seal is intact) to rinse your teeth after brushing.

What to do if you have diarrhoea

The main concern when suffering from diarrhoea is to prevent dehydration, so drink plenty of fluids (but not alcohol, which dehydrates). Oral rehydration salts are an excellent remedy for dehydration.

PROTECTING YOURSELF AGAINST MOSQUITO-BORN DISEASES

Mosquitoes can transmit diseases including West Nile virus, Zika virus, chikungunya, dengue fever, yellow fever and malaria. Mosquitoes are most common in country areas and near water and are more active at night.

The best protection against disease is to avoid being bitten, by using effective insect repellent, such as those containing DEET or picaridin; covering up when outdoors, especially at dawn or dusk, and staying in an air-conditioned hotel room or accommodation with mesh-screened lanais, balconies, pool

areas, doors and windows. If this is not possible, use an insecticide-impregnated mosquito net.

In those areas of the world where travellers are at risk of catching malaria through mosquito bites, you need to take prophylactic medicine before you go. Check with the Centre for Disease Prevention and Control (CDPC) or your doctor which tablets you need for the countries you are visiting. The course normally starts a few weeks before you depart for your trip and continues for 4 weeks afterwards.

These can be bought from a pharmacy – ready-made in individual sachets – before your trip, and then made up as and when needed. If you don't have any such salts, you can easily make some from water, salt and sugar. Use ½ level tsp of salt and 6 level tsp of sugar and add these to 1 litre (1¾ pints) of boiled, purified or bottled water. Be careful not to mix in too much salt or sugar – it's better for the solution to be too dilute than too concentrated.

For each loose motion passed give 60-120ml (4-8 tbsp) of the solution to babies (but seek medical help as soon as possible), 120-250ml (4-8fl oz) to small children, 500ml (17fl oz) to older children and 1 litre (1¾ pints) to adults, plus plenty of bottled or boiled water.

In addition, zinc supplements may help to reduce the severity and duration of diarrhoea. In adults, an anti-diarrhoeal drug called loperamide (brand name Imodium) that can be bought over-the-counter should help to "dry up" the diarrhoea. This should not be given to children under two except on medical advice. For children over two, be sure to use the correct child dose.

In any case, if you are suffering from a high fever, there is blood in your stools, or the diarrhoea persists for more than four days, then it is advisable to seek medical help as soon as you can.

THE RISK OF BLOOD CLOTS
Reduce the risk of clots on long-haul flights by following these tips:
- Drink plenty of non-alcoholic fluid.
- Wear elasticated stockings to thigh level.
- Walk up and down the aisle for a few minutes at least once every two hours.
- Be aware that pregnancy, recent operations, obesity and the contraceptive pill can all increase the risk.
- Perform foot and ankle exercises while seated.

PRACTISE SAFE SEX
Sexually transmitted infections may be contracted on holidays or trips abroad, especially if you have sex without

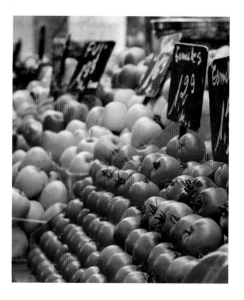

△ If you buy fruit from a stall make sure that you peel it or wash it with bottled water.

appropriate precautions. The best form of protection against diseases such as hepatitis B, HIV and gonorrhea is condoms, although they do not offer complete protection. Take plenty of condoms with you if you think you're going to be sexually active while away; in some countries, condoms are not as reliably made or are not as easy to buy.

DEALING WITH TRAVEL SICKNESS
Some people are prone to motion or travel sickness regardless of the mode of travel, but boats are particular culprits. If you suffer regularly from motion sickness, there are drugs to prevent it. Acupressure bands (also suitable for children), may help to quell nausea. Try these tips, too:
- Keeping your eyes on the horizon or on a fixed point.
- Staying in the fresh air, rather than cooped up indoors.
- Sitting in the front passenger seat of a car rather than the rear seat.

GETTING THROUGH JET LAG
When flying across time zones, your natural body clock can find it difficult to readjust to the local time. This jet lag is a common problem. Symptoms of jet lag include: extreme tiredness, difficulty concentrating,

loss of appetite and constipation. It can take several days to adjust completely. Try to fit in with local times but rest when you feel you need to. Early light exposure at the new morning time is helpful in adjusting to the new time zone.

USEFUL MEDICINES FOR A TRAVEL FIRST-AID KIT
The following suggestions for travel medicines are given only as a guide. If travelling to a remote area, it is wise to discuss malaria treatment and antibiotics for traveller's diarrhoea with your physician before you leave.

Don't forget to take sufficient supplies of your regular medications and always carry them in your hand luggage. It is advisable to take copies of your prescriptions and to check local laws at your destination before you travel – in some places certain prescription medications, such as some sedatives or painkillers, are illegal, and even some over-the-counter medications may be banned in some countries. Penalties may be severe, including arrest and imprisonment.

➤ Oral rehydration salts are helpful if diarrhoea causes dehydration.

➤ Antihistamines are useful for insect bites and itchy rashes. They are also useful in travel sickness.

➤ Hydrocortisone cream (1%) can be bought over the counter and is helpful for allergic skin rashes, insect bites and sunburn. Aloe vera gel is also useful for sunburn.

➤ Antifungal creams are good for itchy rashes (which are often due to a fungus) in hot sweaty places, such as between the toes or in the armpits.

➤ Antidiarrheal tablets to help prevent and control diarrhoea.

➤ Painkillers – such as paracetamol or ibuprofen – may be helpful for quelling headaches, toothache or pain from minor injuries should as joint sprains.

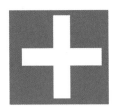

SKILLS CHECKLIST FOR
OUTDOOR SAFETY

KEY POINTS

- Prevention is far preferable to cure, especially in outdoor activities when it may take considerable time to obtain assistance ☐

- Don't be tempted to push yourself beyond your abilities ☐

- Always supervise children in hazardous situations ☐

- Always carry a basic first-aid kit and a cellphone ☐

- Get as much information as possible before you set out ☐

- Move about regularly when flying in a plane ☐

SKILLS LEARNED

- How to have fun while minimizing risk ☐

- Recognizing the value of researching your sport or activity and location ☐

- Checking out your equipment, first-aid kit and maps ☐

- Obtaining in advance specific medicines for various medical complaints ☐

- How to avoid a bout of diarrhoea – the most common travellers' complaint ☐

USEFUL INFORMATION

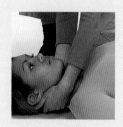

CONTENTS

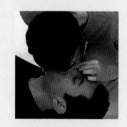

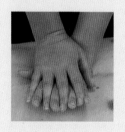

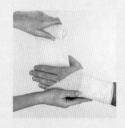

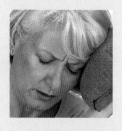

Useful addresses

UNITED KINGDOM

Action for Sick Children
10 Ravenoak Road
Cheadle Hulme
Stockport, SK8 7DL
Tel: 0161 486 6788
email: gill@a4sc.org
www.actionforsickchildren.org.uk

Alcoholics Anonymous (AA)
Helpline Tel: 0800 9177650
email: help@aamail.org

Allergy UK
Planwell House
LEFA Business Park
Edgington Way, Sidcup, Kent
DA14 5BH
Helpline Tel: 0132 2619898
email: info@allergyuk.org
www.allergyuk.org

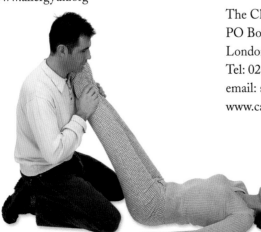

The British Epilepsy Association, known as Epilepsy Action
New Anstey House
Gateway Drive
Yeadon
Leeds LS19 7XY
Tel: 0113 210 8800
Helpline Tel: 0808 800 5050
www.epilepsy.org.uk

British Heart Foundation
Compton House
2200 The Crescent
Birmingham Business Park
Birmingham B37 7YE
Tel: 0300 330 3311
email: heretohelp@bhf.org.uk
www.bhf.org.uk

British Red Cross
44 Moorfields
London EC2Y 9AL
Tel: 0344 871 1111
email: contactus@redcross.org.uk
www.redcross.org.uk

British Safety Council
70 Chancellors Road
Hammersmith
London W6 9RS
Tel: 020 3510 8355
email: customer.service@britsafe.org
www.britsafe.org

The Child Accident Prevention Trust
PO Box 74189
London E14 1SQ
Tel: 0207 608 3828
email: safe@capt.org.uk
www.capt.org.uk

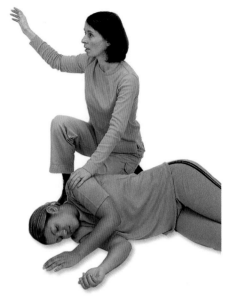

ChildLine
Freepost 1111
London N1 0BR (no stamp needed)
Tel: 0800 1111 (Freefone)
www.childline.org.uk

The Lullaby Trust
Information tel: 0808 802 6869
Bereavement support tel: 0808 802 6868
www.lullabytrust.org.uk

Cry-sis
BM Cry-sis
London WC1N 3XX
Helpline Tel: 08451 228 669
www.cry-sis.org.uk

Headway: The Brain Injury Association
Bradbury House
190 Bagnall Road
Old Basford
Nottingham NG1 1EW
Helpline Tel: 0808 800 2244
email: enquiries@headway.org.uk
www.headway.org.uk

The Confederation of Healing Organisations
Tel: 0300 302 0021
email: admin@the-cho.org.uk
www.the-cho-org.uk

Medic Alert Foundation
327-329 Witan Court
Upper Fourth Street
Milton Keynes MK9 1EH
Tel: 01908 951045
email: info@medicalert.org.uk
www.medicalert.org.uk

Meningitis Now
Fern House
Bath Road
Stroud
Glos GL5 3TJ
Helpline Tel: 0808 80 10 388
email: info@meningitisnow.org
www.meningitisnow.org

Narcotics Anonymous (UKNA)
Helpline Tel: 0300 999 1212
www.ukna.org

Asthma UK
18 Mansell Street
London E1 8AA
Tel: 0300 222 5800
email: info@asthma.org.uk
www.asthma.org.uk

National Childbirth Trust (NCT)
Alexandra House
Oldham Terrace
London W3 6NH
Helpline Tel: 0300 330 0700
email: enquiries@nct.org.uk
www.nct.org.uk

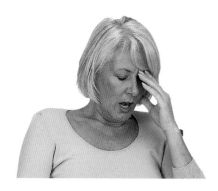

Family Lives
Tel: 0808 800 2222
www.familylives.org.uk

Resuscitation Council (UK)
5th Floor, Tavistock House North
Tavistock Square
London WC1H 9HR
Tel: 020 7388 4678
www.resus.org.uk (gives latest guidelines)

Royal Society for the Prevention of
   Accidents (RoSPA)
28 Calthorpe Road, Edgbaston,
Birmingham B15 1RP
Tel: 0121 248 2000
email: help@rospa.com
www.rospa.com

St John Ambulance
St John's Gate
Clerkenwell
London EC1M 4DA
Tel: 0870 010 4950
www.sja.org.uk

Samaritans
(to write a letter)
Chris
Freepost RSRB-KKBY-CYJK
PO Box 9090
Stirling FK8 2SA
Freephone tel: 116 123
email: jo@samaritans.org

Spinal Injuries Association
2 Trueman Place, Oldbrook
Milton Keynes MK6 2HH
Freephone tel: 0800 980 0501
email: sia@spinal.co.uk
www.spinal.co.uk

The Stroke Association
240 City Road,
London EC1V 2PR
Tel: 0303 3033 100
www.stroke.org.uk

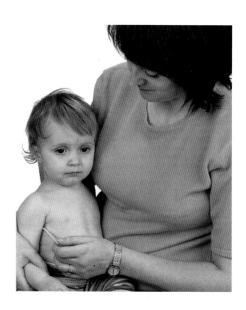

USA

American Red Cross
National Headquarters
431 18th Street, NW
Washington DC 20006
Tel: 0202 303 4498
www.redcross.org

National Safety Council
1121 Spring Lake Drive
Itasca
Illinois 60143-3201
Tel: 0630 285 1121
www.nsc.org

Occupational Safety and Health
   Administration
US Department of Labor
200 Constitution Avenue NW
Washington DC 20210
Tel: 1-800 321 6742
www.osha.gov

National Safekids Campaign
1301 Pennsylvania Avenue NW
Suite 1000
Washington DC 20004
Tel: 0202 662 0600
www.safekids.org

CANADA

Canadian Red Cross
National Office
170 Metcalfe Street
Suite 300
Ottawa
Ontario K2P 2P2
Tel: 0613 740 1900
www.redcross.ca

St John Ambulance Canada
1500 Lansdowne Street West
Peterborough ON K9J 2A2
Tel: 0705 745 0331
www.sja.ca

Canada Safety Council
1020 Thomas Spratt Place
Ottawa ON K1G 5L5
Tel: 0613 739 1535
email: csc@safety-council.org
canadasafetycouncil.org

Parachute Canada (formerly Safe Kids)
150 Eglinton Avenue East Suite 300
Toronto ON M4P 1E8
Tel: 1-888-537-7777
email: info@parachutecanada.org
www.parachutecanada.org

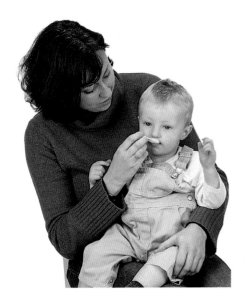

AUSTRALIA

Australian Red Cross
155 Pelham Street
Carlton
Victoria 3053
Tel: 1800 733 276
email: contactus@redcross.org.au
www.redcross.org.au

St John Ambulance Australia
PO Box 292
ACT 2600
Tel: 1300 360 455
www.stjohn.org.au

National Safety Council of Australia
17 McNaughton Road
Clayton
Victoria 3168
Tel: 1800 655 510
email: training@nsca.org.au
www.nsca.org.au

Kidsafe Australia
Kidsafe House
Tel: 07 3854 1829
email: info@kidsafeact.com.au
www.kidsafe.com.au

NEW ZEALAND

New Zealand Red Cross
Level 3, Red Cross House
69 Molesworth St, Thorndon
Wellington 6144
Tel: 0800 RED CROSS (733 2767)
email: firstaid@redcross.org.nz
www.redcross.org.nz

St John Ambulance National Office
Tel: 0800 STJOHN (0800 785 646)
email:info@stjohn.org.nz
www.stjohn.org.nz

Safekids Aotearoa
Level 5, Cornwall Complex

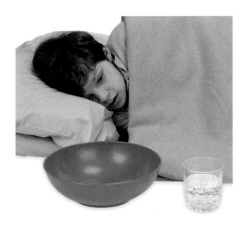

40 Claude Road
Epsom, Auckland 1023
Tel: 09 630 9955
www.safekids.nz

SOUTH AFRICA

The South African Red Cross Society
62 Blanton Street
Lynwood Glen, Pretoria 0081
Tel: 27 10 020 2516
email: redcross@redcross.org.za
www.redcross.org.za

St John Ambulance
19 Woolston Road
Westcliff
Johannesburg
Tel: 011 646 5520
www.stjohn.org.za

Childsafe
Safe Kids South Africa
Red Cross Children's Hospital
Klipfontein Road
Rondebosch 7701
Cape Town
Tel: 021 685 5208
email: info@childsafe.org.za
www.childsafe.org.za

*Note: all address details pages 250–252
correct at time of going to press.*

Index

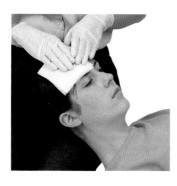

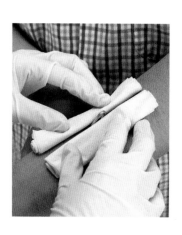

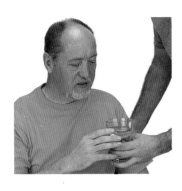

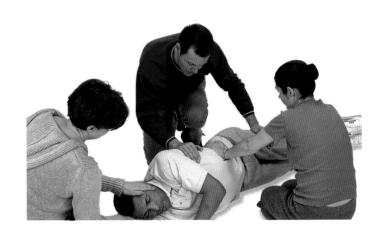

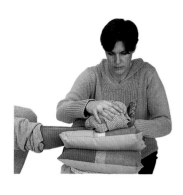

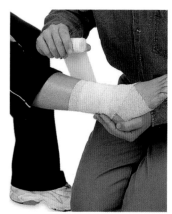

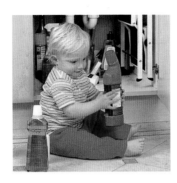

Acknowledgements

The publishers would like to thank the following people for their assistance in the making of this book:

The models:
Peter Akinola, Neil Barnes, Sue Barraclough, Heather Batchelor and Angus (18 months), Aaron Beha-Parks, Lesley Betts, Neil Bradbury, Jim Britton, Natasha Brown, Iva Buckova, Matthew Charlton, Rachel Chilcott and Tabitha (18 months), Valerie Ferguson, Jack France (18 months), John France, Tom France (6 years), Irene Halton, Jane Harris, Hannah Higgins, Lydia Hitchings, Simona Hill, Oliver Hitchings, Louise Hughes, Brian Jackson, Emma Jackson, Sam Jones, Pippa Keech and William (aged 7), Dallas Kidman, Ralph Leming, Helen Lowe, Debra Mayhew and Jamie Austin (18 months), Emily MacQueen, Denise Olive, Alan Powell, Joanne Rippin, David Spicer, Helen Sudell, Vivien Tobies, Melanie Ward, Evie Wyld. Thanks to Dammers Model and Promotion Agency, Bristol, for providing some of the models listed above.

Others:
Two Wheels Service, Bath, for the loan of a crash helmet. Pat Coward, for compiling the index.

Photographic acknowledgements

The publishers would like to thank the agencies listed below for their kind permission to reproduce the following images in this book:

l=left; r=right; t=top; b=bottom; c=centre

p67bc Medical-On-Line/Mediscan; p71t Garry Watson/Science Photo Library; p121t image courtesy of Meningitis Trust © 2003; p133b Jim Selby/Science Photo Library; p137b Marcelo Brodsky/Latin Stock/Science Photo Library; p242br Robert Harding Picture Library Ltd; p243bl Sinclair Stammers/Science Photo Library; p244b Robert Harding Picture Library Ltd. Shutterstock: p27bl; p35br; p71tr; p75b; p114b; p180b, p199.

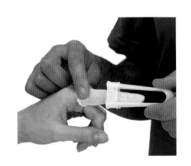

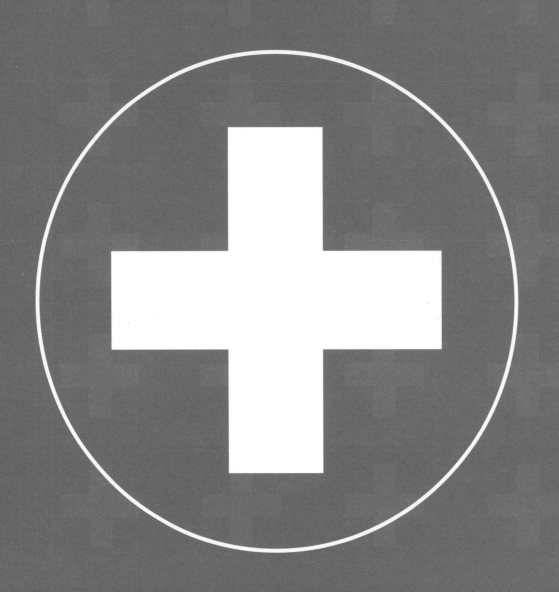